ENLARGED AND ILLUSTRATED EDITION.

HOMŒOPATHIC

DOMESTIC PHYSICIAN.

CONTAINING THE

TREATMENT OF DISEASES;

WITH POPULAR EXPLANATIONS OF

ANATOMY, PHYSIOLOGY, HYGIENE AND HYDROPATHY:

ALSO

AN ABRIDGED MATERIA MEDICA.

BY J. H. PULTE, M. D.,

SIXTH EDITION.

ENLARGED WITH SPECIAL HYDROPATHIC DIRECTIONS, AND

ILLUSTRATED WITH ANATOMICAL PLATES

TWENTY-THIRD THOUSAND.

CINCINNATI:
MOORE, WILSTACH, KEYS, & CO.,
NEW YORK ;— IVISON & PHINNEY. PHILADELPHIA ; MATTHEW & HOUARD,
BOSTON ;—OTIS CLAPP.
1856.

CINCINNATI:
C. A MORGAN & CO., STEREOTYPERS,
HAMMOND ST.

WM. OVEREND & CO., PRINTERS.

PREFACE TO THE FIFTH EDITION.

DURING the past year, the progress of Homœopathy has been great, beyond that of any former; the number of its adherents, professional and non-professional, has vastly increased, and the area of its usefulness extended to the farthest limits of civilization; everywhere, the popular mind seems to be more than ever aroused in favor of medical reform, by introducing homœopathic medication.

No one can deny, that the works on Domestic Practice have been highly useful in effecting these desirable results; their increasing demand, at least, shows the necessity of their important mission, widely disseminating, as they do, the beneficent doctrines of our beloved healing-art, and facilitating their application.

In view of these facts, the Author deems it his imperative duty, to make his work on Domestic Practice still more worthy of the confidence and patronage, so liberally bestowed upon it at home and abroad.

The present, or fifth American edition, has been materially improved, especially in those parts relating to the treatment of diseases; for which purpose, the Author has revised every chapter, making such additions, as by his own, and the experience of others, he considered beneficial for domestic practice. To the materia medica he added a condensed list of the most significant symptoms of *Apis Mellifica,* thus facilitating the use of a remedy, which is becoming more important every day.

In order to discuss more fully the various relations of a sound physical and moral development of Females, together with a more minute description and treatment of their diseases, the Author, to accomplish this highly important object, has since issued a separate work, under the title of "WOMAN'S MEDICAL GUIDE," intended to be a supplement to his "DOMESTIC PHYSICIAN."

THE AUTHOR.

CINCINNATI, *October,* 1853.

PREFACE TO THE THIRD EDITION.

The whole work has been carefully revised, and such alterations and additions made as it was thought would render it more practically useful. In the conscientious desire of condensing in it as much as possible of *practical usefulness*, the author has developed still farther, what was summarily touched upon in the previous editions, the use of Water as an auxiliary to the strictly medicinal treatment of disease.

This, it is generally admitted, when properly applied, materially aids the effects of Homœopathic remedies, and though the author feels that Hydropathy is but the handmaid of Homœopathy, yet the introduction of the different beneficial modes of applying water into a work of this description cannot fail to meet with the approbation of those for whose use it is prepared.

Those who are entirely unacquainted with the application of water in disease, will find in the treatise on Hydropathy such general explanations, as are necessary to guide them ; while under the head of the different diseases, in which it may be beneficially applied, the more specific directions will be found, following the remedial treatment.

The additions made on this subject amount, in the aggregate, to more than thirty pages of matter.

The author has introduced into the present edition, in that part devoted to anatomy, such illustrations as he hopes may in some degree contribute to a readier comprehension of the wonderful structure of the human body, and by so doing aid in a better understanding of disease itself.

THE AUTHOR.

CINCINNATI, *March*, 1852.

PREFACE TO THE FOURTH EDITION.

The rapid sale of two large issues of the third edition (two thousand copies in three months), has convinced the author, that the improvements, introduced by him there for the first time, have met the wants and received the approbation of the public ; he feels it, therefore, more than ever his duty, not to relax his efforts, to perfect the work still farther, and to make it keep pace with the progress of the science itself.

* * * * * * * * *

To the list of medicines has been added a new remedy, the *Apis Mellifica*, which has already proved so efficacious in various diseases, coming under domestic practice, that its speedy introduction into this work was considered of the greatest importance ; for the provings of this new remedy we are indebted to the Central New York Homœopathic Society. It has an extensive range of action, particularly in dropsical affections, Erysipelas and Catarrhs, suppression and translation of acute eruptions, etc. In the list of medicines, it is mentioned at the end, so as not to disturb the numerical arrangement, adopted in former editions.

THE AUTHOR.

CINCINNATI, *September*, 1852.

PREFACES TO THE FIRST AND SECOND EDITIONS.

Of late years a great deal of attention has been bestowed upon the preparation of popular works on the treatment of diseases, by the medical profession, as well by members of the Homœopathic as of other medical schools. This shows, evidently, that the hitherto backward world of medical science has been caught at last, with the proper spirit of modern progress, whose distinguishing feature in scientific matters consists, undoubtedly, in the tendency to popularize abstruse sciences and make them useful and accessible to the many.

Homœopathy has not been in the rear as regards these popular treatises, many valuable volumes having been issued from the press within a short time which have facilitated in a great degree the domestic use of the homœopathic medicines. This service, rendered by the profession to the public in a liberal and generous spirit, has been amply rewarded by the latter, in extending all over the country, more rapidly, the blessings of our beloved healing art, and establishing its title, as a benefactor of mankind, more firmly in the hearts of the people.

The author well recollects that the first "domestic physicians" which appeared, were looked upon with distrust by some of the profession. But the people in general hailed them as welcome friends in their domestic afflictions, where counsel is so often needed at times when medical aid cannot be obtained.

At this time scarcely one homœopathic family is without one or more books on domestic practice, which is a sufficient evidence of their practical utility.

Thus have these messengers of mercy and usefulness traveled with, and often ahead of, the regular practitioners of Homœopathy—the silent, but efficient missionaries of truth, declaring it everywhere by facts and conquests over disease, won by the people themselves. The profession in general seems now to regard them as necessary allies in the great work of reforming the medical state of the world, and bestows a great deal of care on their constantly increasing perfection, by making them more practical and definite, progressing in their improvement as the science itself progresses.

In this spirit the present volume is written and given to the public by the author, who has attempted to embody in it the results of a practice of more than sixteen years.

In the pathology of the work he has followed mostly the views of Hufeland, who is generally practically useful, and of Schœnlein, who is precise and scientific.

In the therapeutics he has endeavored to consult the best authors of our school, carefully comparing their views with his own results, which are embodied in this work.

To increase its general usefulness, popular treatises of Anatomy, Physiology, Hygiene, and Hydropathy, have been added; branches and parts of medical science as a whole, which, when properly understood and digested by the people, will in a great degree aid in promoting the salutary results expected from the use of a domestic physician. Beside this, a condensed extract of the Homœopathic Materia Medica, given at the close of the book, enables the reader to correct his prescriptions, and enlarge his general knowledge of the homœopathic science. Thus it is hoped that, by these additions, the work is rendered more perfect in a twofold manner: first, by giving a more extended knowledge of the human system and its laws through the treatises on Anatomy and Physiology; and, secondly, by making the reader acquainted with those practical branches of medicine, Hygiene and Hydropathy, of which, particularly, the latter has, within the last few years, very much engrossed the attention of the profession and of invalids. In this respect the author himself does not hesitate to declare that he considers Hydropathy, applied within her proper limits, the handmaid of Homœopathy, and that these two, combined in this relationship, are destined to conquer the medical world.

* * * * * * * * *

Beside many corrections and revisions, which almost any work after its first appearance still needs, the reader will find whole articles on diseases, which were not treated of in the first edition; to the list of medicines *Aloes* has been added, as this remedy was considered particularly useful in many diseases coming under domestic treatment: it has been put at the end of the list of medicines, so as not to interfere with the arrangement in the numbers, as given in the first edition.

The author, thankful for the favorable reception accorded to his work by the public, would express his grateful acknowledgments to those of his professional brethren, who favored him with suggestions for improving this second edition; they will find that their wishes have been fulfilled. Similar favors from the profession, for the future, will be thankfully received by the author, for by such co-operation alone will it be possible to arrive at the greatest degree of usefulness and perfection.

CINCINNATI, *April*, 1851. THE AUTHOR.

TABLE OF CONTENTS.

CHAPTER III.

Cutaneous Diseases.

CHAPTER IV.

Fevers.

CHAPTER V.

Affections of the Mind.

CHAPTER VI.

Affections of the Head.

CHAPTER VII.

Affections of the Eyes.

CHAPTER VIII.

Affections of the Ears.

CHAPTER IX.

Affections of the Nose.

CHAPTER X.

Affections of the Face, Lips, and Jaws.

CHAPTER XI.

Affections of the Teeth, Gums, and Mouth.

CHAPTER XII.

Affections of the Throat.

CHAPTER XIII.

Affections of the Windpipe and Chest.

CHAPTER XIV.

Affections of the Stomach and Bowels.

PART II.

I. ANATOMY AND PHYSIOLOGY.

II. HYGIENE AND HYDROPATHY.

LIST OF MEDICINES.

THEIR SYNONYMES AND ANTIDOTES.

1 ACONITE. Aconitum Napellus (plant). *Antidotes*—Camphor, Nux vom., Wine, Vinegar.

2. ANTIMONIUM CRUD. Antimony (mineral). *Antidotes*—Hepar sulph., Mercury, Pulsatilla.

3. ARNICA. Arnica Montana (plant). *Antidotes*—Camphor, Ignatia, Ipecac.

4. ARSENIC. Arsenicum album (mineral). *Antidotes*—For poisoning with it: rust of iron. For its dynamic effects: China, Hepar Sulph., Ipecac., Nux vom., Veratrum.

5. AURUM. Aurum metallicum. Gold. (Metal.) *Antidotes*—Belladonna, China, Cuprum, Mercury.

6. BELLADONNA. Deadly nightshade (plant). *Antidotes*—Coffea, Hyoscyamus, Hepar sulph., Pulsatilla.

7. BELLADONNA^{cc}. Is the two hundredth potency of Belladonna.

8. BRYONIA. Bryonia alba (plant). *Antidotes*—Aconite, Chamomile, Ignatia, Nux vomica.

9. CALCAREA CARBONICA. Carbonate of lime. *Antidotes*—Camphor, Nitric acid, Sulphur.

10. CAMPHORA. Camphor. *Antidotes*—Opium, Nitri spiritus.

11. CANTHARIS. Spanish fly (animal). *Antidote*—Camphor.

12. CAPSICUM. Spanish pepper (vegetable). *Antidote*—Camphor.

13. CARBO VEG. Carbo vegetabilis. Wood charcoal. *Antidotes*—Arsenic, Camphor, Lachesis.

14. CAUSTICUM. Caustic of the alkalies. *Antidotes*—Coffea, Colocynth, Nux vomica.

15. CHAMOMILE. Chamomilla (plant). *Antidotes*—Aconite, Cocculus, Coffea, Ignatia, Nux vomica, Pulsatilla

16. CHINA. Cinchona. Peruvian bark (vegetable). *Antidotes*—Arnica Arsenic, Belladonna, Calcarea carbonica, Carbo veg., Ipecac. Sulphur.

17. CINA. Wormseed (vegetable). *Antidotes*—Ipecac., Veratrum.

18. CINA^{cc}. Is the two hundredth potency of Cina.

19. COCCULUS. Indian berries. Coccle (vegetable). *Antidotes*—Camphor, Nux vomica.
20. COFFEA. Coffee berries (vegetable). *Antidotes*—Aconite, Chamomile, Nux vomica.
21. COFFEA^{cc}. Is the two hundredth potency of Coffea.
22. COLCHICUM. Meadow Saffron (plant). *Antidotes*—Nux vomica, Cocculus, Pulsatilla.
23. COLOCYNTHIS. Colocynth (vegetable). *Antidotes*—Camphor, Causticum, Coffea, Chamomile.
24. CONIUM. Hemlock (vegetable). *Antidotes*—Coffea, Spiritus Nitri.
25. CROCUS. Saffron (vegetable). *Antidote*—Opium.
26. CUPRUM. Cuprum metallicum. Copper (metal). *Antidotes*—Belladonna, China, Ipecac., Mercury, Nux vomica.
27. DROSERA. Round-leaved Sun Dew (vegetable). *Antidote*—Camphor.
28. DULCAMARA. Bitter Sweet. Woody Nightshade (plant). *Antidotes*—Camphor, Ipecac., Mercurius.
29. EUPHRASIA. Eye Bright (plant). *Antidote*—Pulsatilla.
30. FERRUM. Ferrum metallicum. Iron (metal). *Antidotes*—Arnica, Arsenic, Belladonna, Ipecac., Mercury, Pulsatilla.
31. GRAPHITES. Plumbago. Pure Black Lead (metal). *Antidotes*—Arsenic, Nux vomica, Wine.
32. HELLEBORUS (NIGER). Black Hellebore (plant). *Antidotes*—Camphor, China.
33. HEPAR SULPHURIS. Sulphuret of Lime. *Antidotes*—Vinegar, Belladonna.
34. HYOSCYAMUS (NIGER). Henbane (plant). *Antidotes*—Belladonna, Camphor, China.
35. IGNATIA. St. Ignatius's Bean (vegetable). *Antidotes*—Pulsatilla, Chamomile, Cocculus, Arnica, Camphor, Vinegar.
36. IODINE. Iodium. *Antidotes*—Arsenic, Camphor, Coffee, Phosphorus, Sulphur.
37. IPECAC. Ipecacuanha (vegetable). *Antidotes*—Arnica, Arsenic, China.
38. JALAPPA. Jalap (vegetable). *Antidote*—Camphor.
39. KALI HYDRIODICUM. Hydriodate of Potassa (mineral).
40. LACHESIS. Poison of the Lance-headed Serpent (animal). *Antidotes*—Arsenic, Belladonna, Nux vomica, Rhus tox.
41. LYCOPODIUM. Club Moss. Wolf's Claw (vegetable). *Antidotes*—Camphor, Pulsatilla.
42. MERCURIUS (VIVUS). Quicksilver (mineral). *Antidotes*—Arnica, Belladonna, Camphor, Hepar sulph., Iodine, Lachesis, Sulphur

43. MURIATIC ACID. Acidum muriatic (mineral). *Antidotes*—Camphor, Bryonia.

44. NATRUM MURIATICUM. Muriate of Soda (mineral). *Antidotes*—Arsenic, Camphor, Nitri spiritus.

45. NITRI ACIDUM. Nitric acid (a mineral acid). *Antidotes*—Calcarea carb., Conium, Camphor, Hepar sulph., Sulphur.

46. NUX VOMICA. Nux vomica (vegetable). *Antidotes*—Aconite, Camphor, Coffea, Pulsatilla.

47. OPIUM. White Poppy (vegetable). *Antidotes* — Camphor, Coffea, Calcarea carb., Hepar sulph., Sulphur.

48. PETROLEUM. Rock Oil (mineral oil). *Antidotes* — Aconite, Nux vomica, Cocculus.

49. PHOSPHORUS. Phosphor (mineral). *Antidotes* — Camphor, Coffea, Nux vomica.

50. PHOSPHORI ACIDUM. Phosphoric acid (a mineral acid). *Antidotes*—Camphor, Coffea.

51. PLATINA. (Metal.) *Antidotes* — Pulsatilla, Belladonna.

52. PULSATILLA. Meadow Anemone (vegetable). *Antidotes* — Chamomile, Coffea, Ignatia, Nux vomica.

53. RHEUM. Rhubarb (vegetable). *Antidotes*—Camphor, Chamomile, Nux vomica.

54. RHUS TOXICODENDRON. Rhus. Sumach. Poison Oak (vegetable). *Antidotes*—Belladonna, Bryonia, Camphor, Coffea, Sulphur.

55. SAMBUCUS (NIGER). Alder (vegetable). *Antidotes* — Arsenic, Camphor.

56. SANGUINARIA (CANADENSIS). Common Blood Root.

57. SECALE (CORNUTUM). Ergot of Rye (vegetable). *Antidotes*—Camphor, Opium.

58. SEPIA. Inky juice of the Cuttle-Fish (animal). *Antidotes*—Aconite, Spiritus Nitri, Vinegar.

59. SILICEA. Silicious Earth (mineral). *Antidotes*—Camphor, Hepar sulph.

60. SPIGELIA (ANTHELMINTICA). Indian Pink (vegetable). *Antidotes*—Camphor, Aurum.

61. SPONGIA. (Marina Tosta.) Burnt Sponge. *Antidote* — Camphor.

62. STANNUM. Pure tin (metal). *Antidotes*—Coffea, Pulsatilla.

63. STAPHYSAGRIA. Stavesacre (vegetable). *Antidote*—Camphor.

64. STRAMONIUM. Thorn-apple. Gympsum weed (vegetable). *Antidotes*—Belladonna, Nux vomica.

65. SULPHUR (mineral). *Antidotes*—Aconite, Camphor, Mercury, Nux vom., Pulsatilla.

66. SULPHURIC ACID. Oil of Vitriol (a mineral acid). *Antidote*—Pulsatilla.
67. TARTAR EMETIC. Tartarized Antimony (mineral). *Antidotes*—Cocculus, Ipecac., Pulsatilla.
68. TABACUM. Tobacco. *Antidotes*—Camphor, Ipecac., Nux vomica.
69. THUJA (OCCIDENTALIS). Arbor Vitæ Tree (vegetable). *Antidotes*—Camphor, Pulsatilla.
70. VERATRUM (ALBUM). White Hellebore (vegetable). *Antidotes*—Ipecac., Arsenic, Camphor, Coffea, Aconite, China.
71. ALOES. *Antidotes*—Vinegar, Vegetable Acids.
72. APIS MELLIFICA. Poison of honey-bee. *Antidotes*—Ars., Canth.

TINCTURES.

1. ARNICA, Tincture.
2. RUTA, Tincture.
3. SYMPHYTUM, Tincture.
4. URTICA URENS, Tincture.

These tinctures are intended for external use only. In preparing them for this purpose, put from four to ten drops in a teacupful of pure water; mix well, and wash with it, or lay cloths, dipped in the mixture, on the parts affected.

NOTICE TO HOMŒOPATHIC PHARMACEUTISTS.

It will be observed that in this "Domestic Physician," *Coffea*, *Belladonna*, and *Cina*, are used in two preparations—the third and the two hundredth. The latter has CC. attached to it, as *Belladonna* CC., showing, in the Roman numerals, the potency. It is expected that the preparations of these latter for the boxes are made in the greatest purity and genuineness. They can be procured all ready in every large city of the Union.

The potencies of all the other remedies are designed for those from the mineral and animal kingdom in the sixth, and for those from the vegetable kingdom in the third potency. The tinctures mentioned in the "List of Medicines" should accompany the boxes.

INTRODUCTION.

To aid in the search for the proper place in the work, where a disease may be found, its different popular names have always been given, and carefully recorded in the index. Should, however, the identification of a disease be difficult or doubtful, it is only necessary to refer, in the book, to the divisions made as to the parts of the system which are affected, such as "Affections of the Head, Chest," etc., where all the ailments of these parts are generally put together. But there will scarcely ever arise a difficulty in this respect; the index has been made very complete, in view of saving the reader time and unnecessary vexation.

If a disease is found, it is expected that everything will first be read which is said concerning it in the article, before a selection of a remedy is made; at the end of each article, the proper direction as to administration, diet, and regimen, is given. Wherever the attention is directed to the perusal of the Materia Medica, in treating on certain remedies, the medicine in question must be looked for in the Materia Medica, and its symptoms carefully compared with those of the patient. If in the directions for diet the reader is advised to adhere to the usual homœopathic diet in chronic diseases, etc., he will find its rules specified in the following pages, under "*Dietetic Rules.*"

It is necessary to give an explanation in regard to several remedies, whose names will be found different in this work from those used in other similar works. Of the various preparations of *Mercury*, only one kind has been used, and whenever this is mentioned, under the name of *Mercury*, the *Mercurius vivus* is understood by it. This was done for the sake of not unnecessarily confusing the reader with two different names for mercurial preparations, which are essentially the same in their effects and use. On that account the *Mercurius sublimat*. has been left out entirely. Its use is, at any rate, confined to one disease only (the dysentery), in the treatment of which the *Mercurius vivus* supplies its place completely.

On the other hand, three remedies, *Coffea*, *Belladonna*, and *Cina*, appear in two different preparations in the book, the one commonly used bearing the simple name, while the two-hundredth potency of these remedies has a $^{cc.}$ attached to them, showing in the Roman numerals the degree of potency. Although a great many more remedies could have been treated in the same manner, it was not thought advisable to burden the book with more therapeutical detail, as it might interfere with its other simple and practical arrangements. These three remedies, however, in their higher potencies, seemed to be almost indispensable, in a useful work of this kind, as their effects, when properly indicated, cannot well be produced by their lower attenuations. We invite particular attention to the use of *Cina*$^{cc.}$, in the nervous worm symptoms, so frequently experienced in children, in nightly attacks, which quickly disappear after the exhibition of one or two doses of *Cina*$^{cc.}$. Every homœopathic practitioner can soon satisfy himself in regard to the efficiency of the highest potencies, by making the above trial.

In regard to our views on the preference of higher or lower attenuations, we would remark, that we consider homœopathically legitimate and practically useful, all potencies, from the mother tincture and first trituration up to the highest dilution, but that we do not use one exclusively or all indiscriminately. Practical observation and theoretical researches have guided us in applying the various attenuations with real benefit, which is not so difficult as many practitioners might believe. There are principles according to which the different potencies of a remedy must be applied in different cases. But to enlarge upon this subject here, would carry us too far; we content ourselves by remarking that, for a domestic family-chest, we would propose, as a general rule, the third potency for all vegetable medicines, and the sixth potency for all mineral and animal medicines. If this rule was once adopted by all writers on homœopathic domestic practice, their several works might be used with benefit without subjecting the public to additional expense in procuring different medicine-chests for the works of different authors.

For a successful treatment of diseases, everything depends, after the selection of the right, or most homœopathic remedy, on the genuineness of its preparation. We would, therefore, advise our readers to procure their medicine-chests from persons whose competency or recommendations can be relied on; and when in their possession, to take good care of them. The vials must not be opened except when used; each vial must receive its own cork again, and no odorous medicinal substances must be allowed to be near by, when a vial is opened or medicine is taken. If a remedy is prescribed to be taken in water, a clean cup or tumbler must be selected, the prescribed quantity of water, either rain or river water poured in, then the medicine added, and, during its solution, well mixed with a clean teaspoon, and afterward covered well. If more medicines than one are prescribed at a time, in water, each one must be dissolved separately in a teacup, and each one receive its own separate teaspoon, which must not be changed during the administration of the medicine.

If a vial is empty, it is *indispensably* necessary, before refilling it, to cleanse it first thoroughly with warm water and dry it perfectly on a stove or in the sun, before the homœopathic apothecary is allowed to fill it. Persons ought to attend to this scrupulously themselves, before presenting them for refilling; because much depends on it, as regards the genuineness of the medicines.

The medicines should be kept in a dry place, where no odors can reach them. A renewal of their strength, if well kept, is not necessary for years; but if the slightest doubt in this respect should arise, it is better to have it renewed.

DIETETIC RULES.

The observance of a strict diet is essential to the success of a homœopathic treatment, not so much on account of the injury done to the system by the use of improper articles, as because these might be antidotal in their effects to the medicine On this account, homœopathists so generally forbid coffee, it being an antidote to most of their remedies. For the same reason, the use of all other things of a medicinal nature is strictly forbidden, such as spices, perfumeries, perfumed waters, soda waters, spiced ices, etc.

It is a general law of nature, to eat and drink only that which can sustain life, without producing any other effects, that is, simple nutriment; and as medicinal and spicy substances, although sometimes nutritious, are irritating and stimulating, the strict law of nature excludes them peremptorily from the daily use (see "Hygiene").

Diet in Acute Diseases.—As dietetic rules are given for each acute disease, separately throughout the book, it is not necessary to mention them in this place.

Diet in Chronic Diseases.— Consult the chapter on "Hygiene" on this subject.

There are certain principles which must guide us, during the treatment of chronic diseases, in selecting the articles of our diet, even from among those which are generally allowed. If the patient has symptoms of fever or irritation, in any part of the system, he must avoid all articles of a stimulating character, such as meats, eggs, and butter. In such cases, he should confine himself to a nutritious vegetable diet, such as potatoes, turnips, rice, barley, etc. If the disease appears mostly in the digestive organs, as a chronic diarrhea, all articles of a relaxing nature are in themselves injurious, such as fruits and other green vegetables, soups of meat, eggs, etc. In cases where constipation is present, the opposite course must be pursued.

Another consideration is, that articles of food, which disagree with the patient, although allowed or wholesome for others under similar circumstances, must be strictly avoided by him.

Aliments Allowed.

Beef and Mutton baked, roasted, or boiled, fresh or smoked Tongue, lean Ham.

Venison and wild Fowl.

Turkeys, Chickens, Pigeons.

Fresh scale Fish, Oysters.

Butter which is not rancid, mild new Cheese, raw or soft boiled Eggs, or eggs in Soups (except in cases of diarrhea). Meat Soups, Broths, seasoned with salt only.

All kinds of light Bread and Biscuit (except Soda-Biscuit and other Bread made with the addition of unusual substances).

Puddings, Dumplings or Noodles of Wheat, Indian, Rice, and Oat-meal, not too heavy, fat, nor spiced.

Cakes composed of Meal, Eggs, Butter in small quantity, and Sugar.

Food prepared of Arrowroot, Tapioca, Farina, Sago, Salep, Oat-meal and the like.

Irish Potatoes, Sweet Potatoes, Turnips, Carrots, Tomatoes, Cauliflower, Spinach and green Peas, or Beans (except in Colic and Diarrhea), Rice Hominy, Pearl Barley, dried Peas, or Beans.

Roasted or boiled, fresh or dried Fruit, as Prunes, dried Currants, fresh, ripe, sweet Apples, Peaches, Strawberries,

Raspberries, Gooseberries, and other sweet berries, and Grapes (except in Colic and Diarrhea).

Water, pure, or sweetened with Sugar, Currant Jelly, Raspberry, or Strawberry Syrup, Toast water.

Milk, in its different preparations, boiled milk, fresh Whey, Buttermilk.

Decoctions of Barley, Malt, Oat-meal, Farina, Rice, dried Fruit. Cocoa boiled with Milk or Water, pure, plain Chocolate, weak black Tea.

Salt moderately used, Sugar.

Ice-creams flavored with Strawberry and Lemons.

Aliments Forbidden.

Old smoked, salted Meat and salted Fish, old rancid Butter and cheese, Lard, fat Pork, Geese, Ducks, Turtles and Terrapins, Fish not having scales, as Catfish, Eels, Lobsters, Crabs, Clams, and Soups, prepared from these articles of food. All food prepared with Blood, and much animal fat. All kinds of Sausages, particularly such as are smoked. The flesh of all young animals. All Soups highly seasoned, Sauces, different kinds of Hash, drawn Butter, Pepperpot.

All kinds of Cakes, or Pastry, prepared with much Fat or Aromatics, Honey. All kinds of colored Sugar-work prepared by the confectioner, red Sugar, sugared Almonds, or Peach-kernels. Nuts of all kinds.

Radishes, Celery, Horse-radish, Garlic, Parsley, Red or Cayenne Pepper, Mustard, Saffron, Nutmeg, Vanilla, Laurel leaves, bitter Almonds, Cloves, Cinnamon, Allspice, Coriander, Fennel, Anise, Coffee, green Tea, spiced Chocolate.

All kinds of spiritous liquors, Brandy, Rum, Whiskey, Gin, Spirits, etc. Liquors, or Cordials, and other drinks, cold or warm, which are prepared with spiritous liquors, or spices.

All artificial and natural Mineral Waters, Mead, Spruce Beer, Soda Beer, Porter, Ale.

N. B. During the homœopathic treatment especial care

should be taken by the patient to avoid allopathic medicine of every description and form, pills, herb-teas, etc., internally and externally; particularly all salves, aromatic waters, hartshorn, smelling bottles, etc.; also, all perfumery, musk, cologne water, or other aromatic substance, tooth-powders containing such ingredients, etc.; especially be careful in using matches, not to inhale the vapor of the burning sulphur; matches must be lit only where the vapor can easily escape in a fire-place, or open hall. Moderate exercise in the open air, as, also, a careful observance of all other hygienic rules (see the article on Hygiene) is strongly recommended.

PART FIRST.

DESCRIPTION AND TREATMENT

OF

DISEASES.

CHAPTER I.

GENERAL DISEASES.

RHEUMATISM.

DIAGNOSIS.—Pains in the muscles and membranes, together with swelling of the surrounding cellular tissue, light redness, and heat; caused by having taken cold.

This is the general appearance of all rheumatic affections; yet their degrees and complications are so numerous, that it would almost require a separate treatise to do justice to such an extensive subject. We confine ourselves, here, to the more practical subdivision of *acute* and *chronic* rheumatism.

Beside, we would remark that rheumatism, particularly in the acute form, can exist in any part of the system, creating there such an inflammation as the affected organ is naturally disposed to, adding to it only its own rheumatic character. For instance: a patient is attacked with rheumatism in the arms or limbs; this at once leaves those muscles, and falls on the pleura, where it generates a *pleurisy,* not of the usual kind, but one which has the rheumatic character—a *rheumatic pleurisy.* In the same manner, we speak of rheumatic pneumonia, rheumatic inflammation of the eye, heart, etc. The best means to detect the rheumatic character, in cases of this kind, is to investigate whether the disease, in its acute form, has appeared after taking cold, by suppressing or disturbing the action of the skin, or, whether, in its chronic type, the changes of the atmosphere influence its severity. In such cases, we refer the reader to the respective chapters, where the diseases of these organs are specially treated.

There exists an intrinsic difference between rheumatism and gout. (See this article.)

To *prevent* attacks of rheumatism and annihilate within us the predisposition to it, we must avoid all sudden changes of temperature and all excesses, which can create local and general debility. We ought to strengthen the system against injurious external influences, by cold washing and bathing, by acquiring regular habits, and following the rules, as laid down in the chapter on "Hygiene."

a. Acute or Inflammatory Rheumatism.

This form of rheumatism, especially, developes itself after taking cold, or after any check of perspiration, sudden and severe enough to unfit the whole skin for its proper function of exhaling the imperceptible gases. First, an uncomfortable sensation and restlessness will appear, followed by chilliness and feverishness in alternation, thirst, constipation, and accelerated pulse; then the rheumatic pains appear in places where they either fix themselves, creating swelling, heat, and redness, or wander to other parts, where they repeat the same process, while those first attacked heal gradually and get well. In acute rheumatism, we sometimes find a dry skin; at other times, a very moist one, drenched with a watery perspiration, which does not relieve the patient. The perspiration, which will relieve the patient, is greasy, thick, glutinous, and smells acrid or sour.

Treatment.—*Aconite*—In the beginning, when the fever is high, the skin dry and hot, with excessive thirst and redness of the cheeks; *shooting* or *tearing* pains, worse at night and by the *touch*, extreme irritability of temper.

If this remedy, after having been applied for eight or ten hours, has mitigated the fever by producing general perspiration, yet the local pains remain in the muscles and joints, give,

Bryonia, in the same manner, when the pains are worse by *motion* or *at night*, when there is headache, fever, swelling of the joints, and gastric derangement, with constipation. Alternates well with *Aconite* or *Rhus*. (See this remedy.)

Belladonna, when *Bryonia* does not relieve, or when the parts are much swollen, *very red, shining*, and the patient is sleepless at night, complaining of dryness in the mouth and throat, and congestion to the head. Both remedies may be given in alternation, with advantage.

Chamomile, when, in the parts affected, there is a sensation of *numbness* or *paralysis*, worse at night, the patient is feverish, restless, agitated, *irritable*, trying to relieve himself by turning in the bed ; the pains often ascend into the head, ears, and teeth, with chilliness and a bruised sensation after sleep.

Arnica: Bruised or *sprained sensation* in the joints of the hands, feet, and in the small of the back, with hard, red and shining swelling; feeling of *numbness* and *crawling* in the affected parts; the pains are aggravated by *motion;* the patient is thirsty and irritable (*alternates well* with *Rhus*).

Nux vomica, in alternation with *Chamomile*, when the parts are numb, *cold air aggravates*, temper is irritable, bowels constipated. The pains are principally located between the shoulder blades; in the small of the back, and in the loins.

Pulsatilla—The same feeling of numbness and paralysis, but *relieved by exposure to cool air*, the patient wants to be uncovered, and is of a mild temper and whining mood, worse in the night; the pains have a great tendency to change places. (*Shifting* or *wandering* Rheumatism.)

Mercury—pains *increased* in the heat of the bed, or *toward morning*—also, when the patient *perspires profusely without being relieved by it*. *Lachesis* suits well after *Mercury*.

Dulcamara—in an attack of rheumatism which immediately follows a severe exposure to cold; the pains set in at night, are worse during repose, with but little fever.

Rhus—principal indication for its use is: *pains worse during rest,* or as if the flesh was torn from the bones; worse in *cold, damp weather.* This remedy, when the latter symptoms are present, alternates well with *Bryonia.* (See Bilious Rheumatic Affection.) It is, also, of great use, when there is *paralytic weakness* or *trembling of the extremities,* on moving them.

N. B. See also the remedies, stated under "Chronic Rheumatism."

If the pains in the limbs should cease suddenly, followed soon by difficulty of breathing, anxiety, weakness, or pains in the region of the heart, with violent palpitation, give *Aconite, Belladonna, Spigelia, Pulsatilla, Arsenicum* or *Lachesis,* as their detailed symptoms under "*Rheumatism of the Heart*" will indicate.

Administration.—Dissolve twelve globules of the selected remedy in half a teacupful of water, and give every two hours a teaspoonful; discontinue after four teaspoonfuls have been given, for eight or twelve hours, during which time the effect must be looked for before another remedy is selected. As soon as the patient is better, all medicine must be stopped, until he gets much worse again.

Application of Water.—In this disease the external and internal use of water is of great service to accelerate the cure, not impeding in the least the specific action of the rightly chosen homœopathic remedy. If the parts affected are very painful, cold bandages may be applied, well wrung out and changed frequently; during this time the patient keeps in bed, well covered, drinking water which is not very cold. If perspiration ensues, the patient may be kept in it from one to two hours, after which he is well washed off with a wet towel and rubbed dry; he must then, however, take a sitting-bath in milkwarm water, in which he remains until he is perfectly cooled off. These simple appliances, repeated as often as circumstances may require, are powerful accessories to the success of specific remedies. If the patient suffers from constipation, give him cold water injections and let him drink cold water freely.

DIET AND REGIMEN.—As regards nourishment, the patient must absolutely abstain from all meat, or soups of meat even long after the convalescence. He can have, however, gruels of farinaceous substances, oatmeal, farina, rice, etc., toast-water and cold water; during the fever, warm or cold lemonade and oranges. Cover the patient well with blankets, as many as his comfort dictates. Around the swollen joints and other parts affected, breast or neck, put wool, just from the sheep, or, at least, unwashed; this is necessary, however, only in case the patient cannot bear the hydropathic applications. This has, frequently, a very good effect. If possible, consult a homœopathic physician.

b. CHRONIC RHEUMATISM, or commonly called RHEUMATISM.

If a person is severely troubled by chronic rheumatism, let him at once apply to a homœopathic physician, who will give him relief, if it is at all in the power of medicine to do so. But, frequently, the reactive force of nature is already so much weakened, that it first requires to be strengthened, which can only be done by a systematic hydropathic treatment. However, in case of rheumatism, where the system is yet strong, the medicines, as detailed below, may be used, and will be found efficacious in a majority of them. Beside the remedies recorded under "Acute Rheumatism," which may also be used for chronic rheumatism, the following are the principal ones: *Ignatia, Thuja, Arnica, Dulcamara, China, Veratrum, Arsenic, Phosphorus, Caustic, Sulphur, Sepia.*

SYMPTOMATIC DETAIL.—*Ignatia : Contusive pains*, or as if the flesh were detached from the bones; worse at night, ameliorated by change of posture.

Thuja : Tearing, *pulsative* pains, as from ulceration under the skin, with a feeling of coldness and torpor of the parts affected. Pains worse during repose, or in the warmth of the bed. Pain in the right shoulder and arm, *better on movement.*

Arnica: Pains as if the parts were *strained* or *bruised,* with a feeling as if *they were resting on too hard a surface;* a tingling in the hand, red and *shining* swelling, worse when attempting to move. (Suitable before or after *China, Arsenic, Rhus.*)

Dulcamara: Pains after getting cold and wet, worse at night, during repose, and without much fever.

China: Pains, worse on the slightest touch, with easy perspiration, the sore parts feel very weak, almost paralyzed.

Veratrum: Pains as if from a bruise; worse by warmth and bad weather; better by walking; very weak and trembling.

Arsenic: Burning, tearing pains, insupportable at night, worse *by cold air,* and mitigated by external heat.

Phosphorus: Tearing and drawing pains, excited by the slightest chill; headache, vertigo, and oppression of the chest.

Caustic: The pains are *insupportable in the open air;* less severe in a room, or in bed; also, when there is paralytic weakness with *rigidity* and *incurvation of the parts affected.*

Sulphur: In almost all cases of chronic, and after a spell of inflammatory rheumatism, when the pains yet linger about. Often after *Aconite, Belladonna, Bryonia, Mercury,* or *Pulsatilla.*

Sepia: For rheumatic affections in tall, slender persons, especially females.

Application of Water.—The use of the wet bandage is in many cases of this disease most grateful and advantageous; it relieves pain and subdues inflammation, dissolves obstructions and accelerates the circulation in the parts affected. The application of the douche, or of ice and snow, is rather dangerous and must not be undertaken without the advice of a physician, who is conversant in Hydropathy; the same may be said of the use of the partial baths, applied to the affected parts, as the reaction, following their use, might increase the inflammation. The dry packing, to excite perspiration, with the following washing or ablution, is good in some cases, particularly where the pains are wandering, but must in a great many cases be dispensed with, as its frequent repetition would exhaust the system too much. The free use of cold water, internally, is strongly recommended.

ADMINISTRATION. — In chronic rheumatism, the remedies ought not to be repeated often; every three or four days, one dose (four to six glob.) is enough. After a remedy has been tried for ten or fourteen days, another may be chosen, if no improvement has appeared.

DIET AND REGIMEN.—The patient must abstain, during the treatment, from all meats, at least, as much as possible; must not expose himself to the changes of the weather, and should wear, on his skin, flannel underclothes, except while using hydropathy; in which case, he can do without them.

RHEUMATIC PAINS OR COLD.

(*In Chest, Stomach, Limbs, etc.*)

These pains appear on different parts of the body, after taking cold, in persons naturally inclined to rheumatic affections. If they manifest themselves in the chest, they resemble a *pleurisy,* for which the same remedies will be suitable; if they appear in the stomach and bowels, they resemble a *colic;* to which article we refer the reader for the suitable remedies; if the pains are in the *head, ears,* or *teeth,* see these headings.

In every case of this kind, the patient must be kept warm, and *should perspire.*

GOUT (*Arthritis.*)

DIAGNOSIS.—The symptoms of this disease are very similar to those of inflammatory rheumatism: consequently, the remedies will be almost the same. It is characterized by pains in the joints, with inflammatory swelling, and a feeling of dislocation; or, in chronic cases, with a swelling of the joints, caused by deposits in them of a calcareous substance, which impedes their movements and causes them to make a cracking noise. There is always connected with an attack of gout, flatulency, acid stomach, and other derangements of the digestive organs. The principal differences between rheumatism and gout are: rheumatism attacks more the muscles and membranes—gout, more the joints; rheumatism is hardly ever complicated with derangement of the digestive organs; gout is never without that—has, beside, permanent swelling of the joints, by calcareous deposit, which rheumatism never has. Rheumatism is caused by taking cold; consequently, depends on external causes; while gout is generated by internal causes, amounting, sometimes, to hereditary predisposition. Both diseases, however, can intermix with each other, one taking the form of the other.

We acknowledge an *acute* and *chronic* form of gout; recommending for both the same remedies, which we recorded under the two forms of rheumatism. We would add only one more remedy to this list; it is

Antimon. crud., when the attack is attended with nausea and a white-coated tongue; pains are worse *after eating*, in the night, after drinking wine, and in the heat of the sun; mitigated during repose, and in the cool air.

To make the selection of remedies easier, we will give a tabular view of them, in the different gouty complaints. Their details will be found under "Rheumatism."

For *inflammatory* gout; *Aconite, Antimon. crud., Bryonia, China, Nux vomica, Arsenic, Pulsatilla, Arnica.*

For the same, with *gastric derangement: Antimon. crud.*

For the *shifting, wandering, flying* gout: *Pulsatilla, Arnica, Nux vomica.*

For gout with *great swelling: Antimon. crud., Arnica, Bryonia, Rhus, China, Sulphur.*

For the gouty *nodes and lumps: Antimon. crud., Bryonia, Calcarea, Carbo vegetabilis, Graphites, Lycopodium, Phosphorus, Sepia.*

For gout in persons addicted to *spiritous liquors: Nux vomica, Aconite, Sulphur, Calcarea.*

For gout in persons called *high livers: Pulsatilla, China, Antimon. crud., Sulphur, Calcarea.*

For those who sometimes *work in the water: Pulsatilla, Sulphur, Calcarea, Dulcamara, Rhus, Sarsaparilla.*

For gout confined to *the big toe* (*Podagra*) *: Pulsatilla, Arnica.*

For the *stiffness of the limbs*, which remains after an attack of gout or *rheumatism*, give *Colocynth.*

Administration, Diet, and Regimen, the same as in "Rheumatism."

Pains in the Small of the Back, Loins, and Neck.

Notalgia. Lumbago.

Diagnosis.—Violent pain in the region of the small of the back and loins, more or less permanent, sometimes periodical, but mostly excited by seemingly external causes. This species of lumbago (*back and loin-ache*) occurs, frequently, after any quick motion of the back, as in rising from a stooping position. The patient is suddenly seized with a violent pain as if produced from an arrow shot into the part; it pins him, as it were, into a fixed attitude, from which he cannot stir without suffering torture, and forces him to keep quiet.

If such a rheumatic pain suddenly affects the muscles of the *neck*, forcing the patient to keep very quiet, commonly called *Kink* or *Crick* in the *neck*, it has the same origin, and requires the same treatment, as *lumbago*. Rubbing the neck with a soft warm hand untiringly for half an hour, frequently cures it effectually.

Although this disease is essentially rheumatic in its character and process, yet its foundation is constitutional; sometimes a predisposition is acquired by overstraining the muscular system by hard labor during exposure to wet and cold, or when there is a disposition to hemorrhoidal congestion of blood (*piles*) to these parts, which may sometimes increase to a real *inflammation of the spine*, the *spinal marrow* (*myelitis*), or go over, if not cured, into a chronic spinal affection.

TREATMENT.—*Aconite* is the principal remedy in the commencement, and does more to relieve the patient at once, than the lancet can accomplish, which the old school always applies in such cases.

Arnica, alternately with *Rhus*, if this disease is really the result of falling, overlifting, or any other mechanical injury.

Bryonia, if the pains in the back are *pressing;* the patient cannot walk erect; worse after the slightest motion, or current of cold air; patient feels chilly; head and limbs ache.

Rhus, in alternation with *Bryonia*, if the patient feels very weak, trembling, has to get up sometimes to ease himself; throws himself about in the night. After external injury, see *Arnica*.

Bellad., after *Aconite* and *Bryonia*, under similar symptoms, but more suitable for fleshy females during the (change of life) critical period; in alternation with *Rhus*, when the feverishness attending the attack is complicated with *restlessness*, dryness of mouth and throat, headache.

Nux vomica, if the parts feel as if tired, or *very much fatigued*, during the attack; pains are worse by *motion* and *turning in bed;* constipation, irritability of temper. Suitable for persons with a disposition to piles, or addicted to spiritous liquors.

Mercury, in alternation with *Nux vomica*, if catarrhalic diseases, influenza, etc., prevail, or a tendency to dysentery; or if the patient feels very weak, *perspires* a great deal without relief, worse at night.

Pulsatilla: Resembling the pains under *Nux vomica, but* caused by obstructions or irregularity of the courses (*menses*) in younger females of a mild, sensitive, or phlegmatic character.

Application of Water.—The use of the wet bandage and cold foot-baths will accelerate the cure of these diseases; in their chronic forms, where the nervous system has suffered much, sitting-baths, cold ablutions, and finally the douche will be necessary. Constipation is relieved by cold injections and drinking freely of cold water.

Administration.—Same as in "Rheumatism."

Diet and Regimen.—Also the same. We would advise those afflicted with this disease, to lie down immediately on a mattress, or something similar, and not attempt to brave it out, as the phrase is; because the medicine will not be able to cure as quickly, and chronic weakness of the back remains, together with a liability to a return of the disease.

Pain in the Hip. Hip Disease.

Sciatica. Coxalgia. Coxagra.

Diagnosis.—Pain in the region of the hip joint, extending to the knee, even to the foot, accurately following the course of the sciatic nerve. Its continual severity may impede the motion of the foot, producing stiffness and contraction, disturbing the rest at night, and thereby inducing general uneasiness and emaciation.

In *sciatica*, or *pain in the hip*, the pain manifests itself only on the outside of the hip and leg, during repose as well as during *motion*, showing its *neuralgic* character; while, in *coxagra* (*morbus coxarius*), the pain appears only during *motion* and in *stepping*, showing its *inflammatory* character; running in front to the knee, protruding and lengthening the leg. It can terminate in suppuration (*white swelling*).

These diseases are of great importance, and ought not to be neglected, but immediately put under the care of a skillful homœopathic physician, as scrofula is either their remote cause, or excited by them, especially in children, in whom they often occasion the so called *spontaneous limping* (*coxalgia infantilis*) and *white swelling*, particularly when badly treated at first by allopathic remedies.

TREATMENT.—The principal remedies in these diseases are those already enumerated under the headings of "Rheumatism" and "Gout." We will give them here again, to facilitate the selection:

In *sciatica* (*ischias*): *Chamomile, Bryonia, Rhus, Arsenic, Ignatia, Nux vomica, Pulsatilla.*

In *coxagra* (*hip disease*): *Colocynth, Belladonna, Hepar, Lachesis, Silicea, Mercury, Sulphur.*

In *spontaneous limping: Mercury* and *Belladonna* in alternation; every few days, a dose: *Rhus, Colocynth, Pulsatilla, Sulphur, Calcarea.*

SYMPTOMATIC DETAIL.—*Aconite*, in alternation with *Belladonna* or *Bryonia*, where the attack is accompanied with a great deal of fever.

Belladonna, in the inflammatory stage (see *Aconite*), when the pain is increased on the slightest movement, with limping, and on the parts affected the skin is red and shining; dryness of the throat; burning fever. After it, *Mercury*.

Bryonia, under similar symptoms as *Belladonna*, but particularly where the parts affected are more painful than red; constipation. After it, *Rhus*.

Rhus: Darting, tearing, or dragging pains in the hip-joint, with tension and stiffness in the muscles; worse during repose, or when rising from a sitting posture.

Chamomile: Pains worse at night in bed, after having recently taken cold; patient is irritable; does not know what he wants.

Mercury: Sharp, cutting, burning pains; worse at *night*, or during *movement;* profuse perspiration *without relief*. After *Belladonna;* before *Hepar*.

Ignatia: Cutting pains, ameliorated by *change of position*, temperament mild, yet vascillating between high and low spirits.

Pulsatilla: Pains worse in the evening or night, and when seated; *relieved in the open air;* temperament phlegmatic; mild disposition.

Nux vomica: Pains worse in the morning; *worse in the open air;* temperament irritable, morose; constipation.

Arsenic: Burning pains, with great restlessness, obliging the patient to move the limb; pains appear *periodically,* or in spells (alternate with *China*); mitigated by external heat; patient wants to lie down, feels very weak; emaciation of the limb after long suffering (in alternation with *Silicea*).

Colocynth. This is the first and principal medicine in hip diseases, acute or chronic, particularly when there is the sensation of a *tight band around the hips and back,* and the pains *run down from the region of the kidneys into the leg; spontaneous limping;* pains are worse lying on the back, or after a fit of anger or indignation.

Hepar after *Mercury,* when this has not relieved.

Silicea, when the disease assumes the chronic form, after *Hepar;* or, where emaciation has taken place, in alternation with *Arsenic,* and, afterward, with *Iodine.*

Sulphur, in chronic cases, where other remedies have not entirely relieved.

Lachesis: Emaciation, with tearing and contracting pain in the joint; *dread of exercise; deeply penetrating suppurations* (in alternation with *Silicea*).

Application of Water.—See "Pains in the Small of the Back."

Administration.—In the *sciatica* (*ischias*), as well as the febrile stage of the *coxagra,* give the medicines as required in the acute form of "Rheumatism" (see this article). In the chronic form (suppurative stage) of *coxagra,* give the remedies as stated in "Chronic Rheumatism."

Diet and Regimen.—The same as in "Rheumatism," but

without outward applications, save cold-water bandages, in any stage of the disease, when the patient can bear them, and feels relieved after them.

Inflammation of the Knee Joint. (*Gonitis.*)

Inflammation and swelling of this important joint, requires the use of *Aconite* and *Belladonna*, *Bryonia*, *Rhus*, *Lachesis*, *Mercury*, one after the other, if the first two have not allayed the inflammation. If suppuration threatens, which is indicated by the swelling not going down after the severest fever is over, give *Sulphur;* in eight days *Silicea*, and consult medical aid.

Administration of *Aconite*, *Belladonna*, and the other remedies, the same as in "Acute Rheumatism."

Diet and Regimen.—Also the same, but without any outward application, save cold water bandages, when the patient feels relieved by them, at any stage of the disease.

Inflammation of the Psoas Muscle. (*Psoitis.*)

Diagnosis.—Pain in the region of the kidneys, hip, and downward to the leg, which cannot be stretched, or drawn near to the abdomen, without pain; increased, also, by turning, when lying and lifting, with a feeling of numbness of the affected side; walking is possible only by hobbling, with the body bent forward. Although not often fatal, yet it is very important in its consequences, as its issues may give rise to lingering diseases. If suppuration takes place, by not preventing it in time, the matter discharges itself in the abdomen, and causes death; or it sinks down farther and farther, until it reaches, sometimes, even the knee, before it escapes; frequently, the spine becomes affected and is rendered carious in such cases. The causes of this disease are, beside external injuries, rheumatism, and piles.

Treatment.—Give, first, *Aconite*, and *Bryonia*, in alternation, every two, three, or four hours, a dose (four glob.);

afterward, *Belladonna* or *Nux vomica,* if not relieved within twenty-four hours, and when the pains increase during motion; *Rhus* and *Pulsatilla,* however, when the pains are worse during rest; *Mercury* and *Chamomile,* when the pains are worse at *night.*

Staphysag., when the pains are beating, indicating incipient suppuration.

Colocynth, when the disease assumes the chronic form.

If possible, consult a physician in this important disease.

Application of Water, in this disease, is confined to the use of the wet bandage, often renewed, on the parts affected; lukewarm sitting-baths, afterward applied, will accelerate the cure.

Administration, Diet, and Regimen, as in "Affection of the Knee Joint."

Cramp in the Legs.

Some persons are habitually addicted to cramp in the legs, from various causes. The first remedy, which every one naturally will resort to, is, to rub the parts taken with the cramp, either with the hands or a rough towel, which, in a short time, will destroy the spasm. Another expedient is, to jump on the cold floor of the room, if the cramp occurs in the calves of the legs, and while in bed; but, if it should occur frequently in the *night,* take

Veratrum, every night a dose (four glob.), for a few nights; or, if it occurs in pregnant females,

Secale, in the same manner.

If the cramps occur more in the day-time, take *Rhus,* in the morning, in the same manner.

Colocynth relieves the remaining stiffness, *also* cramps, occurring in the *night.*

Sulphur, Lycopodium, and *Sepia,* may be taken in intervals of four or six days, to prevent the return of the cramps.

Diet and Regimen, as in all chronic diseases.

4

SWEATING FEET.

This is a complaint with which a great many persons are afflicted. It is generally connected with a qualitative corruption of the secretions, by which a bad smell is emitted, thereby rendering the complaint very disagreeable. It can be easily suppressed by alum and sugar-of-lead ablutions; but he who ventures to do so, risks being taken with blindness, deafness, asthma, consumption, etc.

Homœopathy possesses remedies, which, when applied rightly, will insure a permanent and safe cure.

TREATMENT.—*Rhus*, inwardly, every third evening, six glob., to be continued for at least four weeks, after which two weeks must elapse before the next remedy may be taken. During the first four weeks, bathe the feet every other evening, in cold water, into which four drops of the mother tincture of *Rhus* (to be had in any homœopathic pharmacy) have been dropped.

Silicea, is the next remedy after *Rhus*, if this has not already ameliorated the complaint; to be taken in the same manner. In this way, alternate with these two remedies, until better, or apply to a homœopathic physician, who has more remedies at his command, which, however, can be chosen, only according to the individual constitutionality of each one's case.

APPLICATION OF WATER.—Cold foot-bath must not be used in this disease; if a person wants to use the hydropathic means, he had better resort to an institution, as in this disease, simple as it seems to be, the greatest caution is necessary in the use of water, and generally a full treatment, to change the constitution of the patient.

GOITRE. (*Struma.*)

This disease consists in a swelling of the thyroid gland, in front of the throat. It is, in the majority of cases, of a scrofulous origin; depends, sometimes, however, on an endemical cause, it occurring most frequently on mountains, especially at their base, and in their valleys.

Treatment.—Take, internally, *Spongia*, every evening a dose (six glob.) and wash externally with a solution of the tincture of *Iodine* diluted in alcohol, every evening, until it disappears.

If this treatment does not disperse the goitre within two months, apply to a homœopathic physician, who has other remedies, suitable for each individual case.

Diet, as usual in chronic diseases.

Sleeplessness. (*Agrypnia.*)

This disease consists in an impossibility to sleep, without any apparent external or internal cause to disturb the sleep. If it continues for months and years, a serious disturbance of all functions must ensue. In infants, particularly, it becomes a distressing circumstance for mothers and nurses, as we often are unable to find out its cause.

Treatment.—*Coffea* and *Belladonna*, two doses in alternation (in children, *Coffea*$^{cc.}$ and *Bellad.*$^{cc.}$), every hour one dose (four glob.) frequently allay the over-excitement of the nervous system.

If this will not do one night, try, on the next,

Belladonna, if caused by congestion of blood to the head.

Hyoscyamus, especially after severe illness.

Ignatia, when caused by *grief, indignation.*

Nux vomica, when from study and meditation in hypochondriacs.

Opium, after fright and fear, or in old people, or where frightful visions appear when closing the eyes.

Pulsatilla, when having indulged too freely in eating.

Aconite, when caused by agitating events and anxiety.

If caused by drinking tea or coffee, see their antidotes in the articles respecting these substances.

In *children*, beside *Coffea* and *Bellad.*, are recommended

Cham., *Jalap*, and *Rheum.*, when it is caused by *colic*. See this article in "Diseases of Children."

APPLICATION OF WATER.—Beside these remedies, a sponge-bath of cold water, every evening when going to bed, is strongly recommended; also a cold foot-bath, before going to bed, if the patient cannot sleep on account of congestion to the head.

NIGHTMARE. (*Incubus.*)

A well known troublesome disease, consisting in a heavy pressure on the precordial region, which impedes breathing, creating thereby many images of fancy, monsters, robbers, bears, etc. It occurs mostly in the first hours of sleep, and, if recurring every night, would certainly injure the general state of health.

It is caused either by an overloaded stomach, congestion of the blood to the abdomen, or to the precordial region, when lying on the back.

TREATMENT.—Persons liable to this disease must first avoid the above-mentioned exciting causes, before the following remedies can have their effect:

Aconite: Especially in women and children, when feverishness, oppression of the chest, anxiety, and inquietude, prevail.

Nux vomica, after drinking spiritous liquors, eating a full meal in the night, or by sedentary habits.

Opium: The principal remedy in severe attacks, snoring, respiration, eyes half open, face covered with cold perspiration, and convulsive movements of the limbs.

APPLICATION OF WATER.—The wet bandage around the chest during the night is strongly recommended, with a cold ablution and dry rubbing in the morning; beside daily exercise in the open air, and the free use of cold water internally.

DIET must be moderate, consisting more of vegetables than meat; constipation is relieved by cold water injections, and the drinking of cold water.

PALSY. (*Paralysis.*)

This affection of the nerves of voluntary motion, is one of those diseases, to remove which, it requires the greatest skill of a physician; and, by bringing it under our notice here, we intend merely to warn our readers not to waste time, health, and money, in using a variety of nostrums which might be recommended for it; but to apply at once to a skillful homœopathic physician, who can effect a cure in a majority of cases. Beside, we will record a few remedies, with which such a cure may be commenced.

If from *debility* caused by loss of fluids, *China, Ferrum, Sulphur.*

If from suppression of an eruption or habitual discharge, *Lachesis, Sulphur, Caustic.*

If from *rheumatism, Bryonia, Rhus, Arnica, Lycopodium.*

If from *apoplexy, Ipecac., Lachesis, Lycopodium.*

If from handling *white-lead,* or exposure to the *fumes of lead, Opium, Bellad., Platina, Pulsatilla.*

If the *facial muscles* are paralyzed, *Belladon., Graphites, Caustic.*

If the tongue, *Bellad., Opium, Stramonium, Hyoscyamus, Lachesis.*

If the *arms, Bellad., Lachesis, Nux vomica, Opium, Lycopodium.*

If the *lower limbs, Cocculus, Opium, Nux vomica, Stannum, Silicea.*

Electricity and *Galvanism* may be used in this disease with the greatest advantage, as also the cold water in bathing and drinking. See "Hydropathy."

APPLICATION OF WATER. — Rubbing with cold water, the wet bandage, and finally the douche are powerful helps in this disease; but their use ought to be sought rather in hydropathic institutions, where the facilities for their application are greater and more regulated.

Delirium Tremens. (*Mania a potu.*)

This terrible disease is almost exclusively confined to drunkards and opium eaters, who are taken especially when exhausted otherwise, with a delirium and frenzy, in which appearances of horrible monsters, animals, figures of all kinds, frighten their imagination, combined with ravings, convulsion fits, and complete inability to sleep. In the long and sleepless hours, they converse incessantly with these supposed realities, by which they wear out their strength more and more.

Treatment.—*Opium* is the specific in this disease, if it is caused by ardent spirits, as this drug is itself able to produce such a disease. Give of it, every hour or two hours, a dose (one or two drops of a diluted tincture of opium), for at least twenty hours, to see its effects. After this, give *Bellad.*, *Nux vomica*, *Sulphur*, one after the other, each, for twenty-four hours, every three or four hours a dose (six glob.), or *Calcarea carbonica*, if frightful images appear as soon as the patient shuts the eyes, or when he talks in his sleep, groans, cries, dreams fantastically and frightfully. If nothing will produce sleep, give *Lachesis* and *Arsenic*, in alternation, every three hours a dose (four glob.).

Let the patient drink freely of *ice water*, as the best stimulus which can be substituted. For solid nourishment, give him hard-toasted bread: as soon as he is convalescent, give him a good beefsteak, bread, and water, on which he has to subsist for a long time. In this way, I have cured very bad cases, and had the satisfaction to see them not only restored to health again, but to usefulness and their friends, as they never relapsed into their former error.

Epilepsy. (*Epilepsia.*)

Diagnosis.—Convulsive motions, with loss of consciousness; falling down, with cries, foaming at the mouth, the thumbs fixed into the palms of the hands. The loss of con sciousness is the most essential symptom, not the violence of the convulsions. The weakest convulsion, with unconsciousness, is epilepsy, while the most violent convulsions, but with consciousness, is *not* epileptic.

Most of the epileptic patients can be cured, but it requires the attendance of a skillful homœopathic practitioner. We refrain, therefore, from mentioning here any more of the treatment of this disease, but that which relates to the attack itself.

TREATMENT.—A patient in an epileptic fit must be placed in a position in which he cannot hurt himself; give him, however, full liberty of his own actions, without holding him, or forcing open his thumbs, which is of no use. Let him smell on *Camphor spirits.* If convenient, put between his teeth a cork or piece of wood, to prevent his tongue being injured. As soon as possible, give him one dose (four glob.) of *Bellad.;* or, if his face is dark and congested, his breathing very hard and snoring, a dose of *Opium* (four glob.).

ST. VITUS'S DANCE. (*Chorea.*)

DIAGNOSIS.—Involuntary motions of single members or the whole body, wandering from one part to the other. The patient retains full consciousness, which is a distinctive feature of this disease from epilepsy. It varies very much in degree; occurs most frequently at the time of the development of puberty, from the seventh to the sixteenth year, more among the female sex, more in moist regions on the sea-coast than in more elevated places. It may occur, also, as an epidemic, and is then infectious, particularly when large crowds meet. It is not a dangerous disease, but troublesome, and may lead to other derangements; ought to be attended to, therefore, immediately, as, in such a case, it can easily be cured.

TREATMENT.—As we recommend our readers to apply, in a case of this kind, to a homœopathic physician at once, we limit our remarks on the treatment to a few remedies, which may be given in the beginning.

Ignatia, every evening a dose (six glob.) for eight days, after it,

Sulphur, every other evening a dose (six glob.) for eight days, and then discontinue for three or four weeks, to await the effect.

Diet and Regimen.—No greasy substances, no coffee or tea, but good plain food. Try to divert the attention of the patient from his disease; never speak of it in his presence.

Tetanus. Trismus. (*Lockjaw.*)

Diagnosis.—Constant spasmodic contraction of one muscle, or all the muscles. According to the parts affected and the direction in which the body is drawn, the disease has received different names; which distinction does not come, however, within the limits of our description, as such severe diseases as these will require medical aid. We intend here to speak more especially of one form of tetanus, called *trismus* or *lockjaw*, which is of frequent occurrence in southern latitudes, and, from its quick termination, requires prompt action, and, therefore, domestic attention.

Lockjaw. (*Trismus.*)

It arises immediately after a wound has been inflicted, in consequence of the violent pain and nervous irritation, in which case it proves fatal in a very short time; or it occurs in the first few days after the infliction of a wound, during its inflammatory stage, or from eight to ten days afterward, while the wound is healing and suppurating, without any pain and inflammation. The exciting causes are, mental affections, taking cold, corrupt air, foreign bodies in the wound, tension, and distraction of single fibers in the wound. The most dangerous are the stitch wounds in tendonous parts, as in the sole of the foot and the palm of the hand. The pulse frequently remains normal, the head free, yet there is great anxiety and oppressed breathing.

Treatment.—Enlarge the wound, if possible, and poultice it with bread and milk. Beside, give the following remedies:

Arnica. In the beginning, externally, in a wash or fomentation; internally, in globules or drops, every two hours a dose (four glob. or one drop).

Belladonna and *Lachesis*, in alternation, in the same dose and time, if the spasms increase. If no improvement, after twelve hours, takes place, give *Opium* and *Hyoscyamus*, in the same manner.

Secale, if the patient feels worse in the warmth.

Ignatia, if the patient grows worse, whenever touched or handled.

Rhus and *Ignatia*, in case the body is bent backward, in the form of an arch. Administer it in the same manner.

Stramonium, in the same form of lockjaw, if the two former remedies were of no avail.

Application of Water.—The action of the homœopathic remedies, in this disease, may be supported by the following hydropathic process. The patient having been put in a bathing-tub, is rubbed well and for a long time with cold water, after which he is brought to bed again and rubbed dry with the hands or dry woolen cloths. In an hour or two this process has to be repeated, if no change has taken place; sometimes it is good to expose the spine to the douche, after which the rubbing with the hands must be repeated again.

Diet and Regimen.—The same as in fevers.

SOMNOLENCY. LETHARGY.

Diagnosis.—A sleep, continued beyond the natural time, for days or weeks. During this time, short intervals of waking intervene, but the patient soon relapses into sleep again. Nourishment can be given only by injecting fluid aliments; otherwise, the functions of life are not disturbed.

In such cases, a physician will be consulted; but up to

the time of his coming, the following medicines may be given.

Opium, if the pulse is full and slow, the breathing snoring, and the face very red, even dark; every three hours a dose, or until better.

Belladonna, if the head is hot and the feet are cold; pulse accelerated and hard.

Lachesis, if the pulse is very weak; beside, *Aconite, Veratrum, Pulsatilla, Phosphoric acid*, one after the other, if necessary.

Application of Water.—That cold water must be a powerful auxiliary in the treatment of this disease, is very evident; its use must be regulated according to the symptoms of the case; cold foot-bath, if the head is hot and congested; sitz-baths, hand and head-baths are variously applicable.

Fatigue, Overheating, and Mental Exhaustion.

Arnica, for a feeling as if the body were *bruised*, after over-exertion of the body, and too long and fast traveling on foot; wash the fatigued limbs in water, with which a few drops of the *Arnica tincture* has been mixed.

Rhus: Pains in the joints. After *Arnica*, if this was not sufficient. In alternation with *Bryonia*, if there are shooting pains in the small of the back on *moving*.

China: Weakness after loss of fluids, or heavy perspirations.

Veratrum, if persons are so fatigued as to cause fainting, in alternation with *Ipecac.* or *Apis mel.*

Coffea and *Camphor*, in alternation, when the system is exhausted by disease, abstinence from food, or violent exercise.

Cocculus and *Nux vom.*, if caused by long night-watching.

Aconite, if, with weakness, there is palpitation of the heart, pain in the side, difficulty of breathing, aching in the limbs from running fast; and then in alternation with *Bryonia*.

Cocculus, if the least exertion causes fatigue, followed by *Veratrum* and *Calcarea*, if necessary.

ADMINISTRATION. — Dissolve twelve glob. of a remedy in half a teacupful of water, and give, every half-hour or hour, a teaspoonful, until better.

If *overheated* by bodily exercise in the summer, take a little brandy and water, and no cold drinks until restored again; or, if possible, take a warm bath for twenty minutes. If the limbs feel sore, rub with *Arnica*, or alcohol in which soap is dissolved.

For *mental exhaustion* by over-study or anxious night-watching, take *Nux vomica;* if very much excited and sleepless, *Coffea;* if with fullness of the head, *Belladonna.*

FAINTING, SWOONING. (*Syncope.*)

Nervous persons, particularly females, are subject to fainting fits, excited by various causes, external or internal. The first thing to be done is, to lay the patient quietly on a bed or couch, where the fresh air is accessible; loosen everything tight about the neck, chest, and stomach, and sprinkle cold water in the face, for a minute or two; during this time some one has procured spirits of camphor, which now may be held under the nose, to be inhaled. This, in most cases, is sufficient to restore the patient for the time, who must now be let alone, to gather strength. If the cause of the fainting can be ascertained, one of the following remedies may be given, to destroy the bad consequences which the attack may have on the nervous system.

If caused by *fright, Aconite, Opium, Sambucus, Staphysag., Veratrum.*

By excessive joy, *Coffea, Aconite, Opium.*

By *anger, Pulsatilla, Platina, Nux vom., Chamomile.*

By *excessive pain, Veratrum, Aconite, Chamomile.*

By the *slightest pain, Hepar.*

By *grief, mortification, Ignatia, Colocynth, Platina, Mercury, Phosphor. acid, Staphysag.*

By *fear*, *Ignatia*, *Pulsatilla*, *Veratrum*, *Opium*.

By *depletion*, *blood-letting*, etc., *China*, *Carbo veg.*, *Veratrum*, when, also, a little wine or brandy and water may be given.

ADMINISTRATION.—Dissolve twelve glob. of the selected medicine in half a teacupful of water, and give, every five or ten minutes, a teaspoonful. If not relieved in twenty or thirty minutes, prepare and give another remedy in the same manner.

APPARENT DEATH.

Whenever a sudden extinction of life appears, our suspicion must be aroused, as regards the real or apparent death of the individual, in as far as we frequently might be able to restore the apparently dead to life again, if we would only take the trouble and have the patience to use the requisite means. And even when these are applied, it is often done in an unsystematic manner.

As most cases of apparent death occur under violent circumstances, such as drowning, hanging, etc., it is quite natural that the minds of the by-standers become agitated and confused, not knowing what is first to be done. This uncertainty and hurry of action, however, cannot produce any favorable results in resuscitating the apparently dead.

It is of the utmost importance to remain self-possessed, to reflect well, and then to do only one thing at a time, until all available means to restore life are exhausted. There are a great many accidents in life, by which its existence is put in jeopardy. We will enumerate them here, and the means which ought to be used. On poisoning, we give a separate chapter.

1. *Apparent Death from Hunger.*

If starvation was the cause of an apparent suspension of life, inject small quantities of warm milk mixed with a very little brandy or Madeira wine; beside, lay cloths, dipped in warm milk and brandy, on the stomach. Do not attempt to give any nourishment by the mouth, until after the patient has commenced breathing again, at which time the warm milk may be given to him, drop by drop, through the mouth. Increase the doses of milk very gradually, until the patient can take a teaspoonful; then a few drops of wine or brandy will be salutary. After a while, give him small quantities of beef-tea, or other broth. Solid food is not allowed, until after the patient has had a sound, healthy sleep: and even then, he has to be very careful in not eating too much at a time, or indulging in anything indigestible.

2. *Apparent Death from Drowning.*

The following cautions ought to be observed:

1. Be quick, but not rough, in all that has to be done.
2. Do not roll the body on casks.
3. Do not hold it up by the feet.
4. Do not rub the body with salts or spirits, nor inject smoke or infusion of tobacco.
5. Do not bleed the patient.

But do the following immediately:

1. Convey the body, carefully, in a raised position, to the nearest house, if possible; or, if not, lay it on a dry, sandy place, in the hot sun.
2. Strip the body, and rub it dry; then wrap it in warm blankets, either in a warm bed, or in heated sand or ashes, until other means of warming the body can be procured, such as bottles of hot water, warming pans, heated bricks, etc., which may be applied successively on the stomach, spine, thighs, under the armpits, and soles of the feet.
3. Wipe and cleanse the mouth, nostrils, and throat, carefully; during this operation the body may be turned on its side, the head bent forward, to allow the water to run out of the mouth; all the water which can run out is in the mouth.
4. Rub, continually and briskly, the whole body with the hands, or with warm cloths. Do not suspend, however, the use of the other means.

5. From time to time, try to inflate the lungs of the patient, by introducing into one of the nostrils the pipe of a pair of bellows, carefully closing the mouth and the other nostril; blow the bellows gently until the chest rises, then set the mouth and nostrils free, and press lightly on the chest, to eject the air from the lungs; after which, the same process must be repeated and continued for some time.

6. Immerse the body, if possible, in a warm bath, at blood heat.

7. Electricity or galvanism may be used.

8. Put a few globules of *Lachesis*, and afterward, *Opium* on the tongue of the patient.

9. Continue this treatment for, at least, four or six hours, even if then no signs of life appear, do not remove the body immediately from its position, but wait until signs of decomposition are manifest.

If, however, the patient recovers and can swallow, give him small quantities of warm wine or brandy and water. Beside, watch him and attend to his further wants carefully.

3. *Apparent Death from Freezing.*

See "Frozen Limbs," page 67.

4. *Apparent Death from Lightning.*

Remove the body into the fresh air, and, immediately, dash cold water on face, neck, and breast. If possible, cover the body all over (except the face) with newly-excavated earth. These means are the best, because water and wet ground are good conductors of electricity, with which the patient's system is surcharged at the time. Inwardly, give him, from time to time, a few globules of *Nux vomica*, of which, also, a solution may be injected.

If the patient recovers, remove him to a light, sunny room, where he should be kept quiet for some time, without mental excitement.

5. *Apparent Death from Hanging, Choking, or Suffocation by Burdens and Pressure.*

Tight clothing must be removed, and the patient placed in an easy, half-erect position; the neck not bent forward too much. Then rub him gently, but steadily, with the hands or warm cloths, and give, inwardly, from time to time, a few drops of the following mixture: five drops of laudanum or tincture of *Opium* in four tablespoonfuls of water; of which, also, injections may be made; five drops of the mixture to each injection. Afterward, apply means for warming the body, such as heated bricks, bottles of hot water, etc.

If this has been continued for an hour or two, and still no signs of life appear, mix a drop of Prussic acid in a tumblerful of water, or pound a bitter almond fine and mix it in a tumblerful of water, and put a few drops of either of these mixtures on the tongue from time to time.

After recovery, treat the patient as stated under the head "Apparent Death from Drowning."

6. *Apparent Death from Noxious Vapors.*

Remove the body into cool, fresh air; dash water over neck, face, and breast, and treat it, in general, as is recommended under the head "Apparent Death from Drowning."

7. *Apparent Death from a Fall or Blow.*

After the sufferer has been placed in a half-erect position on a bed or couch, put on his tongue a few globules of *Arnica*, and wash the parts which have been hurt by the fall or blow with a solution of the tincture of *Arnica* and cold water (twelve drops of the tincture in half a pint of water); also give injections of the same mixture. Then examine carefully the patient's condition as regards fractures of bones or other injuries, and do not allow him to be bled, as this expedient is, to say the least, always of a doubtful character, and entirely superseded by the above treatment.

Continue steadily the use of *Arnica,* internally and externally; if the patient has been bled, a dose (four glob.) of *China* may be given, if much blood has been taken.

8. *Apparent Death from Violent Mental Emotion.*

See the article on "Fainting, Swooning," page 51.

CHAPTER II.

CASUAL DISEASES.

I. External Injuries.

As this subject commands such a wide sphere of action, including as it were the whole art of surgery, it would be impossible to do it justice in a treatise like this, except we were able to condense it in a lucid manner, showing the application of a few medicinal agents and mechanical appliances, and pointing at those principles, on the strength of which they are used. Thus, every one can easily be prepared to do, if not all, what could be done right; at least, not to do wrong, in cases where circumstances require him to do something.

In the term "external injuries," are comprehended,

1. *Fractures of Bones.*
2. *Dislocations of Joints.*
3. *Wounds and Bruises.*
4. *Sprains and Concussions.*
5. *Burns and Scalds.*
6. *Poisoned Wounds, Stings of Insects, etc.*
7. *Frozen Limbs, etc.*

1. Fractures of Bones.

It is all-important from the first, to know whether a fracture has taken place, and to what extent. Its immediate reduction is not so necessary, as this can be done, just as conveniently and better, after the first wound-fever has disappeared.

The fracture of a bone is presumed to have taken place, when the force and direction of the injury or accident were sufficient to accomplish it. Its certainty, however, is established, when on closer examination, we find the injured limb shorter, in some measure deformed, unable to move, when the patient feels stinging pains on the injured place, and when we can hear on handling this spot, a crepitation, that is, a grating noise, which is produced when the two broken surfaces of the bone are rubbed together.

There are a number of terms to indicate the nature and extent of the injury sustained by a fracture.

It is called a *simple* fracture, when the bone is broken without any severe contusion or external wound.

A *compound* fracture is attended by an external wound or protrusion of the broken bone through the skin.

Complicated is a fracture, when the bone is either broken in more than one place or is attended by other severe injuries, such as lacerations of flesh, ligaments, larger blood-vessels, etc. In a *transverse* fracture the bone is broken in a perpendicular direction to its axis, while in the *oblique* fracture this is not the case. If the bone is broken into several pieces, the fracture is called a *comminuted* fracture.

TREATMENT.— Put the patient in a comfortable position; move the broken limb or part as carefully as possible, and compare its formation with the corresponding healthy one. If it is possible, without much exertion, to straighten its form, do so, even if temporary extension of the broken parts would be required to bring them together; then put a compress around the broken parts, on top of which place four strips of pasteboard or shingles, which are to be kept in their places by a circular bandage, not fastened too tight. Over the whole pour, from time to time, a mixture of cold water and *Arnica tincture* (twelve drops of the tincture to half a pint of water, well mixed); put the limb in a comfortable posture, by pillows, etc.; keep the fractured parts wet, and give, internally, a drop or two of *Arnica tincture* every six or eight hours.

After the second or third day of the injury, when by the use of the *Arnica* the bruises and contusions of the limb have healed, prepare and use the tincture of *Symphytum* in the same manner as directed under *Arnica*. The use of *Symphytum* accelerates the adhesion of the broken parts.

The attention of a surgeon must be sought, at any rate; but, if he cannot be had, a repetition of the above bandaging on the third, sixth, and twelfth day, etc., will be sufficient to insure the healing of the fractured parts.

In fractures of the skull, do nothing more than apply cold water and *Arnica*, as above stated, until a surgeon arrives.

2. Dislocations of Joints.

Compare the dislocated part with the corresponding healthy one, and consider, quietly, without being confused, whether it can easily be brought back, for which purpose a few trials may be made. If, however, this should be too hazardous, desist from any further attempts, but use cold water and *Arnica*, as stated in "Fractures of Bones," and wait for the arrival of a competent surgeon. If bandages are necessary, their use must be to confine the joint for some time in the same position after it becomes set.

3. Wounds and Bruises.

Wounds are either *incisive, lacerated, contused, punctured*, or *gunshot* wounds, according to the various instruments which have inflicted them.

Our object is to heal them as quickly as possible, as circumstances will allow. This is done, by bringing their edges immediately in close contact and keeping them there by adhesive plaster or sutures, which is the quickest mode of healing wounds, particularly those of the *incisive* kind. In some wounds the edges cannot be brought together, because the flesh is lacerated or bruised. Cases of this kind have to heal by means of suppuration, by which healthy granulation is produced, gluing as it were the parts together. This process applies to all the other kinds of wounds, including the *punctured* and *gunshot* wounds. One important consideration must always be kept in view: never to allow the surface of a wound to heal or close before it is certain that its deeper parts have firmly adhered. This can be prevented by introducing lint to the bottom of the wound, renewing it as often as necessary, at least once a day, and cleaning it with lukewarm water.

The first thing to be done, in attending to a wound, is to clean it, by cold water, from all foreign bodies which may be in it. Splinters must be extracted carefully, and the hemorrhage stopped, which, in most cases, ceases after the application of cold water mixed with a few drops of *Arnica tincture* (see "Fractures"); if it does not stop, however, or if the blood gushes out of the wound in jets, and is of a bright red color (arterial blood), try to compress the wound with lint dipped in arnica-water, overlaid with a sponge; and if this does not succeed, compress with the fingers the artery above the wound (on a place nearer to the heart), which can be found on the inside of a limb, indicated by the beating of the artery; if this cannot be done, bind around the whole limb, above the wound, a handkerchief, as tight as is necessary to stay the hemorrhage. If the patient has lost a great quantity of blood, give him some good wine and a few doses of *China;* he will feel stronger in a short time. When this is done, dress the wounds, either with adhesive plaster (if they are cut or incisive wounds), or loosely with lint kept constantly wet by cold water mixed with *Arnica tincture* (see "Fractures"). Give, internally, a few drops of *Arnica tincture* in water, and place the patient in a comfortable position.

Contused and bruised wounds allow of a certain degree of

compression, by adhesive plaster, after the inflammation has left, to make the edges adhere more closely; this can be done afterward.

Another important consideration is, to keep healing wounds well cleansed, by means of allowing the secreted matter to escape easily in the lint spread over the wound to keep off the air. Every day a suppurating wound ought to be cleansed and bathed freely in lukewarm water. If a wound inflames, becomes hot, swollen, and painful, put a warm bread-and-milk poultice over it, until it feels easier; internally, give *Chamomile, Belladonna*, and *Hepar*, alternately, every two hours a dose (four glob.).

If a *wound fever* sets in, give *Aconite, Chamomile, and Belladonna*, in alternation, in the same manner.

If *lockjaw* should appear, see page 48.

N. B. Although *Arnica tincture* is recommended above in *all* kinds of wounds as the proper outward application, yet *Calendula tincture* is best after *Arnica*, in all contused and lacerated wounds.

If a wound suppurates too freely, or secretes unhealthy matter, give *Hepar* and *Silicea*, in alternation, every evening a dose (four glob.), until better.

4. Sprains and Concussions.

These are caused by falls, lifting of heavy weights, jerks, false steps, etc. Bruises, wounds, or fractures, which may attend them, have to be treated first. If the patient is free from them, however, put him at once in a comfortable position, and use, externally, a mixture of cold water and *Arnica tincture*, particularly when the parts are *black and blue* (*bloodshot*); after it, *Rhus* in solution, when the *joints, membranes* and *tendons*, are more affected. This latter remedy is also suitable for the bad consequences of lifting too heavy weights (*strains*).

Internally give *Bryonia* and *Rhus* in alternation, every four hours six globules, until the patient feels relieved from the stiffness and soreness in the limbs.

Diet, must be light, no meat or stimulating drinks are allowed; gruels and lemonades are recommended.

5. Burns and Scalds.

Slight degrees of these injuries heal quickly by holding the scalded parts to the fire (if that is possible), or fomenting them with warm alcohol, or covering them with a plaster of Castile soap. But burns and scalds increase in importance and danger, in proportion to the depth and extent of the injury, which, if very great, threatens the life of the patient. If more than one-half of the surface of the skin is deeply scalded, the sufferer will seldom recover.

A great many remedies are recommended for burns and scalds, but their usefulness must be determined according to the quickness with which they can be procured, their easy applicability, and, lastly, their specific effect on the burns, as such.

Treatment.—The best remedy in slight cases is already mentioned above. In severer cases, and even the worst, use *Castile soap*, scraped and mixed with water to a thick lather; spread it on strips of linen or cotton cloth, to the thickness of the sixth of an inch; then spread it over the wound, taking care to cover with soap every burned part, and keep it moist for awhile with cold water, which may be dropped on top, very sparingly, from time to time. Let these plasters remain until they drop off themselves; or, if matter forms underneath, remove them and dress the wounds with a salve made of equal parts of sweet oil or linseed oil and lime-water, which is a very good remedy in the beginning, if it only could be had quick enough.

Another remedy, easy off access, is *raw cotton*, with which the burned parts must be covered, pressing it lightly on the wounds.

If a person has inhaled hot steam, or has burned his throat with hot liquids, give him, of a solution of Castile soap in whisky or alcohol (which can be made very soon, by scraping soap into the liquor and shaking the bottle well), every five or ten minutes, two or three drops in water, lengthening the intervals as the patient gets better.

N. B. Every steamboat ought to be provided with a bottle of spirits of soap, decidedly the best remedy for these internal burns, as it acts specifically on the injured nervous system and composes immediately.

Another remedy is the tincture of *Urtica urens* (*stinging nettle*), of which each homœopathic medicine-chest contains a bottle. Apply it in a manner similar to the *Arnica tincture* (twelve drops to a pint of water). For internal burns, put three drops of it in a teacupful of water, and give, every five or ten minutes, a teaspoonful, until better.

If the burns ulcerate, wash them with a solution of twelve globules of *Caustic* in half a teacupful of water, three times a day, and give, internally, *Hepar* and *Silicea*, alternately, every evening a dose (six glob.) until better.

Diet and Regimen.—The diet must be light, as in fevers; but when ulceration takes place, give stimulating diet, beef, etc., even brandy and water. If a *diarrhea* ensues during the healing of the burns, do not disturb it by giving medicine for it (except it be too excessive), as it is a critical discharge, the intestines supplying by their action, the interrupted functions of the skin. When dressing the wounds, open the blisters which have formed, remove as much of the skin as can be done easily, and take care that the patient is not exposed to currents of air during this operation, which must not last a longer time, nor be oftener repeated, than is necessary; but, if the patient should have taken cold, in consequence of which the wounds pain very much and become inflamed, red, swollen (a kind of erysipelas in the scalded parts), give *Aconite* and *Belladonna*, in alternation, every two hours a dose, and dress the wounds with dry lint; but if the wounds were already suppurating when this took place, give *Chamomile, Bellad.*, and *Hepar*, in the same manner, and dress the wounds with a warm poultice of bread and milk, until suppuration commences again and the fever leaves.

6. POISONED WOUNDS. BITES AND STINGS OF INSECTS — *Bees, Spiders, Bugs, Musquitoes, Snakes, Mad Dogs.*

In injuries from the above-named animals, except the two last (which are treated of below), cover the injured part with wet or damp earth, immediately, and then wet it afterward with a mixture of cold water and *Arnica tincture* (twenty parts to one). Internally, give *Arnica* and *Camphor*, every three or four hours a dose (four glob.), until better.

In the treatment of wounds inflicted by *venomous snakes* and *mad dogs*, and of their immediate or distant consequences, *hydrophobia*, etc., there exists yet a great deal of uncertainty and diversity of opinion. The old school has at least retired, as it seems, from further investigation on the subject (their last trial was that of using Chloroform and Ether); and it befits homœopathists the more to promote farther investigations, as they alone possess the true means to shorten the labor in discussing the merits of a proposed remedy. As experiences in this class of diseases occur so rarely, the observations and opinions will be slow in forthcoming. We prefer to give those of Dr. Hering, as follows:

The best remedy against the bites of *venomous serpents, mad dogs*, etc., is the application of *dry heat* AT A DISTANCE. Whatever is at hand at the moment, a red-hot iron or live coal, or even a lighted cigar, must be placed as near the wound as possible, without, however, burning the skin, or causing too sharp pain; but care must be taken to have another instrument ready in the fire, so as never to allow the heat to lose its intensity. It is essential, also, that the heat should not exercise its influence over too large a surface, but only on the wound and the parts adjacent. If oil or grease can be readily procured, it may be applied round the wound, and this operation should be repeated as often as the skin becomes dry; *soap* or even *saliva* may be employed, where oil or grease cannot be obtained. Whatever is discharged in any way from the wound ought to be carefully removed. The application of burning heat should be continued in this manner until the patient begins to shiver and to stretch himself; if this takes place at the end of a few minutes, it will be better to keep up the action of the heat upon the wound for an hour, or until the affections produced by the venom are observed to diminish.

Internal medicines must be judiciously administered at the same time. In the case of a BITE FROM A SERPENT, it will be advisable to take, from time to time, a gulp of *salt and water*, or a pinch of *kitchen salt*, or of *gunpowder*, or else some pieces of *garlic*.

If, notwithstanding this, bad effects manifest themselves, a spoonful of *wine* or *brandy*, administered every two or three minutes, will be the most suitable remedy; and this should be continued until the sufferings are relieved, and repeated as often as they are renewed.

If the shooting pains are aggravated, and proceed from the wound toward the heart, and if the wound becomes bluish, marbled, or swollen, with vomiting, vertigo, and fainting, the best medicine is *Arsenic*. It should be administered in a dose of four globules in a teaspoonful of water; and if, after this has been taken, the sufferings are still aggravated, the dose should be repeated at the end of half an hour; but if, on the contrary, the state remains the same, it should not be repeated until the end of two or three hours; if there is an amelioration, a new aggravation must be waited for, and the dose ought not to be repeated before its appearance.

In cases in which *Arsenic* exercises no influence, though repeated several times, recourse must be had to *Belladonna*; *Senna* also frequently proves efficacious.

Against chronic affections arising from the bite of a serpent, *Phosphor. ac.* and *Mercury* will generally be most beneficial.

For the treatment of persons bitten by a *mad dog,* after the application of dry heat, as directed and described above, see "Hydrophobia," below.

If morbid affections or ulcerations exhibit themselves in consequence of a bite from a rabid *man* or *animal, hydrophobine,* administered in homœopathic doses, will often render essential service.

For wounds that are envenomed by the introduction of animal substances in a state of putrefaction, or of pus from the ulcer of a diseased man or animal, *Arsenic* is generally the best medicine.

Lastly, as a PREVENTIVE against bad effects, when obliged to touch morbid animal substances, envenomed wounds, or ulcers of men and animals under the influence of contagious diseases, the best method that can be pursued is the application of *dry burning heat at a distance.* To effect this purpose, it will be sufficient to expose the hands for five or ten minutes to the greatest heat that can be borne; and after this, it will be proper to wash them with soap.

The use of *Chlorine* and muriatic acid, in similar cases, is well known.

HYDROPHOBIA.—Apply *distant heat* to the recent wound, as described under "Poisoned Wounds," or until shudderings appear; and continue this practice three or four times a day, until the wound is healed, without leaving a colored cicatrix.

At the same time the patient should take, every five or seven days, or as often as the aggravation of the wound requires it, one dose of *Belladonna* or *Lachesis,* or also of hydrophobine, until the cure is completed.

If, at the end of seven or eight days, a small *vesicle* shows itself *under the tongue,* with feverish symptoms, it will be necessary to open it with a lancet or sharp-pointed scissors and to rinse the mouth with salt and water.

If the raging state has commenced before assistance can be procured for the patient, the medicines ought to be carefully administered according to circumstances, especially *Bellad.* or *Lachesis;* or else, again, *Cantharides*, *Hyoscyamus*, *Mercury*, or also *Stramon.* or *Veratrum.*

7. Frozen Limbs, etc.

If limbs, ears, fingers, nose, etc., are frost-bitten, rub them with snow, or put them in the coldest water, and then, by degrees, let the water be warmer, until a natural feeling returns again. If the person is in a state of insensibility from being frozen APPARENTLY TO DEATH, undress him carefully (cut the clothes off from him) and cover him all over with snow, leaving the mouth and nostrils free. As the snow melts, renew it. If no snow can be had, put him into a bath of water, cold as ice, in which he may lie from ten to fifteen minutes; afterward, continue to rub with snow, or cover him with bags containing pounded ice. If in this way, the body has thawed by degrees, and the rigidity of the muscles relaxed, dry the body carefully, and place it in a cold bed in a cool room, and begin to rub, under the bedclothes, with the warm hands only, all over. In this way continue for hours.

If signs of life show themselves, inject a little camphor and water; also, put a drop of spirits of camphor on the tongue, from time to time.

If more signs of life appear, give warm black coffee (without milk), in injection and in small quantities by the mouth, until he can take more by the latter.

If severe pains in the whole body appear, give *Carbo veg.* (twelve glob. dissolved in half a teacupful of water), every fifteen or twenty minutes a teaspoonful, in alternation with *Arsenic*, if necessary, until better.

The patient must avoid the heat of fire or of a stove for some time.

II. Poisons.

Of the poisonous substances which can be introduced into the system, those are the most deleterious and pernicious which have the readiest facility of assimilation; consequently, the animal poisons rank first, then come the vegetable, and, lastly, the mineral poisons.

The animal poisons show their effects immediately on the nervous system, through the blood. The poison of snakes, for instance, while introduced into the stomach, is of no dangerous consequence. The vegetable poisons must be carried into the blood by digestion before their effects become dangerous. The mineral poisons kill only by corroding the surface, with which they come in contact, creating inflammation, which has a great tendency to pass quickly over into gangrene or mortification;* their bad effects on the system, afterward, are more lasting.

In cases of poisoning, the first thing to be done is, to *eject the poison as soon as possible* from the system, by provoking vomiting,† or, to *neutralize its action* by means of suitable antidotes.

* This peculiarity of the mineral poisons, to kill only by corrosion of the mucous membranes of the intestines, renders their use as remedial agents in diseases quite safe and expedient, as they can easily be divested of this poisoning or corroding quality, by reducing their crude bulk (which alone can corrode or inflame) by trituration and subsequent dilution, without diminishing in the least the curative effects of these minerals. For instance: one grain of *Arsenic*, in its crude state, would kill; yet, if triturated with one hundred grains of sugar-of-milk, one grain of this mixture would have lost all corroding or poisonous power, retaining, at the same time, all the curative quality, and this in a more developed form. In this way, Homœopathy can avail itself of all the healing effects of the most deadly poisons, with the greatest ease and safety; while Allopathy stands trembling and in fear before these dreadful agents, not knowing how to tame their useless fury, or to harness these wild medicinal steeds to the car of Esculapius.

† That, in such cases, Homœopathists make use of emetics and other violent means to eject poisons from the stomach, is not a proof that

To produce *vomiting*, the following means may be resorted to, in preference to the so-called *emetics*, which the allopathic school has hitherto employed:

1. *Tepid water*, in large quantities and often repeated.
2. *Snuff* or *mustard*, mixed with *salt* on the tongue.
3. *Tickling* of the throat with a feather or fine straw; or, lastly,
4. *Injections* of tobacco smoke into the anus through a pipe-stem.

To *neutralize* or *mitigate* the injurious effects of poison, the following means may be used as each case requires, which will be shown below under the heading of each poison named.

1. *White of Egg*, dissolved in water, and thus drank in large quantities, is of the greatest efficacy in poisoning by *metallic* substances, particularly *Corrosive sublimate, Verdigris, Tin, Arsenic, Lead, Mercury, Sulphuric acid,* particularly when there are violent pains in the stomach and bowels, with or without diarrhea.

In all cases in which the poison imbibed is unknown, the white of an egg is first given when violent pains in the abdomen are present.

---

they resort to allopathic means, as allopathists, quite sophistically, would make people believe. It only shows that, in cases of this kind, the homœopathic law cannot come into operation until these substances are removed, which act, as it were, as external injuries all the time, while they are buried in the stomach. In the same way, Surgery might be pronounced insufficient in its doings, because a surgeon can not heal a wound as long as the knife continues to lacerate and even enlarge the wound.

It is evident that external injurious substances (and such are all poisons) must be removed, just as a burning coal or a stinging blister, before the injuries done to the system can be repaired by the proper homœopathic agents; and this is done by Homœopathy more safely and quickly than by Allopathy, as the knowledge of antidotes is further advanced by the former, which is of the utmost importance in curing the after-effects of the poison.

2. *Soap* (*white household soap*), one part dissolved in four parts of hot water, is given in all cases where the white of an egg, when indicated, was insufficient.

In cases of poisoning by *alkaline* substances, it must be *omitted* as injurious.

3. *Vinegar* (made from wine or cider) diluted with water, as a draught or in injections, alternately with slimy things, is the principal remedy against *alkaline* substances, but is very injurious in cases of poisoning by minerals (the very opposite of *soap-water*).

4. Sugar, diluted and given in water, can be administered in cases of poisoning by *mineral*, as well as *alkaline* substances, and is, therefore, one of the most valuable remedies in domestic practice, as it can be most easily procured.

5. *Milk* and *Olive oil* are substances not so well calculated to envelop poisons in the stomach, as slimy, mucilaginous drinks, made of pearled barley, linseed, or rice ; yet they may be used with advantage against *alkaline* substances, and *corrosive acids*, such as *Nitric* and *Sulphuric acid.*

6. *Mucilaginous* drinks, in draughts and injections, are very useful against *alkaline* poisons, particularly in alternation with vinegar. They are made of barley, rice, linseed, farina.

7. *Coffee — strong black coffee* — taken very warm, is the principal remedy for all *narcotic* poisons, such as *Opium, Nux vomica, Belladonna, Stramonium* (Jamestown weed).

8. *Camphor* is principally efficacious against all *vegetable* poisons of an acrid, *corrosive* nature ; also, against *Cantharides* (Spanish fly).

The following table shows the proper and successive application of the above-named remedies in cases of poisoning with the different substances alluded to.

Table of Antidotes to the most Powerful Poisons.

POISONS.	ANTIDOTES.
I. ANIMAL POISONS.	
a. *Cantharides* (Spanish fly)	*Camphor,* internally or by smelling; externally, use white of eggs and gruels.
b. *Poisonous fish, clams, muscles, etc.*	*Charcoal, Sugar and water, Black coffee, Camphor.*—For eruptions and swelling of the face, *Bellad., Rhus.*
c. *Poison of fat* in half putrefied meat (*Sebacic acid*), as it appears often in cheese, sausages, etc.	*Vinegar and water,* internally and externally as a gargle, *Lemon juice, Black coffee, Black tea.* For the remaining symptoms, *Bryonia, Phosphoric acid, Creosote.*
II. VEGETABLE POISONS, in general.	Require mostly *Camphor,* by smelling, and *Black coffee* in a drink.
a. *Opium* (*Laudanum, seeds of Poppy*), *Stramonium* (*Gymson weed*), *Nux vom., Tobacco,*	*Narcotics,* require particularly *Black Coffee* and *Vinegar* diluted with water.
b. *Gamboge, Euphorbia,* and all other burning, corrosive vegetable substances which produce violent pains,	Require mostly *Soap-water* and *Milk.*
c. *Sumach* (*Poison vine*)..........	No external application, but, internally, *Bellad., Bryon., Rhus.*
d. *Camphor* and *Saffron*,..........	*Black coffee,* until the patient vomits; afterward *Opium.*
e. *Spirits of Turpentine*,..........	*Opium, Bellad., Bryon.*
III. MINERAL POISONS.	
a. ACIDS—*Prussic* or *mineral acids, Sulphuric, Muriatic, Nitric, Phosphoric acid,*	*Spirits of Hartshorn.* Tepid *Soapsuds; Magnesia; Chalk,* powdered and mixed with water; *Wood ashes* mixed with water; *Potash* or *Soda.*
b ALKALINE SUBSTANCES—*Pot* and *Pearl ashes, Lapis infernalis, Salt,* and *Oil of tartar,*	*Vinegar, Lemon-juice,* and other acids; *sour milk,* mucilaginous drinks and injections.

POISONS.	ANTIDOTES.
c. METALLIC SUBSTANCES—*Arsenic,*	*Soapsuds; white of eggs with water; Sugar water; Milk; Rust of Iron.*
Corrosive sublimate, Copper, Verdigris,	*White of eggs in water; Sugar-water; Milk; Starch from Wheat flour.*
Lead..........................	*Epsom salt; Glauber salt.*
Lunar caustic,.................	*Common salt,* dissolved in water.
Tin,..........................	*Sugar, white of eggs and milk.*

III. MEDICINAL DISEASES.

The abuse of medicines, prescribed often by allopathic physicians, and taken in large quantities, for a long time, produces, frequently, artificial diseases, well known under the name "Medicinal Diseases." The most obstinate and deleterious of these maladies are those produced by vegetable drugs, as their readiness to assimilate with the human system is far greater than that of minerals. From this it is evident how foolish or deceptive the conduct of those physicians is, who pretend to use in their practice only "vegetable medicines," as if this kingdom of nature did not contain the most noxious and violent poisons.

In the following table, the drugs are put together with their antidotes, which may be given as the indications mentioned may require. In administering them, it must be understood, that all these cases are more of a chronic nature; consequently, the repetition of doses is not required to be made so often, say from half a day to two, three, or more days, until improvement takes place, or another remedy has to be selected.

Medicinal diseases are not so easily cured as natural ones, because the reactive force of nature (so important in the treatment of diseases in general) cannot altogether be relied on in cases of this kind.

List of Drugs causing Diseases, and their Remedies.

DRUGS.	REMEDIES.
1. *Opium, Laudanum, Paregoric,*	*Coffea, Ipecac., Belladonna, Nux vomica, Mercu.*
2. *Mercury, Calomel.*	*Hepar sulph., Nitric acid.* Against *salivation* and *sore mouth; Hepar, Nitric acid, Carbo veg., Sulphur.* Against ulcers in the throat; *Carbo veg., Nitric acid, Bellad., Lachesis, Sulphur.* Against *nervous weakness; China, Hepar, Lachesis.* Against *nervous excitability; Chamomile, Pulsatilla, Carbo veg.* Against *sensitiveness to changes of the weather; Carbo veg., China.* Against *rheumatic pains, Neuralgia; Carbo veg., China, Lachesis, Sulphur.* Against *ulcerations* and *swellings of glands, Buboes; Carbo veg., Hepar, Lachesis, Nitric acid, Sulph., Thuja.* Against *dropsical affections; China, Dulcamara, Hellebor., Sulph.*
3. *Quinine Peruvian bark.*	Against *rheumatic pains; Arn., Puls.—Dropsical swellings; Arsenic, Ferrum.—Congestions* to the head and bowels; *Bellad., Mercury.—Fever, intermittent; Ipecac., Pulsat., Carbo veg., Arsenic.*
4. *Sulphur.*	*Puls., Merc., Chin., Sep.*
5. *Magnesia.*	*Colocynth, Ars., Rheum., Puls.*
6. *Arsenic.* (Fowler's solution.)	*China, Ferrum, Ipecac., Verat., Nux vom.*
7. *Lead* (used in ointments and in washes, as *sugar-of-lead water, etc.*)	*Opium, Bellad., Platina, Nux vom.*
8. *Iodine.*	*Bell., Phos., Hep., Spong., Chin., Ars.*
9. *Rhubarb.*	*Chamomile, Colocynth, Mercury.*
10. *Chamomile.*	*Aconite, Ignatia, Pulsat.*
11. *Cantharides*—(Spanish fly.)	*Camphor, Aconite, Pulsat.*
12. *Asafœtida.*	*China, Mercury, Pulsat., Caustic.*

CHAPTER III.

CUTANEOUS DISEASES.

THE skin, as the external covering of the whole body, is, on account of its exposure and extent, liable to many and various diseases—from the slightest redness, or rash, to the most inveterate itch and leprosy. The importance of its preservation is, therefore, obvious. We divide the diseases of the skin into,

1. *Acute Eruptions, Eruptive Fevers, etc.*
2. *Chronic Eruptions* and *Ulcers.*

1. ERUPTIVE FEVERS.

Rash.

DIAGNOSIS. — Frequently, after taking cold, particularly with a disordered stomach, persons are troubled with a rash on different parts of the body, which appears in red spots, of the size of a pin-head, scarcely visible; however, more so in a warm bed; with intolerable itching, particularly at night, preceded by shivering toward evening, disturbing sleep, and followed by feverishness during the night.

In such cases, the common practice heretofore has been, and is yet, where homœopathy is not known, to put scorched flour on the parts affected. This is not, however, without danger, and ought not to be resorted to immediately. It would be better first to give some of the following remedies, which will relieve, without driving the disease to internal parts.

Treatment. — If the itching is intolerable, with either shivering or heat, restlessness, sleeplessness, give *Aconite*, every hour one dose (four glob.). If not better within two or three hours, give *Chamomile*, every two hours a dose (four glob.). If perspiration follows this treatment, keep it up as long as necessary, and give, the next day, a dose of *Sulphur* (four glob.).

Diet and Regimen.—The diet ought to be very light—farinaceous substances, gruels, toasted bread and toast-water—but no meat, or soups of meat. The patient must be kept in a dry, warm room.

Nettle Rash — Hives. (*Urticaria.*)

Diagnosis.—A disease similar to the former in origin and appearance, only that the red spots, with a whitish tinge, appear in groups, somewhat elevated, and itch and prick intolerably. They resemble that eruption caused by contact with nettles. Hence the name, nettle-rash. Sometimes the body is covered with these spots, and then the patient feels sick, has no appetite, with a feeling of fullness in the pit of the stomach.

Treatment. — When caused by indigestion, particularly from rich and fat food, give *Pulsatilla*, morning and evening (four glob.). When caused by taking cold, and accompanied with diarrhea, bitter taste in the mouth, and slimy coated tongue, give *Apis mellifica* alternately with *Dulcamara* (four glob.). When caused by taking cold in damp, wet weather, exhibiting itself with pains in the limbs, shivering, and headache, give *Bryonia* and *Rhus*, alternately, every three or four hours a dose (four glob.), followed, in twenty-four hours, by a dose (four glob.) of *Sulphur*, if necessary. If not better the third day, give, evening and morning, a dose (four glob.) of *Carbo veg.* When these remedies are of no avail, or there is a burning sensation, with itching, great restlessness, and even an uneasy feeling, give two doses of *Arsenic*, in alternation with *Apis mellifica*, and, the next day, of a solution of *Urtica urens* (one drop in six tablespoonfuls of water), every three hours a teaspoonful.

Sometimes this rash strikes in suddenly, when the patient feels oppressed, sick at the stomach, and weak. In such a case, give immediately, *Ipecac.* (four glob.); in an hour afterward, *Bryonia* (four glob.), and, after that, in two hours, if not better, *Arsenic* (four glob.). At the same time, cover the patient well, to produce perspiration, which will also be promoted by warm drinks, particularly warm lemonade, if he has no diarrhea at the time.

If a person is troubled with this disease for a longer time than common, or liable to it on the slightest occasions, let him take *Calcarea*, every four days a dose (four glob.), in the evening, and, if not better, in four or six weeks, *Lycopodium*, *Sulphur*, *Carbo vegetabilis*, *Nitric acid*, in the same manner.

No external application whatever, should be made, as the disease might suddenly strike in, producing serious or even fatal consequences.

Diet must be simple; no meat nor heating drinks; nothing but water, black tea, gruels, dry toast, baked apples, and stale bread.

Erysipelas, or St. Anthony's Fire.

Diagnosis.—It is characteristic of this disease, that it appears suddenly, on different parts of the body, with heat, redness, swelling, tingling, and other painful sensations; in severer cases, the heat becomes intense on the parts affected; the surface almost shines, the pains become burning and shooting, and the skin rises in blisters filled with water (*erysipelas bullosum*).

In such cases, an intense fever is present, with its concomitant gastric nervous symptoms, such as a quick, full, wiry pulse; high fever, preceded by shivering or chill; tongue coated, white or dry brown; great thirst; pains all over the body; scanty and deep-colored urine; intense headache, with sleepiness or wakefulness ; very sensitive to noise and light.

The nearer to the brain this disease appears, as on the face, the ears, or the scalp of the head, the severer the symptoms of the head will be, and consequently, the more dangerous is the attack, so that delirium often ensues.

In the so called "wandering erysipelas" (*erysipelas erraticum*), the morbid spot disappears from one place, changing into a yellowish hue, to reappear again on another, in the form of redness and heat, so that it frequently wanders from the left side of the face, around the ear and neck to the right side, before the whole disease disappears. In such cases, the face is very much swollen and disfigured, closing, for a time, the eyes, nose, and ears. If the scalp of the head is attacked, the hair often falls off afterward.

Causes. — In most cases, exposure to cold immediately after the system has been heated or excited by over-exertion or mental emotions, particularly with a previous derangement of the stomach ; or, in females, during menstruation. Some persons are predisposed to it. Certain kinds of food, at certain seasons, will also produce it, such as lobsters, oysters, and other shell fish ; also the abuse of alcoholic liquors.

Treatment.—All outward applications ought to be avoided as dangerous—at any rate, all which are greasy. In the use of wet bandages cover the parts well. Salves and ointments are very dangerous. If the itching and burning is too violent, we may mitigate it a little, by applying powdered starch made of wheat flour, but not until after having given some of the following medicines internally. The internal remedies are the most important.

If the fever is very high, pulse full, skin dry, give first a few doses of *Aconite*, one every two hours (four glob.), followed by *Belladonna*, two doses, one every four hours (four glob.), which, in less severe attacks of this disease, is alone sufficient. In such cases, the patient improves after twelve or sixteen hours, and no more medicine is needed; he simply remains at home a few days, until there is no more danger of taking cold.

In severer cases, however, when after the above treatment the symptoms do not abate, give *Lachesis*, two doses, every three hours one (four glob.), particularly if the patient complains of dryness in the throat and pain in swallowing; also, coughs without raising; or *Apis mellif.* in alternation with it.

If no better after this, or if there be great sensitiveness to noise and light; the rash expanding in radiation; shining redness on its surface, which is very sensitive to the touch; sometimes raised in blisters; give *Belladonna* and *Rhus tox.* in solution (twelve glob. in half a teacupful of water, each cup having its separate teaspoon), every two hours a teaspoonful, alternately, until four teaspoonfuls of each are taken. Then wait twelve or more hours. If the patient is then very drowsy, give a dose of *Opium* (four glob.); or, if very wakeful and restless, give *Coffea*$^{cc.}$ and *Bellad.*$^{cc.}$ alternately, every hour a dose (six glob.), for three or four hours, and wait again twelve hours; after which repeat *Belladonna*, and *Rhus tox.*, in solution as above. If the symptoms are yet the same, give two doses of *Hepar*, every three hours one (four glob.), when the skin looks less shining and inflamed, but heat, pain, and swelling, are the same.

The above treatment suits severe cases of erysipelas of the face, head, or ears, with high fever, and, also, the vesicular form, where it appears in blisters, and the "wandering erysipelas." In the latter, however, where we cannot expect so rapid a termination of the disease, *Pulsatilla* is often successful, particularly when the skin is more of a bluish red, or the internal or external ear is attacked; also, in those cases which originated from eating noxious articles, such as oysters, clams, etc. If erysipelas appears on the joints, give *Bryonia*, three doses, every six hours one (four glob.), alternating with *Rhus*, and followed by *Sulphur* after thirty-six or forty-eigh hours, one dose (four glob.), if necessary.

If it appears on the scrotum, *Arsenic* is necessary, administered in the same manner as *Bryonia.* If the vesicles become gangrenous or of a dark color, the patient is weak, or black diarrhea sets in, *Arsenic* and *Carbo veg.* ought to be given alternately, every three hours one dose (four glob.), until a homœopathic physician takes charge of the patient.

Sometimes a swelling of the affected parts, showing the pressure of the finger, combines itself with erysipelas (*erysipelas œdematodes*). This requires *Rhus tox.*, in alternation with *Apis mellif.*, twice a day (four glob.) for three or four days.

If erysipelas terminates in ulceration of the parts affected, give *Rhus* and *Sulphur* alternately, every evening a dose (four glob.) for four days, and, afterward, a dose of *Silicea* for two evenings, and wash the ulcer three or four times a day with lukewarm water, in half a teacupful of which twelve globules of *Silicea* are well dissolved.

The disposition to this disease will be taken away by the alternate use of *Rhus*, and *Graphites*, every four days a dose (four glob.), if continued for four or six weeks. Beside this, however, change the mode of living, if it was too luxurious; avoid highly-seasoned or salted food, drink freely of cold water, and wash and bathe frequently and systematically.

Application of Water, as an auxiliary to the homœopathic medication, is confined to the use of the wet sheet, to produce perspiration; this accomplished, a great step in the cure of erysipelas has been gained; no direct application of the cold water on the parts affected, is advisable, except where the burning pain is intolerable, when a wet bandage may be applied, but well covered; too long-continued constipation, treat with injections and drinking of cold water.

Diet.—During this disease, the diet should be as in fevers, very light; dry toast, gruels, and black tea; warm lemonade is very good and refreshing, if no diarrhea prevails; stewed prunes may also be allowed, particularly in convalescence.

If, at any time during this disease, the bowels are confined, even for four or six days, it will not exert, in the least, a detrimental effect upon the patient; on the contrary, it is better than the opposite state.

Avoid taking cold during the convalescence, as it is often followed by dangerous results, dropsies, etc. If, at any time during the attack, the erysipelas suddenly disappears, and the brain, in consequence, becomes affected, which shows itself in drowsiness, difficulty of breathing, and spasmodic twitchings, give *Cuprum*, in solution (twelve glob. in half a teacupful of water), every half hour a dose, until a homœopathic physician takes charge of the patient.

Before we leave this subject, let us here remark, that erysipelas, as such, is *no infectious* disease whatever, and has lost its dread entirely, since homœopathic remedies have been used in the treatment of it.

Eruptive Fevers with an Infectious Epidemic Character.

We now come to a class of eruptive diseases which appear, generally, as epidemics, and are infectious. These are *measles, French measles, scarlet rash, scarlet fever, chicken-pox, varioloids* and *small-pox.* Their epidemic appearance depends upon the general laws of disease growing out of the changing conditions of the seasons and atmosphere. As a general rule, we can say that persons are attacked only once in their lifetime with these diseases, though some few exceptions may happen. Their contagiousness does not commence, as is generally believed, during the fever period, or when the eruption first appears; but *only after* the pustules are well filled, or drying up, that is, from the seventh day onward, to three or four weeks, as long as the system throws out through the skin the infectious matter. Before the seventh day of ither of the above diseases, no infection can take place, for the same reason as no vaccination is possible out of a pustule before that time. The infecting matter must be first fully ripe in the system before it can affect another; be, therefore, rather more careful during the convalescence of a patient, or after his death (when the contagion is in its highest state of perfection), than in the beginning of his sickness. This is the case, as well in measles as in scarlet fever, varioloids and small-pox.

Measles. (*Morbilli.*)

In adults, this disease generally assumes a severer character than in children, because it developes in them more readily those constitutional germs of diseases which often lie hidden in the system a long time, such as consumption, sore eyes, etc. In children, its attacks are rarely dangerous, except when other causes render it complicated, or it is badly treated.

Diagnosis.—For the first three or four days the patient seems to have taken a cold ; he has a dry, hoarse cough, and sometimes a sore throat ; his eyes water constantly, and cannot bear the light ; these symptoms and more or less feverishness (the catarrhal fever) precede and accompany the eruption of the measles, which appear in small red spots of irregular shape and size (the skin between them preserving its natural color), the first day on the temples, face and neck, the second day, on the breast, or stomach and back, and the third day on the arms and limbs. In mild cases they disappear after the fifth or sixth day in bran-like scales.

This is the regular course of the disease ; whenever it varies from it, the attending symptoms become more dangerous, particularly if the eruption appears irregularly in regard to time and disappears quickly.

Treatment.—*Aconite* and *Pulsatilla* are the principal remedies, and are regarded almost as specifics, which, in milder cases, without complication, they prove to be.

Administration.—Dissolve of each remedy twelve glob. in two teacups half full of water, each (put to each a separate spoon), and give alternately every two, three, or six hours, a teaspoonful (children under two years, half a teaspoonful), beginning with *Aconite;* and if the patient remains, or becomes more comfortable, lengthen the intervals still more. If, at any time, there is great restlessness and sleeplessness, introduce a dose of *Coffea*cc., repeating it as often as necessary, particularly in the night.

If the cough is very dry and hoarse (resembling croup), give a dose (four glob.) of *Hepar* in alternation with *Coffea* (if the patient is very much agitated and irritable), at intervals of one or two hours.

If, however, the cough excites severe pain in the upper part of the breast and sides (complication with bronchitis and pneumonia), *Aconite* and *Bryonia* (dissolved in water and administered the same as *Aconite* and *Pulsatilla*) are necessary.

If the measles strike in at once, and look pale, or if sickness at the stomach and feebleness ensue, give *Ipecac.* and *Bryonia* alternately every hour or half hour a dose (four glob.), and if the skin looks bluish brown, give *Arsenic* and *Apis mell.* in alternation every hour or two hours a dose, until better. If the head is affected in children, give *Cuprum* every half hour a dose (three glob.), twice or three times; and if not better in three hours, give *Belladonna* and *Hellebor.* in solution (twelve glob. of each to half a teacupful of water) every hour, alternately, a teaspoonful until better.

Application of Water in this disease, is, in general, the same as in scarlatina, where the detailed treatment is given. If the cough affects the breast very much, a wet bandage may be applied, well covered; the water for drinking must not be too cold.

Disorders consequent upon Measles. — If sensitiveness to light continues too long after the eruption is out, give *Belladonna,* morning and evening one dose (four glob.); this same remedy, applied similarly, suits, if the head is affected (*congestion of the head*), in alternation with *Stramonium.*

Constipated, or not too open bowels, are not injurious

during or after this disease; if a mucous diarrhea ensues give *China, Mercury, Pulsatilla, Apis mellif.*, every six hours, until better. If not better, give one or two doses of *Sulphur*—every six hours one dose (four glob.). If the diarrhea is watery, and connected with typhoid symptoms, loss of consciousness, dry tongue, give *Arsenic* and *Phosphorus* in the same manner.

If *earache* ensue, give *Pulsatilla*, every two or three hours a dose; if this is accompanied by running of the ear, give after *Pulsatilla* a dose (four glob.) of *Sulphur* on two successive evenings, and if not better in two or three days, give *Carbo veg.* in the same manner.

If the glands below and in front of the ear swell (*parotitis*, or mumps), give *Arnica* and *Rhus* every four hours or six hours a dose (four glob.), till better.

The remaining *cough* requires principally *Pulsatilla, Sulphur, Bryonia, Drosera, Hyoscyamus*, whose symptoms must be compared in the "*Materia Medica.*" See also under "*cough.*" Burning and itching of the skin requires *Chamomile, Nux vomica, Arsenicum*, and *Sulphur*.

DIET must be light—as gruels, water (children milk and water), toasted bread; and only gradually more nourishing.

N. B. Do not allow the children to go out of the room too early, or even to go to the door or window, or play on the floor; we cannot be too careful to avoid taking cold.

As a preventive of measles, give *Aconite* and *Pulsatilla* every third day a dose (four glob.), alternately, during the epidemic; it may prevent an attack, and will certainly mitigate its severity.

French Measles.

In this disease, which resembles the former, but is milder in every respect, it is only necessary to mitigate the fever and restlessness, if there is any, with alternate doses (four glob.) of *Coffea* and *Aconite*, one every two, three, or six hours, after which, the eruption soon disappears.

Diet and Regimen the same as in measles, but when complicated with *catarrhal* symptoms, give a dose or two (four glob.) of *Pulsatilla;* and when the head is congested, give a couple of doses of *Belladonna* in alternation with *Aconite.*

Scarlet Rash.

This disease is different from scarlet fever, in as far as the redness of the eruption is darker, and the finger, on slight pressure, leaves no white imprint, beside there are numerous small granular elevations, felt under the skin, sometimes distinctly seen. There is another distinctive difference from scarlet fever; this latter appears, invariably, first on the face, next on the body, and lastly on the extremities. Such a regularity is not found in scarlet rash—it may appear irregularly or at once over the whole body. It is frequently and mostly seen in combination with scarlet fever, which is known by its smooth redness on the surface.

Treatment.—If it appears alone, it is not a dangerous disease, and yields easily to a few doses of *Aconite,* every three or four hours one dose (four glob.), and in alternation with *Coffea,* if there is great restlessness and irritability.

If it is combined with scarlet fever, the symptoms sometimes become very severe; see, for their treatment, the next article, "Scarlet Fever." In case it disappears suddenly, *Ipecac.* and *Bryonia* should be given, every half hour, or hour, a dose (four glob.), twice or three times, at the same time covering the patient well; but when congestion to the head appears, with drowsiness, give *Opium* (four glob.), or, if the patient starts on closing the eyes, *Belladonna* (four glob.), once or twice in four hours.

Application of Water, the same as in "Scarlet Fever."

Diet the same as in measles, and the same caution as regards taking cold afterward.

N. B. This disease does not strictly *prevent* patients from having the real scarlet fever afterward, although it often diminishes their liability to it, as I have had occasion to observe in many instances. It bears the same relationship to scarlet fever, as French measles (or measle-rash, as we may call it) does to ordinary measles.

Scarlet Fever. (*Scarlatina.*)

A well-known scourge to the world of children, and dreaded by the allopathic physician more than any other. It is not the least triumph of the glorious Hahnemann to have found the true specific against this disease, diminishing its terrors, and furnishing a remedy, which the allopathists have adopted to a great extent.

DIAGNOSIS.—After a fever of more or less severity, characterized by a very quick pulse, and sometimes accompanied with sore throat, headache, thirst, and stupor, or uncommon liveliness, the eruption appears in the form of bright red (scarlet) blotches indefinitely marked, on which, when pressed by the finger, a white spot remains, which soon becomes red again, from the center to the circumference. If it is not combined with scarlet rash, no grains can be found in the skin by rubbing over it with the hand; it appears, the first day, on the face and neck, the second on the breast and region of the stomach, and the third day, on the arms, hands, and limbs. But more frequently it appears in combination with scarlet rash (see this article), in which case it assumes a more dangerous and destructive character.

If this disease exists alone, it generally terminates in five or six days, the skin coming off in large pieces.

TREATMENT.—*Belladonna* is the specific for this disease, which is cured by its use alone, except in complicated cases.

The symptoms requiring its use, are dry burning fever, quick pulse, starting on closing the eyes for a few minutes, great thirst, dry, red, or whitish coated tongue, urine scanty and highly colored, scarlet eruptions on the face, or over the entire body. Sometimes this external redness does not appear, but instead of it the throat is more or less affected, in which case the tongue has always a reddish gloss. Yet, even this wandering of the scarlatina from the outside skin to the mucous membrane of the throat, does not materially increase the danger of the case, if the glands only do not enlarge too much. Under all these circumstances, as indeed always at first, give *Belladonna* in the following manner: Dissolve twelve globules in half a teacupful of water, and give of this solution every two, three, or four hours, a teaspoonful for four or six times. If the disease gets worse soon after giving *Belladonna*, discontinue its use, or let the patient smell of spirits of camphor a few times and do not recommence the use of *Belladonna*, until the child gets worse again; this, however, will not generally be found necessary.

In this manner continue to use the *Belladonna* for three or four days, until the scaling process commences, when it is only necessary to keep the patients away from the slightest draught: it is by far the safest to keep them in bed closely for four or five days after the fever has left, when a dose of *Sulphur* (four glob.) may be given to complete the cure.

But if the case is a complicated one from its beginning, or becomes so in its progress, other remedies beside *Belladonna* are needed. Cases of this kind ought to be treated by a homœopathic physician; yet, where none is to be had, the following prescription will be found beneficial:

If there is great restlessness and sleeplessness, irritability, whining, and tossing about, give *Coffea* and *Belladonna* in solution (twelve glob. in half a teacupful of water), alternately, every hour a teaspoonful; or, if there is violent fever, with *dry heat*, full and quick pulse, congestion of the head, occasional delirium or lethargy, with starting when awaking, and dry, short, painful cough, give *Aconite* and *Belladonna* in solution, alternately, in the same manner.

If the patient is better under this treatment during the daytime, but in the night these symptoms appear more or less, particularly restlessness and sleeplessness, give *Coffea*$^{cc.}$ and *Belladonna*$^{cc.}$, every hour alternately (four glob.), until the patient is more composed.

If, with great drowsiness and tossing about, the tongue is very dry, thirst great, with swelling of glands on the neck increasing, skin shining on the face and neck, head thrown backward, and almost constant delirium, give *Rhus* and *Belladonna* in solution in the same manner as above, every hour a teaspoonful, alternately, for six or eight hours, followed by *Coffea*$^{cc.}$ and *Belladonna*$^{cc.}$; if very restless during the night, as above, this prescription repeated every day for three or four days, secures, in most cases, a favorable issue; perspiration sets in, and then one or two doses of *Sulphur* (four glob.) are necessary to complete the cure.

If this disease is combined with scarlet rash, as it mostly is at present, the symptoms become more severe, the throat is affected inside and the glands swell outside, sometimes to a great extent. We call this the *malignant scarlet fever*. In such cases, when ulceration of the glands commences, indicated by a very offensive smell, and a great quantity of mucus running from the mouth, give *Mercury* (twelve glob. dissolved in half a teacupful of water), every two hours a teaspoonful, for six or eight times alone, or alternating with *Belladonna*, if the patient starts or jerks on closing the eyes, cannot swallow liquids easily, has violent thirst, with sensitiveness to light.

If no improvement takes place within twelve hours, give *Sulphur* in solution the same as *Mercury*, twice or three times, and then wait six or eight hours, giving in the meanwhile, only an occasional dose (four glob.) of *Coffea*$^{cc.}$ and *Belladonna*$^{cc.}$, alternately, if the patient is very restless.

If no better at the end of that time, restlessness still increasing, the saliva excessively fetid, with grating of teeth, give *Arsenic* and *Lachesis* alternately in solution, in the same manner as *Mercury*, and after that, in the same manner, give

Nitric acid and *Lycopodium*, particularly when the stupor of the patient increases and lethargy sets in.

If, in this condition, the breathing resembles snoring, with burning heat of the skin, whether dry or covered with perspiration, give *Camphor* and *Opium* in solution (twelve glob. of each, separately dissolved in half a teacupful of water), every half hour a teaspoonful, alternately; give of each three or four times, and after that, if there is no improvement, give *Cuprum* (twelve glob. in half a teacupful of water), in solution, every hour a teaspoonful.

If, at any time, during this disease, a kind of *stranguria* (difficulty of urinating) ensues, give *Cantharides* (four glob.) once or twice, and in alternation with *Coffea*, if there is great restlessness and irritability, if not better, give *Conium* in the same manner.

If croupy symptoms appear, give *Aconite* and *Hepar sulph.*, alternately, every hour a dose (four glob.), until better.

Application of water. — In all eruptive fevers the use of water as a remedy has proved to be very beneficial, and is particularly so in combination with homœopathic medication. In very severe cases of Scarlet Fever we would recommend its use, especially when the fever is intense and the reactive force of the system impeded, or when a repercussion of the eruption has taken place. We insert the treatment as directed by Dr. Munde, a very experienced hydropathist, who treated thus hundreds of Scarlet Fever patients successfully; it supports Homœopathic medication very much.

The patient is wrapped in a wet sheet and well covered with blankets; he remains in this position, until perspiration ensues, when he is washed off in milk-warm water; if the throat is inflamed, a cooling bandage is placed on it during the perspiration and renewed every five minutes. If the first packing does not promote perspiration, the wet sheet is renewed until perspiration ensues. In this perspiration he remains until the heat in the head and throat increases or difficulty of breathing ensues, when he is unpacked and washed off, as stated above. This whole process is repeated as often as the fever reappears in a high degree. Sometimes a sitting-bath of milk-warm water of one half or three-fourths of an hour duration is applied, if the pains in head and throat are severe. As soon as the perspiration appears, the patient may be considered to be out of danger.

In case the scarlet strikes in suddenly, the patient is sponged off in cold water all over, and if spasms had ensued, cold water is dashed over him in larger quantities, until the spasmodic action ceases; he is then wrapped, without being dried or rubbed, in woolen blankets, and, if possible, as much cold water given, internally, as he can drink; in most cases a general perspiration will ensue, the eruption reappears and the patient is saved.

Diseases consequent upon Scarlet Fever and Scarlet Rash.

Earache and Ulceration in the Ear.—For severe pains in the ear, give *Belladonna*, *Pulsatilla*, and *Hepar sulph.*, alternately, every two hours one dose (four glob.), until better.

For the running of the ear (otorrhœa), give *Calcarea* six times, every evening and morning one dose (four glob.), wait three or four days, and if no better, give *Silicea* in the same manner. For the swelling of the glands below, and in front of the ear (*mumps*), give *Carbo veg.* and *Rhus*, alternately, every four or six hours a dose (four glob.), until two doses of each are taken.

If a child after this disease evinces symptoms of *dropsy of the brain* (head hot, extremities cold, vomiting on moving, with or without diarrhea, sleeps with eyes half open), give *Belladonna* and *Hellebor.*, in solution (twelve glob. in half a teacupful of water) every two hours, alternately, a teaspoonful until it gets more lively again and the above symptoms disappear, when a dose (four glob.) of *Sulphur* will be serviceable.

In case of *dropsical swelling* of the whole body, give first *Hellebor*. and *Belladonna* in the same manner as above, and afterward *Bryonia* and *Hellebor.*, alternately, then *Apis mellif.*

In such cases *Arnica, Arsenic, Phosphor. acid* and *Sulphur* are also useful; commence with *Arnica*, of which two doses may be given, one in the evening and one in the morning (four glob.); and then wait one day until signs of improvement show themselves. If these do not appear, give the other remedies one after another in the same manner. Keep the patient always covered during this treatment.

For soreness of the nose and face, with swelling of the glands under the chin, give first *Mercury* twice, every evening a dose (four glob.), then wait two or three days, and if necessary, give one after the other, *Hepar sulph., Silicea, Sulphur.* and *Calcarea*.

If the scarlet strikes in suddenly, the eruption assuming a livid bluish hue, and the child becomes drowsy, with hurried breathing, give first *Bryonia* and *Belladonna*, a couple of doses, every half hour a dose (four glob.), and then if no better give *Cuprum* in solution (twelve glob. in half a teacupful of water) every fifteen or thirty minutes a teaspoonful. If not better in two hours, continue the same with *Camphor* in alternation, and cover the patient well.

Diet and Regimen the same as in measles; examine closely "N. B." at the end of article on "Measles."

As a *preventive* against scarlet fever, give, during the prevalence of the disease, to every child a dose (four glob.) of *Belladonna*$^{cc.}$ every other evening.

N. B. It is hardly necessary to urge the necessity of the advice and attendance of a homœopathic physician in this disease, if one can possibly be obtained.

It frequently occurs, that before the eruption comes out, convulsions set in which seem to threaten the life of the patient. In such a case give *Belladonna* and *Cuprum* in alternation (twelve globules of each dissolved in half a teacupful of water) every ten or fifteen minutes, half a teaspoonful, until better; *Tartar emetic*, if the convulsions are accompanied with vomiting and diarrhea, cold, clammy skin, and hurried respiration; beside, treat the patient as directed under the heading "Convulsion" in "diseases of children." As soon as the eruption appears more distinct, the congestion to the head, and with it the convulsion, ceases; cases of this kind, commencing apparently so unfavorably, terminate nevertheless most favorably, as the worst of the disease appeared in the beginning, where the patient had more power to overcome it.

Chicken-Pox. (Varicella.)

DIAGNOSIS.—This eruption is often mistaken for small-pox or varioloid, particularly when a small-pox epidemic is raging. We will give the differences between them. Before the chicken-pox appears, the patient is only sick from twenty-four, to forty-eight hours, and then he has, generally, fever and headache, with bilious rheumatic symptoms, without the severe swimming in the head and the backache, which never fail to appear before the small-pox breaks out. Instead of that, he complains of stranguria and tenesmus (see glossary), which is not the case in small pox.

The chicken-pox appears irregularly on different parts of the body at once, while the small-pox and varioloid always appear on the face first. Again, the pustule of the chicken-pox appears at once in the form of a bladder, not as in small-pox and varioloid, in the form of a point like the head of a pin. When the chicken-pox is developed, the pustule has but one cavity, without any inner divisions, containing the clear liquid, and without a dent on the top of it; while the pustule of the small-pox contains the liquid in divisions, like an orange, and has a dent on top. The liquid of the chicken-pox very seldom becomes turbid or mattery, as is the case in small-pox, but dries up in a spongy crust, without leaving a mark; the crusts of small-pox are hard, and oftentimes leave marks. Chicken-pox is not contagious in the same manner as small-pox; it depends, for its propagation, more on individual predisposition, strengthened by atmospheric influence.

TREATMENT.—For the fever, prior to the eruption, give *Aconite* and *Belladonna* every two or three hours, alternately, a dose (four glob.), until three doses of each are given. If the patient complains of *bilious rheumatic* symptoms, give *Bryonia* and *Rhus*, alternately, every two hours a dose (four glob.), until three doses of each are given.

If there are *bilious nervous* symptoms, give *Belladonna* and *Rhus*, alternating in the same manner.

If tenesmus is present, give *Mercury*, every two hours one dose (four glob.). If there is stranguria, give *Cantharides* and *Conium*, alternately, every two hours a dose (four glob.), until three doses of each are given, or the patient is relieved. If the eruption is very considerable, give two doses of *Antimon. crud.*, every twelve hours one (four glob.).

DIET AND REGIMEN as in measles.

N. B. In children severe symptoms of the head may appear, for instance, convulsions (see this article) or the eruption might strike in; in the latter case, treat it as stated in measles striking in. (See article "Measles.") Chicken-pox may occur more than once in a lifetime.

Small-Pox. (*Variola.*)

This disease has four important stages, which we will first describe, giving their treatment afterward.

First. *Febrile Stage.* — This commences, generally, from seven to fourteen days after the exposure to the contagion, with a chill more or less severe, after which, intense fever sets in with severe pains *in the head and small of the back*, aching in the bones and general soreness; dry, hot skin, great thirst, cough, oppression in the stomach, sometimes vomiting of bile; light hurts the eyes, with swimming of the head; the mind wanders, is flighty, anxious expression of countenance and great prostration of strength.

Second. *Eruptive Stage.*—After the febrile stage has lasted from forty-eight to seventy-two hours, the eruptive stage commences, by the appearance of small red pimples on the forehead and face of the size of pin-heads, after which the severity of the fever symptoms abates gradually. On the first day the eruption appears on the face; the second, on the breast and body; and the third, on the limbs and arms—this stage, therefore, lasts three days.

Third. *Stage of Suppuration.* The pustules now grow to perfection, as large as a bean cut in two; the liquid inside is contained in cells like an orange, on top is a little dent, and around them a red circle. This stage lasts three days; but as the pustules first appear on the face, then on the breast, and lastly on the extremities, they are already in perfection on the face when they are still filling on the breast and growing on the extremities.

Thus, a wise Providence has divided the burthen in three parts, which would otherwise be unbearable.

At the end of this period, the liquid in the pustules is turbid and mattery.

Fourth. *Stage of Desiccation.*—On the eighth or ninth day the eruption begins to dry up; some of the pustules burst, and with the formation of scabs desiccation commences and progresses until the tenth day, at which time, in favorable cases, the fever has entirely disappeared, the swelling of the face has diminished, the scabs have fallen off the upper part of the body, leaving marks of a reddish-brown color.

This is the regular and favorable course of the disease where the pustules are not so numerous as to run together; but where the small-pox is *confluent*, the danger of the case and its duration are considerably increased.

TREATMENT.—*Febrile Stage.*—During the chill and the first six hours of the fever, give *Aconite*, every two hours a dose (four glob.). If severe headache (congestion), with sensitiveness to light, and delirium, are present, alternate with *Belladonna*, in the same manner.

If, afterward, severe backache ensues, with pains in the bones and general soreness (bilious rheumatic), give *Bryonia* and *Rhus*, alternately, every two or three hours a dose (four glob.), for twelve or sixteen hours. This is generally sufficient.

If, however, there is vomiting, give one dose (four glob.) *Tart. emet.*

If the headache increases to insensibility, stupor ensues, and snoring-like breathing, give one or two doses of *Opium*, every two hours one (four glob.).

If the patient is very restless, sleepless, and irritable, give *Coffea*$^{cc.}$ and *Belladonna*$^{cc.}$, every hour a dose (four glob.) until better.

Treatment of the second or eruptive stage. — If the delirium, which may have lasted up to this time, does not disappear entirely when the eruption comes out, or if the eruption does not appear sufficiently or not at all, give *Stramonium*, in solution (twelve glob. in half a teacupful of water), every two hours a teaspoonful, for twelve hours.

If the lungs suffer, at this stage, with a hoarse, rattling cough, give *Tart. emet.*, a few doses, every two hours one (four glob.); if with great oppression on the chest, give *Ipecac.* in the same manner.

In children, this stage requires particular attention, and *Belladonna*, in alternation with *Stramonium*, should be given, every two hours a teaspoonful of each (ten glob. in half a teacupful of water), until the eruption is out.

If, however, this stage progresses finely, without severe symptoms, give nothing but *Tart. emet.* and *Thuja*, in alternation, every three hours a dose (four glob.), until six doses of each are taken. These remedies have the specific power to mitigate the eruption, from the similar eruption they produce on the healthy. Still more powerful acts, in this respect, the *Varioline*, shortening the disease perceptibly and divesting it of its dangerous progress.

TREATMENT OF THE THIRD STAGE.—*Suppuration.*—If this stage has a great deal of fever, give *Mercury*, every three hours a dose (four glob.) until four doses are taken, particularly when there is abundant saliva in the mouth. The swelling of the eyes only requires ablutions of warm water and milk.

If, however, in this stage, the skin between the pustules becomes of a livid hue or dark brown, and the pustules themselves are watery and flabby (black small-pox), give *Arsenic* in solution (twelve glob. in half a teacupful of water), every two hours a teaspoonful, alternating, in the same manner, with *China*, if diarrhea ensues. After these remedies, a dose of *Sulphur* (four glob.) will be of service.

This treatment is also serviceable, if, in the confluent form, typhoid symptoms occur, with brown, cracked tongue; in which case give, in the absence of diarrhea, instead of *China*, *Rhus* in alternation with *Arsenic*.

Striking in of the eruption happens in this stage more than in any other, and ought to be treated with *Cupr.*, as directed in "Scarlet Fever" (see this article).

TREATMENT OF THE FOURTH STAGE.—*Desiccation.*—In the beginning of this stage, give a dose (four glob.) of *Sulphur;* if the patient is tolerably comfortable, he does not require anything more than cleansing the skin by frequent ablutions with tepid water, and a careful attention to diet.

If, however, the diarrhea continues, give *Mercury* in alternation with *Sulphur*, every three or four hours a dose (four glob.) until better.

The itching at this period is alleviated by a couple of doses of *Sulph.*, evening and morning one dose (four glob.).

If the patient has reached this period in a typhoid state, he must be treated accordingly. (See "Typhus.")

APPLICATION OF WATER.—The wet sheet, as applied in scarlet fever, is in this disease of great service, as also the application of the wet compress under the head and neck, if the eyes and ears suffer a great deal. The wet sheet is repeated every day, as also the ablutions in milk-warm water after the sweating process ; sometimes it is necessary to repeat it twice a day, if the disease has assumed a nervous, putrid character. Constipation is relieved by injections and drinking of cold water.

DIET AND REGIMEN.—The room of the patient should be kept well ventilated, not too warm, and almost dark, during the whole time.

The diet should be more cold than warm ; for instance, water, ice-cream as much as wanted, lemonade, oranges (the latter three not in diarrhea), gruels, dry toast; also, well-stewed prunes and roasted apples ; animal food is not allowed, even long after convalescence.

Diseases which may occur after small-pox, such as consumption, diarrhea, inflammation of the eyes, etc., see under their proper heads.

As a *preventive* against this disease, vaccination is well and favorably known ; for how long a time, however, this may prevent small-pox, is yet a matter of speculation. It varies, certainly, in different individuals; the shortest period may be seven years ; the longest is not known.

I consider vaccination and revaccination from time to time, our duty and a safeguard against the encroachments of this fearful disease upon society.

N. B. See introduction to "Eruptive Infectious Fevers," p. 80.

Varioloid, or Modified Small-Pox. (Variolois.)

This disease is similar, in all respects, to the former, yet not the same. It is decidedly milder, and requires no mention of a different treatment from that given under "Small Pox." (See this article.)

N. B. A person who is well vaccinated may, when exposed to small-pox, take the varioloid; and, thus far, vaccination, which is a protection against small-pox, seems not to prevent the varioloid, although one who has had the small-pox will very seldom take the varioloid. The varioloid rarely leaves scars on the skin.

2. Chronic Eruptions.

To give a detailed description of all the varieties of cutaneous diseases coming under the above head, would be of no advantage for domestic practice, as most of these chronic skin diseases require the most skillful discrimination of an attending physician; for the reason that their causes and character are too deeply connected with the patient's constitution (in each case, perhaps, differently so); and, thus, it is almost impossible to generalize them and their treatment, within the limits of a medical guide-book like this. We will describe some of the most familiar ones, advising the reader, at the same time, to apply to a homœopathic physician immediately on finding his own treatment insufficient, because all chronic cutaneous affections require immediate and proper treatment.

Irritation of the Skin.—Itching. (*Pruritus.*)

A fine rash under the skin, scarcely perceptible, and colorless, produces a very disagreeable and distressing itching, particularly at night, when undressing, or in bed after getting warm. It is caused, mostly, by exposure to the extremes of heat and cold, and appears, consequently, in the height of summer, as well as in winter. Sometimes, the eating of too much fat or greasy food produces it: if so, the diet ought to be changed.

Treatment.—Wash, every evening before going to bed, with water and plenty of Castile soap, without drying it off. If this does not relieve within four or six days, try brandy or alcohol, in the same manner (but take care not to come in contact with a light). If this does not give any relief, wash with water mixed with *Spirits of Camphor*. Internally, administer as follows:

If the irritation is worse in the warmth of the bed or near the fire, particularly after scratching, give *Pulsatilla*, every evening a dose (six glob.), and, also, if fat food may have caused it.

If it commences after going to bed, and resembles flea bites all over the body, the pain shifting from one part to another, *Ignatia*, given in the same manner, will be of service.

Mercury suits, when it continues through the whole night, and after scratching bleeds easily and freely; in this case alternately with *Sulphur*, every other evening, one dose (four glob.) for a week.

If an intolerable *burning* accompanies the irritation, amounting almost to feverishness, take *Bryonia* and *Rhus*, alternately, every six hours a dose (four glob.) for twenty-four or thirty-six hours; two days after take *Hepar sulph.*, evening and morning a dose (six glob.). If not better in four or six days after, take *Carbo veg.*, evening and morning, one dose (six glob.).

If it commences when undressing, take *Nux vomica* and *Arsenic*, in alternation. If old people are troubled with it, give *Opium* and *Secale*, alternately, every evening a dose (four glob.). If it renders the patient *very restless*, so that he perspires, take *Colocynth*. If it is caused by summer heat, take *Lachesis* and *Lycopodium*, alternately, every evening a dose (four glob.).

If it is accompanied with *fine stitches*, like needles, take *Thuja*, every evening a dose (four glob.), for two evenings.

If it does not yield to one of the above remedies, take *Silicea*, every third evening a dose (four glob.), until four doses are taken. If then not better, take *Sulphur*, in the same manner.

If this irritation shows itself around the anus or the private parts (*prurigo*), its cause is rather a constitutional one, and requires *Calcarea, Lycopodium, Sulphur, Nitric acid, Sarsaparilla,* and *Sepia.* If it is around the anus, *Dulcamara, Nitric acid, Petrol., Sulphur, Lycopodium, Graphites.* If on the *scrotum, Thuja.* If on the *pudendum, Calcarea, Carbo, Conium, Sepia, Sulphur, Nitric acid.*

Administration.—In using these remedies, begin with the first—put twelve globules in four tablespoonfuls of water, and take, evening and morning, a teaspoonful. After it is taken, discontinue four days; then take the next in the same manner, if not better. Beside this, wash frequently in cold water.

Chilblains.

Diagnosis.—Chilblains mostly appear on hands and feet which have been frost-bitten, and are extremely painful if they burst and ulcerate.

Treatment.—If the parts begin to swell, assuming a dark, reddish-brown color, with itching and beating, worse in the evening or at night, take *Pulsatilla,* in solution (twelve globules in half a teacupful of water), morning, noon, and evening a teaspoonful, and occasionally wash the parts affected in a teaspoonful of the solution.

In a few days afterward, take *Sulphur,* evening and morning, a dose (four glob.). If the parts have a bright red color, and itch more in the warmth, take *Nux vomica,* in the same manner. If these remedies do not relieve, give *Phosphorus* alone or in alternation with *Hepar sulph.,* if ulceration has commenced.

If the parts are very painful and burning, take *Chamomile* alone, every three or four hours, a teaspoonful, or alternately with *Arsenic,* in the same manner, if not relieved soon.

If the swelling is hard and shining, take *Arnica* internally, and wash externally with two drops of the tincture to a teaspoonful of water, the same as *Pulsatilla.*

If the swelling still increases, and appears of a bluish red, take *Belladonna*, in the same manner as *Chamomile.*

Diet.—Abstain strictly from pork, and all irritating substances, such as pepper, and too much salt and salted meats.

If ulceration sets in, dress externally the parts with poultices or other mild applications, until relieved.

Excoriations. (*Intertrigo.*)

If they appear during the summer, in adults, give *Arnica, Carbo veg., Nux vom., Lycopodium, Sulphur,* beginning with *Arnica,* every evening a dose (four glob.) for two days, and then wait two days for its effect—taking the next in the same manner, and so on until better.

Chafing of bed-ridden patients (*bed sore*) requires *Arnica* (ten drops of the tincture to half a teacupful of water), externally applied, with cloths dipped into the mixture. At the same time place a soft, tanned deerskin under the sheets of the bed, the hairy side down.

If the affected parts look bluish, and there is danger of mortification, give *China* internally, in alternation with *Carbo veg.,* every four or six hours a dose (four glob.), and wash externally, with a solution of *Silicea* (twelve globules in half a teacupful of water), several times a day.

Disposition to fester.—There exists in some persons a disposition of the skin to fester, if the slightest injury has taken place, or ulcers do not heal. In such a case, give of the following remedies every week, on two succeeding evenings, one dose (four glob.), until better, *Chamomile, Hepar sulph., Lachesis, Silicea, Sulphur.*

Chapped hands (*rhagades*), from *working in water,* require *Calcarea, Hepar sulph., Sepia, Sulphur,* administered in the same manner.

Cracked skin, from cold in the winter, requires *Petrol., Sulphur,* in the same manner.

RINGWORM. (*Herpes circinnatus.*)

This eruption appears in small rings on various parts of the body; within them the skin looks healthy as usual; at least, this is the case at first. They are more apt to appear in summer.

TREATMENT.—Dissolve *Sepia* (twelve glob.) in half a teacupful of water, and give for three days, morning and evening a teaspoonful, and wash with part of the solution; repeat the same for eight or ten days, if necessary.

If this treatment should be insufficient give internally *Rhus* and *Sulphur*, alternately, every other day a dose (four glob.), and if not improved after twelve or fourteen days *Calcarea*, succeeded by *Causticum*, four doses of each every week, one dose (six globules).

TETTER. (*Herpes.*)

This term comprehends a great many varieties of the same disease, which, when present, show a constitutional disorder that ought to be treated by a homœopathic physician. The tetter may appear on any part of the body—hands, face, lips, the ears, etc., and requires different remedies accordingly; but the easiest direction which can be given for practical purposes, in a domestic way, is to be guided by its discharging quality.

Dry tetter requires *Dulcamara, Sepia, Silicea, Sulphur.*

Running tetter—*Dulcamara, Rhus, Graphites, Calcarea, Lycopodium, Sulphur.*

Bleeding tetter—*Arsenic, Carbo veg., Rhus, Mercury, Sulphur.*

Ulcerating tetter—*Mercury, Sulphur, Rhus, Sepia, Lycopodium.*

Violently itching tetter requires principally: *Nitric acid, Phosphorus,* and *Graphites;* if it itches worse in the warmth, *Clematis;* if worse in the evening, *Alumina* and *Staphysagria.*

ADMINISTRATION.—In using these remedies for a tetter,

having one of the above qualities (its locality on the body does not make so much difference), take a dose (six glob.) of the first-named remedy, on two consecutive evenings, and repeat this every week for four weeks, then discontinue for two weeks, taking the next remedy in the same manner, if the tetter shows no improvement during that time. In case of amelioration, however, take no more medicine unless worse again.

Keep the air off the tetter by a simple cover.

Application of Water, in very obstinate cases of this disease, is sometimes required; its use, however, must be directed in an institution, to which we recommend patients of this kind to resort.

Diet as in chilblains.

Itch. (*Scabies.*)

Not every eruption or pimple that itches is the itch; a malady so much dreaded in a family, that everything is welcome, and indiscriminately used, which will tend to eradicate this loathsome disease; and thus salves and ointments without number are used, but not without danger. Even if apparently cured by these salves, it is only driven *into* the system, laying the foundation for innumerable diseases afterward. Therefore, never do anything of this kind, under any consideration. First, be sure that it is *the real itch,* which is contagious. Frequently, it is only a disease described in the article on "Itching."

Diagnosis.—The real itch appears in pointed vesicles, filled with a transparent serous fluid, mostly about the wrists, between the fingers, and around the joints. The itching increases in the evening, especially in the warmth of the bed. It never appears on the face.

Treatment.—*Sulphur* is the specific for it. Take, every evening, a dose (ten glob.), for eight days; at the same time, wash the parts with half a pint of water, into which is put a grain of powdered *Sulphur*, twice a day, morning and evening, shaking the mixture well before using. Repeat this treatment if, after a week, no improvement has taken place; but, then, alternately with *Mercury* internally, as above.

If, after another week, there is no improvement, and the eruption is yet small and dry, take *Carbo veg.*, for eight days, every other evening a dose (six glob.), and, afterward, if necessary, *Hepar sulph.*, in the same manner; but if, during this time, pustules have made their appearance, give *Caustic*, in the same manner.

The *pustular* or *humid* variety generally spreads more over the body, and also appears frequently on the back, shoulders, arms, and thighs. In this form *Sulphur* and *Lycopodium* are necessary, given, as stated above, in "*Sulphur* and *Mercury*," for eight days; then wait eight days, and, if no better, take *Caustic*, and, after it, *Mercury*, in the same manner.

Sepia, internally and externally, applied in the same manner as *Sulphur*, has frequently been beneficial when nothing else seemed to have the desired effect.

When the pustules are large, and turn yellow and blue, take *Lachesis*, for several evenings a dose (six glob.).

When the itch has been suppressed by external applications, and dangerous results threaten, give *Sulphur* and *Arsenic*, in alternation, every evening a dose (six glob.).

In obstinate cases, apply to a homœopathic physician.

Application of Water internally and externally is, in this disease, of the greatest benefit; bathing and washing daily are essential; beside, the patient can perspire in the wet sheet twice a day with a cold sponge-bath after it. If possible, he ought to take a sitting-bath of half an hour's duration, before going to bed. Drinking of cold water is recommended.

Milk-crust. (*Crusta lactea.*)

This disease, as, in fact, all chronic eruptions of any extent, ought to be treated by a skillful homœopathic physician; yet we will here insert as much of the treatment as will warrant its rational commencement and often favorable termination.

Diagnosis.—It consists of numerous small, whitish pustules, appearing in clusters upon a red basis, first on the face, the cheeks and forehead, but spreading, afterward, over the whole head and other parts of the body. The redness and swelling frequently increase, and, with it, the itching becomes intolerable, particularly if a large part of the face and head is covered with the eruption. In such cases, the glands on the neck and under the ears enlarge in consequence.

Children, from four to eighteen months of age, are liable to it.

Treatment.—*Rhus* is the principal medicine, of which is to be given, every fourth evening a dose (four glob.), in alternation with *Hepar sulph.*, in the same manner, so that the child takes one or the other of the medicines every other evening.

If the child at any time is very restless, and the itching seems to be very aggravated, particularly at night, give *Aconite* and *Chamomile*, alternately, every two hours a dose (two glob.) until better.

If the running of the eruption suddenly dries up, and the child becomes drowsy, sleeps with eyes half open, has a hot head and cold feet, give *Belladonna* and *Hellebor.*, as directed under the head of "Measles." Externally, apply nothing but a little sweet cream, or wash occasionally with weak soapsuds.

If these remedies do not relieve within three or four weeks, apply to a homœopathic physician, who has in his possession an isopathic remedy, called "*Tinein*," which seldom fails to effect a speedy and safe cure.

Scald-head. (*Ring-worm of the Scalp.*) (*Tinea capitis.*)

There are several varieties of this disease; but for practical purposes, the distinction of dry and running scald-head is sufficient.

Diagnosis.—It appears, generally, on the hairy part of the head, in numerous yellowish pustules, finally forming a thick crust covering the head and neck of children from two to fourteen years of age: bad as it is, and obstinate to cure, yet its sudden disappearance, after the application of violent external means, creates worse internal disorders, and frequently even death. It is highly contagious; be careful even with the articles of clothing, particularly on the patient's head; let no other child come in contact with them. It generally lasts a long time, and ought to be treated by a skillful homœopathic physician.

Treatment. — First institute the treatment given under "Milk-crust," and continue it for four weeks; if no amelioration takes place during that time, give, if the eruption is of the *dry kind, Calcarea carb.*, every third evening a dose, (six glob.) for two weeks, and then, if there is no sign of improvement, give *Sulphur* in the same manner. If it is the *running scald-head,* give *Lycopodium,* and afterward *Sulphur,* in the same manner. If scrofulous symptoms appear, such as swelling of the glands on the neck and throat, give *Bryonia* and *Dulcamara,* alternately, every six hours a dose (four glob.) until better. If the discharge of the eruption is very corrosive, causing ulcers, give *Arsenic* and *Rhus* in alternation, every evening and morning a dose (four glob.), and wash with a solution (twelve glob. in half a teacupful of water) of each medicine, applying it to the edges of the scab, while giving it internally.

Application of Water.—See "Tetter."

Diet and Regimen.—The usual homœopathic diet must be adhered to strictly. (See "Introduction.")

The hair ought to be removed in the beginning of this disease.

Corns. (Clavi pedis.) Induration of the Skin.

Corns on the Feet.—If they will not disappear after several cuttings and applications of *Arnica* tincture (six drops mixed, with two tablespoonfuls of water, or *Arnica plaster*) an internal treatment must be resorted to for their eradication.

First, take *Antimon. crud.*, every evening a dose (six glob.), if the pains are more pressing, and as if *needles* were running through the corn. If the pain is of a burning nature, take *Calcarea carb.*, every other evening a dose (four glob.). If they are inflamed, take *Lycopodium, Sepia, Silicea* in the same manner, taking every week another remedy if necessary. If they are particularly troublesome in wet weather, take first *Bryonia* and *Rhus*, alternately, every two hours a dose (four glob.), for eight hours, and then twelve hours afterward a dose of *Sulphur*.

Induration of the skin.—Sometimes the *skin indurates* (gets *callous*) on the *hands and feet*, becomes painful and peels off—in such cases, take *Graphites* internally, every second evening a dose (four glob.), until four doses are taken, and use externally the same remedy (twelve glob. in half a teacupful of water well shaken) three times a day.

Warts. (*Verrucæ.*)

Neither cauterize nor cut these excrescences; it is too dangerous; a better remedy is the application of the tincture of *Rhus* on the wart three times a day. They will quickly disappear. If they do not disappear within four or six weeks, resort to the internal use of the following remedies:

Causticum, if the warts are fleshy or seedy.

Antimonium crud., if they are flat, hard or brittle.

Dulcamara, if they are on the back of the fingers.

Calcarea, if on the sides.

Administration.—Take of a remedy every other evening a dose (four globules), for eight days.

Whitlows on the Fingers. Felons. (*Panaris.*)

This disease exists in the form of an abscess, more or less

deeply seated, on the end of the finger, attended with severe pain and considerable swelling.

In the beginning, its formation may frequently be prevented by dipping the finger quickly into water almost boiling, or by wrapping around it finely-powdered wood soot made wet with alcohol, or by washing the finger with a mixture of a drop of creosote in half a teacupful of water. But if this does not avail, keep warm bread-and-milk poultice around it all the time until it opens, and take internally, *Mercury*, *Hepar sulph.*, and *Silicea*, alternately, every six hours a dose (four glob.), for two or three days.

After it opens, wash the finger three times a day in water, in half a teacupful of which twelve globules of *Silicea* are dissolved, or keep the bandage around the finger wet with this solution.

ULCERS.

We can only give their general treatment here, as their origin and appearance are too various to be discussed in a work on domestic practice. They arise, mostly, from a diseased condition, which must be first changed by systematic internal treatment, before the external sign of it, the ulcer, can heal. When it is forced to close itself by violent external means, the disease, of which it was the expression, attacks internal parts, and the danger is thus increased, as the dignity of the organ affected is greater.

Be careful, therefore, in using salves and ointments.

DIAGNOSIS AND TREATMENT.—First. An ulcer may be deep, presenting a *hollow excavation*. In this case fill it once or twice every day with dry scraped lint, previously cleaning it well with warm water, and tying it up with a bandage. This promotes healthy granulation, and the hollow gradually fills up. Internally give *Lachesis*, *Hepar*, and *Silicea*, alternately, every second day a dose (four glob.), until four doses of each are given, or improvement is perceptible.

Second. An ulcer may be *flat*, *superficial*, sometimes presenting *proud flesh;* in this case dress it with finely-powdered loaf sugar, or with a bandage dipped in cold water and changed from time to time. Internally, *Petroleum, Lycopodium,* and *Silicea,* in the same manner as above.

Third. An ulcer may be *fistulous:* in this case try to compress, if possible, the farthest ends of the fistula, or fill them with dry lint to excite healthy granulation, always trying to heal up the deepest cavity first. Give *Antimon. crud., Calcarea carb., Silicea,* and *Sulphur,* in the same manner as above.

Fourth. An ulcer may be *callous,* with thick, hard, broken margins. In this case fill the bottom with dry lint, and dress around the margins with simple cerate. Give *Arsenic, Pulsat., Lycopod.,* and *Sulphur,* in the same manner as above.

Fifth. An ulcer may be *carious,* proceeding from the bone; dress outside with simple cerate, and give *Mercury, Sulphur, Calcarea carb.,* and *Lycopodium* in the same manner as above.

Sixth. An ulcer may be *varicose,* caused by swelling of the veins, for instance, on the lower limbs; dress outside with simple cerate and lint, or cold-water bandage, and give *Pulsatilla, Lycopodium, Lachesis,* and *Sulphur* in the same manner as above.

We have another condition of the ulcer to take into consideration, in order to determine what medicine has to be given.

First. Ulcers may be *painful;* in this case give:

a. When accompanied by a burning or drawing sensation, *Arsenic, Rhus,* and *Sulphur* in the same manner as above.

b. When *beating, eating,* or *pressing, Mercury, Lachesis, Lycopodium* and *Sulphur* in the same manner.

c. When *itching, Hepar sulph., Pulsatilla,* and *Sulphur* in the same manner.

Second. An ulcer may be *without pain;* in this case give *Phosphor. acid, Carbo veg., Sepia,* and *Sulphur* in the same manner.

Third. An ulcer *smells offensively;* in this case give *Carbo veg.*, *Arsenic*, *Pulsatilla*, and *Sulph.*, in the same manner.

Fourth. It *spreads* very much, *increasing in size;* in this case give *Mercury*, *Lachesis*, *Hepar sulph.*, *Silicea*, and *Sulphur* in the same manner.

Syphilitic ulcers require *Mercury*, *Nitric acid*. *Lachesis*, and *Thuja* in the same manner.

APPLICATION OF WATER.—See "Tetter."

Abscesses. Tumors. Swelling of Glands.

When a congestive or inflammatory swelling is not dispersed or absorbed, it changes gradually into an abscess; matter forms which finally discharges through an opening of the sore, either prepared naturally, or artificially by a lancet.

TREATMENT.—Before an abscess opens, it may be very painful; in this case, poultice it with bread and milk, and take internally, *Belladonna*, *Lachesis*, and *Mercury*, alternately, every three or four hours a dose (four glob.), until better.

If it is a long time *maturing*, without being very painful (*cold swelling*), take *Hepar sulph.*, *Iodine*, and *Sulphur*, every other evening a dose, alternately, and poultice it when it comes near breaking.

After an abscess has opened, wash it frequently during the day with a solution of twelve globules of *Silicea* in half a teacupful of water, and take internally *Silicea*, every other evening a dose (four glob.), until three doses are taken.

If it be desired to open an abscess with a lancet, select the lowest part, if it be also the softest, which latter place is *always* to be chosen first. In other swellings, particularly when they appear hard, with stitches through them, or soft, without much pain, apply nothing externally, until after having consulted a homœopathic physician. Meanwhile, take internally *Calcarea carb.*, every three or four days a dose in the evening (four glob.), until six doses are taken; afterward, *Sulphur* in the same manner.

Enlarged and indurated *glands* on the neck, etc., require *Mercury* and *Dulcamara,* every evening, alternately, a dose (four glob.); when suppurating, *Hepar sulph.* and *Silicea,* every third evening a dose (four glob.), alternately, until four doses of each are taken.

Boils. Malignant Boils. Carbuncles.

These are painful, hard tumors, of a pyramidal form, and deep red color, generated sometimes by a constitutional tendency, very often, however, as critical discharges after acute or eruptive fevers, or terminating chronic eruptions, such as itch, etc. They suppurate slowly, and discharge, on breaking, a little pus mixed with blood, exhibiting a core which is gradually discharged.

TREATMENT.—The best applications externally are poultices made of bread and milk or flax-seed; all other things, such as roasted onions, soap and sugar, are too irritating, and enlarge the suppurative sphere. Internally take first *Arnica* evening and morning a dose (six glob.), and if the boil gets very painful and red, take *Belladonna* and *Mercury,* alternately, every three or four hours a dose (four glob.). If matter has formed, take *Hepar sulph.* every four hours a dose (four glob.), until the tumor breaks.

The predisposition to boils may be removed by taking *Sulphur,* every week one dose (six glob.), for six weeks. If a boil becomes *blue,* and *increases* very fast (*malignant boil*), take *Lachesis* every three or four hours a dose (four glob.) in alternation with *Arsenic.* Let the treatment be the same if typhoid fever ensues, and the patient is very weak, restless, and sleepless (*Carbuncle, Anthrax*), and mortification threatens.

A boil is called a *carbuncle,* when it is hard, of a livid hue, and after its breaking does not present a central core, but numerous openings, through which offensive matter and blood is discharged. *Carbuncle* or *Anthrax* is always a dangerous disease particularly when seated on the head. If it is on the back, wash with a solution of *Silicea;* if on the chin, with a solution of *Nitric acid* alternately with *Carbo veg.:* particularly if salivation attends the disease. If the pain in the ulcer is *burning*, wash with a solution of *Arsenic*, and give internally *Arsenic* and *Carbo veg.*, if *stinging*, give *Apis mellif.*

Scirrhus. Cancer.

We mention these diseases here, not to give their treatment, because the seriousness of their character would not allow of their being treated domestically; but it is necessary to warn patients of this kind against all those who pretend to cure them with the knife or cauterizing applications. They always end fatally under such treatment, and with increased misery. At the same time, we would advise them not to despair, but to apply immediately to a skillful homœopathic physician, who possesses the only means which can rationally afford relief, and which sometimes effect a complete cure.

Indurations under the skin, in glands, on the lips, nose, etc., with stitching pains through them, should receive attention, from the fear that they might be of the *scirrhus* nature; if so, and if not attended to in time, they will become open cancers.

In such cases, relief is possible, but only by the timely advice of a skillful physician. Meantime, take *Belladonna*, every third evening a dose (four glob.), until four doses are taken.

In open cancers, the distressing burning pains are relieved by *Arsenic*, in solution (twelve glob. in half a teacupful of water), every two or three hours a teaspoonful, until four or six are taken.

CHAPTER IV.

FEVERS.

The term *fever* is frequently misunderstood; people intending to express by it the disease itself, while, in reality, *fever is the reaction of the vital powers against a disease;* and, as every action in nature can be of a threefold kind, either not powerful enough for its purpose, or just powerful enough, or, lastly, too powerful, the fever, also, as an action of nature, allows these three divisions.

Accordingly, we have simple *irritative fevers*, where the effort of nature to remove the disease is just sufficient; or, *inflammatory fevers*, where this effort is greater than is necessary; or, lastly, *torpid fevers*, where the effort is not sufficient to accomplish the removal of the disease.

In all forms of acute disease, fever of one of the above kinds is present to a greater or less extent. It is obvious that one form of fever may, under circumstances favorable to the change, merge into another; for instance, a simple irritative fever may become an inflammatory one, if the patient is over stimulated; or a torpid one, if his vital energy is too much depressed.

How dangerous, therefore, must be the use of allopathic remedies in fevers, as, when a little too strong or too weak, they lead to such awful consequences! But, in Homœopathy, this result is altogether obviated, as the remedial agent used, neutralizes, by its specific action, the disease of which the fever was only an attendant symptom.

Thus we see, in pneumonia, under allopathic treatment, that the fever frequently returns with great violence, although the patient, shortly before, had been depleted to exhaustion. The reason is, that the cause of the fever, the pneumonia, had not been removed by the depletion; the reactive force or vital energy to overcome the disease was merely diminished, and, therefore, the system rouses itself up again to a second attempt; if checked or depressed again, it must finally sink to rise no more; it must fall into the *torpid* or *typhoid* form. Not so, under the homœopathic treatment, where the disease itself is specifically reached and as it were absorbed; for when the disease is removed, no effort of nature is necessary, and, consequently, the fever disappears of itself.*

The action of the unaided vital force of nature, during the fever, is in two directions—by the *nervous*, and by the *vascular* system—to bring about a crisis, sufficient for the extermination of the disease; but if it fails in establishing a sufficient crisis, nature has to surrender, and death ensues, either by paralysis of the nervous system (paralysis properly so called), or paralysis of the vascular system (mortification).

The less the disease, therefore, the less needs be the crisis; and we aid nature, indeed, if we take away the disease, but not if we take away her vital power to overcome it. Herein lies another important difference between the two medical systems; and it is easy to see how salutary the homœopathic, and how destructive the allopathic treatment of fevers must be.

* The best illustration of the *modus operandi* of the homœopathic medicines, or what is meant by specific action generally, is found in the effect of the dynamic agents of nature on each other. Positive and negative electricity, being similar, but not identical in their nature, neutralize or absorb each other; while positive and positive, being identical, repel each other, having no affinity to each other. In the same manner, two similar diseases absorb each other to the zero point, this state is where neither exists, and, therefore, health.

In most cases, Homœopathy takes away the disease so entirely, by its specific method, that no crisis at all appears. If it, however, takes place, it manifests itself by diarrhea, perspiration, or other secretions, or by an eruption; after which, the skin becomes moist and the pulse regular.

DIAGNOSIS.—The symptoms by which the presence of the three forms of fever may be known, are given in the following characteristics:

First. *Irritative form.*—Shivering, preceding a moderate heat; skin natural or a little moist; pulse not very much accelerated, but fuller, stronger, and not hard; urine a little more reddish than common, and with a sediment after the fever leaves.

Second. *Inflammatory form.*—Great lassitude precedes a short but severe chill (which frequently does not appear, however), followed by an intense heat; skin dry and burning; eyes sparkling; tongue dry; thirst intense; pulse quicker, hard, and full; urine red and scanty.

Third. *Torpid form.*—The greatest lassitude prevails during its presence; the patient feels very weak, although he may be very hot at times; at others, the temperature is very much diminished; the skin is now very dry and inclined to crack; then, again, covered with clammy perspiration.

At one time, the tongue is dry and black; at another, either natural or covered with a tough mucus. There is often an absence of thirst, although the tongue is dry; and then, again, thirst is intense, with a moist tongue.

The pulse shows the same anomaly, being sometimes full, with a low temperature of the body; and again, at other times, small and weak, with a high fever-heat of the system.

TREATMENT.—As we have only given here the general character of the three kinds of fever that combine themselves with local diseases of the different organs, we must, also, generalize their treatmen there, and refer, for details, to the affections of the respective organs where fever manifests itself. For instance: fever of the lungs, *pneumonia*, inflammatory, or torpid (*typhoid*), see "Affections of the Lungs."

The essentials in the treatment of all fevers are as follows:

Quiet and rest of body and mind, as much as possible; cool and even temperature of the patient's room, say from fifty to sixty degrees, according to comfort; pure air and thorough ventilation, without producing it by draughts passing on or over the patient. Let the patient lie on mattresses, and be covered with quilts, light, but sufficiently warm.

As the patient himself does not desire solid food, we ought not to give it; but, when thirsty, we must never refuse drink. The best drink is cold water, as much as the patient desires, if it agrees with him; frequently give toast water, barley or rice water, or lemonade, except when the patient has a diarrhea, or is taking *Aconite*, with which no acid will agree.

In convalescence, baked apples and stewed prunes are very salutary, if there is no diarrhea at the time; the latter, however, should be partaken of sparingly.

We will now treat of several other general forms of fever as they occur.

Common or Ephemeral Fever.

(*Febris Simplex.*)

Diagnosis. — Shivering, followed by heat, restlessness, thirst, quick pulse; its termination is generally within twenty-four or thirty-six hours, by profuse perspiration.

It is mostly caused by exposure to sudden changes of temperature, and will then terminate in from twenty-four to forty-eight hours; but where it is the forerunner of other more serious diseases, such as scarlet fever, measles, etc., it will be superseded by them.

Treatment.—*Aconite*, in solution (twelve glob. to half a teacupful of water), every two hours a teaspoonful, until perspiration ensues.

Diet and Regimen.—Cover the patient well, and let him

drink cold water, which promotes perspiration. Bathing the feet in warm water before lying down is allowed, but it should be done near the bed.

N. B. If pains are felt in different parts of the body, see respective headings, and treat accordingly.

General Inflammatory Fever. (*Synocha.*)

Diagnosis.—See "Fevers—Inflammatory form."

Causes.—This form of fever is frequently caused by sudden checks of perspiration and exposure to high degrees of temperature or its sudden change. It also originates by external injuries or lesions. Plethoric and young persons are most liable to it.

It frequently runs into typhus fever, particularly when treated allopathically.

Treatment.—*Aconite* must be given first, the same as in common fever. See preceding article.

But, if, after six hours, there is no improvement, give *Belladonna;* especially when the *head is hot with violent pains in the front part; red face, sensitiveness to light; sparkling* eyes ; *noise distresses;* very restless or drowsy ; great thirst; delirium.

Administration.—the same as *Aconite* above, or alternating with it, until better.

But, if, with the general symptoms of inflammatory fever, there is *swimming in the head* on rising or moving; some delirium ; *oppression at the pit of the stomach; vomiting after drinking; constipation;* aching pains in the limbs and small of the back; oppression of the lungs; give *Bryonia;* and, if the weather is damp and rainy at the time, give *Rhus*, in alternation with *Bryonia*, in the same manner as above in *Aconite* and *Belladonna*, until better.

Application of Water, in the form of the wet sheet, and a covering of blankets, beside drinking of cold water, is recommended as an auxiliary to the homœopathic medication.

Diet and Regimen—the same as under the head of "Common Fever."

Nervous or Typhoid Fever. (*Typhus.*)

These names signify the same disease, the various grades of which are distinguished by prefixing the appropriate word in an adjective form, as a *malignant* typhoid fever; a malignant typhus, or, a malignant nervous fever; all three of which signify the same.

Although we could not advise any one to treat a fever like this on his own responsibility, with no other guide than a work on domestic practice, unless in cases of absolute necessity, it is, nevertheless, advisable to give a sufficient account of the disease and its remedies, to enable the inquirer to distinguish it from others, and commence its treatment with the right remedies.

The progress of the disease may frequently be arrested by early and proper treatment in its commencement. To the realization of this important point our particular attention will be directed, as in the prevention of disease is seen the great advantage of domestic practice.

Diagnosis.—The real nature of typhus consists in an alteration of the blood, which becomes thick, decomposed, and carbonized; but as such a qualitative change of the blood cannot take place at once, the disease begins slowly, but is sure in its progress, unless arrested by the proper homœopathic remedy.

The first indications are, general lassitude, chilliness, followed by occasional feverishness, and, sometimes, pain in the head, chest, or abdomen, followed by drowsiness. Then appear the symptoms given under the heading "Fevers—Torpid form." Beside these, one characteristic symptom of real typhus is, a pain in the abdomen near the right hip, sensible to heavy pressure; here, in the intestines, ulcerations of the glands invariably take place in real typhus; hence the pain only on pressing heavily. Under such symptoms, it runs its course, if not checked by good homœopathic treatment, perhaps to convalescence, by frequent critical efforts, in about twenty-eight days.

The best crisis is perspiration which comes on gradually; or, sleep, in the place of delirium and restlessness. Bleeding of the nose is less favorable; and a still less favorable crisis is the swelling of the glands in front of, and below the ear; or, it ends in death, either by paralysis, or mortification. (See "Fevers.")

Causes. — In general, any depressing influence on the vital powers of the body may produce typhus, but, particularly, over-exertion of the body or mind; excesses of any kind; long and imprudent exposure to cold or damp weather; bad air, water, and mode of living; crowded population in filthy streets and small apartments; exhausting blood-letting in inflammatory diseases; or, lastly, a real typhus contagion, which is generated in one form of the disease. (See below, "Contagious Typhus.")

Preventives. — The best preventive is, to avoid the above described causes of the disease, and to take, if already threatened with it, *Bryonia* and *Rhus*, every evening alternately a dose (four glob.), for eight days, or until better. Keep quiet and in the house; follow the diet prescribed in fevers generally; keep the feet warm and head cool; drink freely of cold water, and take no allopathic remedies, such as pills, etc., *under any consideration.*

Different Forms of Typhus.

First. According to the *time of its appearance,* typhus is:

a. *Primary idiopathic*, or *true and contagious typhus;* or,

b. *Secondary*, following another disease, and *pseudo-typhus;* that is, fevers with apparently typhoid symptoms.

Second. According to its *locality*, typhus is .

a. Typhus of the *brain* (*typhus cerebralis*), *typhoid brain fever*, and *congestive fever* ;

b. Typhus of the *lungs* (*typhus pulmonalis*), *typhoid lung fever*;

c. Typhus of the *bowels* (*typhus abdominalis*), *abdominal typhoid*, and *yellow fever*.

N. B. In either of these three forms, those characteristic symptoms of real typhus (pains, on pressure near the right hip, in the intestines), as mentioned above (see "Diagnosis"), never fail to appear, even if the brain or lungs are primarily affected.

Third. According to its *qualitative* appearance, typhus is :

a. *Versatile* (*typhus versatilis*), with *excited* nervous action ;

b. *Stupid* (*typhus stupidus*), with *depressed* nervous action ;

c. *Putrid* (*typhus putridus*), with tendency to *organic dissolution*.

For practical purposes we follow the distinctions made under the "third" or last division, as it is only the *qualitative* differences in typhus that make different remedies necessary. The stupid form is oftener found in the typhus of the brain ; the versatile, in typhus of the lungs; and the putrid, in typhus of the bowels. Yet there are exceptions.

TREATMENT.—At the commencement of all three forms, if there is headache, giddiness, chilliness with alternate heat, rheumatic pains in the limbs and arms, sometimes a slight cough with pains in the back, with or without diarrhea, sickness at the stomach or vomiting, restlessness at night, furred tongue ; give *Bryonia* and *Rhus*, every two hours a dose (four glob.), until three of each are taken. Make the patient lie down, well covered, and await the reaction for twenty-four hours ; giving nothing, during that time, except one or two doses of *Coffea*$^{cc.}$ and *Bellad.*$^{cc.}$, if he is very restless during the night. As soon as the patient perspires and the symptoms gradually disappear, the typhus, as such, is checked, and its return is prevented by giving, on the third day, evening and morning, a dose (four glob.) of *Sulphur;* during which time the patient still keeps his room, and diets as recommended in fevers.

If, however, the disease progresses, and the real typhus symptoms appear more and more, give as follows:

If inflammatory symptoms appear, such as full, hard pulse; hot, dry skin; violent thirst; give *Aconite,* two or three doses, every two hours one (four glob.); and alternate with *Belladonna,* in the same manner, if to the above symptoms are added violent congestion of the head or lungs, with severe headache; sensitiveness to light and noise; starting after closing the eyes, and wild expression of countenance. Wait eight or twelve hours for the effect.

If no change for the better takes place, but, on the contrary, the symptoms increase in violence; give *Bryonia* and *Rhus* again, alternately; but now only every four hours a teaspoonful of their respective solutions (twelve globules in half a teacupful of water), with which continue until four of each are taken, or until better.

After this time, the disease may have changed, so as to make one of the following remedies necessary.

Phosphor. acid. Great exhaustion, flighty when awake, always lying on the back in a drowsy state; giving either no reply to a question, or replying incoherently, loquacious, delirium, or low muttering, picking the bedclothes, black lips, dry, hot skin; frequent, copious, watery and involuntary diarrhea, sometimes bloody; give alternately with *Rhus,* in the same manner as *Bryonia* and *Rhus* were above directed to be given.

Arsenic. If, with these symptoms, there is *extreme prostration of strength,* falling of the lower jaw, open mouth, dull and glassy eyes, burning thirst, profuse diarrhea, pulse barely perceptible; alternate *Carbo veg.* with *Arsenic,* if to the above symptoms is added rattling respiration, cold perspiration on the face and extremities, and very offensive evacuations, to be given in solution as above, every half hour a teaspoonful. These remedies suit principally in the *putrid* form of the disease.

In the *stupid* form, however, after *Bryonia* and *Rhus* have been given, the following remedies may be found necessary.

Opium. When there is great drowsiness, with snoring breathing, open mouth, low mutterings, picking the bed-clothes, lethargy, all discharges passing involuntarily, give every hour a dose (four glob.), until better, if not, give *Phosphor. acid* as above.

Lachesis. Under the same symptoms as those under *Opium*, particularly if the tongue is *very red* and shining, as if varnished; in the same manner as above.

Lycopodium. Under similar symptoms as *Lachesis*, and then in alternation with it, in solution, every two hours a teaspoonful, until a change takes place; but particularly if there is a strongly marked *redness of the cheeks*, constipation, and screaming, especially on awakening, *dryness of the tongue without thirst*.

In the *versatile* form, after *Bryonia* and *Rhus* have been given, the following medicines may be necessary, as,

Hyoscyamus. When there is a desire to escape; twitchings, and grasping at persons that are near; hot, red face, with bluish cheeks, sparkling eyes, dry, brownish tongue; alternately bland and furious delirium, involuntary evacuations; give every three hours a dose (four glob.), alternating with *Belladonna* in the same manner; or, in alternation with

Stramonium. If to these symptoms are added frightful fancies, loquacious delirium, staring eyes, spasmodic action, convulsions, and aversion to liquids; no stool or urine, and loss of consciousness.

There are several other remedies, which, under various circumstances, are important in the treatment of this disease. *Arnica, Arsenic, Camphor, China, Veratrum, Cantharides, Coc-*

culus; see in "Materia Medica" their pathogenetic symptoms, and give them if similar with the state of the patient.

N. B. If at any time the patient is very sleepless, give *Coffea*$^{cc.}$ and *Belladonna*$^{cc.}$, every hour a dose (four glob.), alternately. If there is clammy, *cold* skin, debilitating and clammy sweats, diarrhea or disposition to it, give *Camphor* and alternate with *Coffea*, if very restless, every half hour a dose until better. During convalescence, *China*, *Mercury*, and *Sulphur* are frequently necessary. (See "Materia Medica," at the end of the book.

Application of Water.—In no disease, perhaps, is the wet sheet, as an auxiliary remedy, of more use than in the different forms of typhus, particularly where the skin is dry and hot. In this state, even frequent ablutions will relieve the patient very much ; the drinking of cold water must be allowed, except during a chill or when the patient lays in a heavy perspiration.

Diet and Regimen the same as under "Fevers."

Congestive fever is a typhoid brain fever, and is treated as already stated, with *Aconite*, *Belladonna*, *Bryonia*, *Rhus*, *Opium*, etc.

The *contagious typhus* is in nothing different from the above, only it is caused by contagion. The attack occurs but once in a person's lifetime and its course is marked with great severity.

The *pseudo-typhus* or *bilious-rheumatic* fever is composed of the incipient symptoms of typhus, and has to be treated accordingly, as stated above, with *Bryonia* and *Rhus*, followed by *Sulphur*, to prevent its running into real typhus. For the treatment of this form, however, compare *Ipecac.*, *Pulsatilla*, *Ignatia*, and *Nux vom.*, in the "Materia Medica" at the end of the book.

The *ship fever* is a species of the *contagious* and *abdominal* typhus ; treat accordingly; compare as in "Yellow Fever."

YELLOW FEVER.

As I never had an opportunity to observe and treat this malignant fever, I thought it advisable to insert here the full article of Doctor Marcy on that subject, who had an opportunity to peruse the notes left by Doctor Taft, whose success in the treatment of yellow fever was astonishing:

This fever is exceedingly uncertain in its course, violence, and duration. It may strike its victim suddenly prostrate, overwhelming, in its severity, the whole system, and thus preventing a single rally of the circulatory vessels; or it may advance mildly, differing but little from an ordinary attack of remitting fever. In some instances it bears a strong resemblance to the higher grades of bilious fever. Much depends upon the peculiar circumstances of the individual attacked. If he is recently from a temperate climate, and unaccustomed to hot regions, he will be more susceptible to the action of the poison, than if he had been previously acclimated.

Medical men have supposed that after a certain period of exposure, the system becomes so completely accustomed to the miasm, that it loses all susceptibility to its influence, and in this manner the process of acclimation is accomplished. There is, doubtless, some truth in this idea, but there are other causes which exercise quite as important an influence in this process. Those persons who abandon a temperate, for a residence in a tropical climate, do so in that physical condition which the requirements, habits, and regimen of the former naturally generate. In a previous chapter we have seen that, in cold regions, where the atmosphere is highly condensed, a large amount of animal food is requisite to supply the system with sufficient carbon and hydrogen to resist and neutralize the action of the inspired oxygen. With these habits, appropriate only where a condensed atmosphere is respired, individuals seek the tropics, with bodies abounding in carbon, and continuing, in most instances, their accustomed regimen of animal food and stimulants, thus burdening their systems with an amount of the elements of nutrition fai greater than the oxygen contained in the rarefied air which they inhale can decompose.

It is probable, therefore, that one of the chief predisposing causes of yellow fever, is the presence of a greater amount of carbon in the system than the inspired air can properly act upon. The exact equilibrium between the supply of the elements of the food and the absorbed oxygen is disturbed; the carbon predominates, and all of those derangements which proceed from a superabundance of this agent, necessarily ensue.

The inhabitants of tropical latitudes have comparatively but little desire for animal food, but prefer farinaceous diet, vegetables and fruits, in this manner naturally securing to themselves a due proportion between the elements assimilated and the oxygen absorbed; while the inhabitants of the north find it necessary to consume large quantities of meat and other articles abounding in the elements of nutrition, in order to preserve a healthy equilibrium. We, therefore, most strongly urge it upon those who remove from cold to hot climates, to adapt their systems by appropriate regimen and strict temperance in all things, for the change, and we confidently predict that they will enjoy as great an immunity from this dreadful scourge as the natives themselves.

Diagnosis.—The premonitory symptoms of yellow fever are giddiness, wandering pains in the back and limbs, slight chills, nausea, and frequent sensations of faintness.

After these symptoms have continued a few hours, a decided reaction occurs; the circulation becomes excited, the face flushed, the eyes red; there are violent pains in the head, back, loins, and extremities; distress of stomach, and vomiting of acid bilious matters; the surface becomes dry and burning hot; mouth and throat dry, with intense thirst, and sometimes delirium.

The duration of this paroxysm is usually about twenty-four

hours, although occasionally it continues two or three days, after which there is a remission of all the symptoms, except a distressed sensation in the stomach, with nausea and vomiting. The patient remains in this state with a considerable degree of comfort for a few hours, when there is a recurrence of many of the former symptoms in an aggravated form. The stomach now becomes extremely painful and sensitive; vomiting is violent and incessant; the fluids ejected are of a darker color; the skin and eyes acquire a yellow tinge, and the mind becomes confused and wandering.

The duration of this second stage varies from twelve to forty-eight hours, with sometimes slight remissions toward the termination of the paroxysm, when the third or last stage sets in. This stage is characterized by the complete development of the dreaded "*black vomit.*" At this period, the powers of the system all sink rapidly; the pulse flags, and perhaps intermits; the tongue becomes dry, black, and shriveled; the breathing irregular and laborious; cramps seize the calves of the legs and the bowels; the whole countenance loses its natural, life-like expression; the extremities become cold; colliquative sweats, diarrhea, hemorrhages, and loss of intellect occur, and, finally, dissolution ends the scene.

This is only a brief outline of the more ordinary symptoms and course of the malady, and will, we trust, serve to aid the inexperienced practitioner in his diagnosis. Each case, however, must necessarily present modifications according to the predisposition, habits, and peculiar circumstances of the individual attacked.

Causes. — When animal and vegetable matters are submitted, for a considerable length of time, to the daily influence of intense solar heat, and a certain amount of moisture in the crowded and filthy streets of cities, or other confined places, a miasm is generated, which, under favorable circumstances, will cause yellow fever. Concerning the nature of this miasm we know nothing; but it is evident that the continued high degree of temperature to which these substances are exposed, and the confinement of their noxious emanations within the walls of crowded cities, develop a more virulent morbific agent than is the case when the same matters are exposed in the open country, or to a more irregular and less intense heat, such as usually occurs in more temperate localities.

There are several other causes which act as powerful predisposing influences, one of the most important of which, as before mentioned, is the too free use of animal food and stimulants. We may also include in this category, irregular habits, mental anxiety, depression of spirits, fear, grief, exposure to night air or to a burning sun, and, indeed, whatever else tends to debilitate the organism.

Treatment.—The remedies most commonly applicable in the treatment of this affection are *Ipecac.*, *Belladonna*, *Bryonia*, *Rhus*, *Arsenic*, and *Aconite*. The other medicines likely to prove serviceable are, *Nux vom.*, *Mercurius*, *Veratrum*, *China*, *Sulphur*, *Cantharides*, *Carbo veg.*, and *Lachesis*. The late and much lamented Doctor Taft, of New Orleans, was eminently successful in his treatment of the yellow fever as it occurred in that city. Some time since, we had the pleasure of perusing a letter from a highly intelligent gentleman of New Orleans, in which he states, that the success of Doctor Taft was so great in this malady as to attract the marked attention of a large number of citizens; and the writer expresses a deliberate opinion, that a new and favorable era would soon have occurred in the management of this formidable affection, if the able and accomplished Taft had survived. The remedies which this physician found most successful, and upon which he chiefly relied, were *Aconite*, *Ipecac.*, *Belladonna*, and *Bryonia*, in the *first*, and sometimes *second* stages; in the second and third stages, in addition to the above, *Rhus tox.*, *Arsenic*, *Veratrum*, *Cantharides*, *Carbo veg.*, *Nux vom.* These medicines were usually employed at the first attenuation, and frequently repeated, either singly or in alternation, as the circumstances of each case appeared to require.

When the first symptoms declare themselves, as dizziness, slight chills, pains in the back and limbs, uneasy sensations at the epigastrium, with nausea, vomiting, and sensation of faintness, *Ipecac.*, at the third attenuation, should be immediately exhibited. This remedy may also be found serviceable during the second and third stages, in alternation with some other article. Should the malady continue to progress, the following medicines should be considered, and, in proper cases, promptly administered.

Belladonna. Glowing redness and bloated appearance of the face; eyes red and sparkling, or fixed, glistening, and prominent; tongue loaded with whitish mucus, or yellowish, or brownish; pulse variable. Dry burning heat; sharp, darting and shooting pains in the head; violent throbbings in the head; burning thirst; painful heaviness and cramp-like pains in the back, loins, and legs; pressure, cramp-like, and contractive pains in the stomach; inclination to vomit, or violent vomitings. During the remission, melancholy; dejection; when reaction comes on, great agitation, with continual tossing and anguish.

Administration.—*Belladonna* is for the most part applicable to the first stage of yellow fever. Twelve globules in half a teacupful of water, every hour or two hours a teaspoonful, until better or another remedy is needed.

Bryonia. Skin yellow; eyes red, or dull and glassy, or sparkling and filled with tears; tongue dry, and loaded with a white or yellow coating; pulse rapid and full, or weak and rapid. Severe pain and burning sensation in the stomach; vomiting, particularly after drinking; burning thirst; pains in the back and limbs; headache, aggravated by movement; eyes painful on motion; sense of fullness and oppression in the stomach and intestines. Anxiety, with dread and apprehension respecting the future; loss of memory; delirium.

ADMINISTRATION. — Same as *Belladonna*, or in alternation with *Rhus*.

Rhus. Surface of a dirty yellow color; eyes glazed and sunken; tongue dry and black; lips dry and brownish; pulse quick and small; loquacious delirium, or coma with stertorous breathing; constant moaning. Distressing pain and burning in the stomach; nausea and vomiting; paralysis of the lower extremities; spasms in the abdomen; want of power over the abdominal muscles; colic; diarrhea; difficulty in deglutition, and pain on swallowing. Intellect dull and clouded; constant uneasiness; delirium.

ADMINISTRATION.—Same as *Belladonna*. (See *Bryonia.*)

Arsenic. Face of a yellowish or bluish color; eyes dull and sunken, with a dark mark under them; sclerotica yellow; nose pointed; coldness of the body, with cold and clammy sweat; lips and tongue brown or black; colliquative sweats; pulse irregular, or quick, weak, small, and frequent, or suppressed and trembling. Sense of extreme debility; dull, throbbing, stunning, or shooting pains in the head; burning or sharp and darting pains in the epigastrium, or in the region of the liver; limbs feel stiff and useless; frequent evacuations, with tenesmus, or painless and involuntary; oppression at the chest, with rapid and anxious respiration; cramps in the calves of the legs; great oppression at the stomach, with violent vomiting, especially after drinking; drawing and cramp-like pains in the abdomen; sensation as if a weight was pressing upon the abdomen. Indifference; weakness of memory; stupidity; delirium, with great flow of ideas; loss of consciousness and of sense; raving.

ADMINISTRATION. — Dissolve in water, as stated in *Belladonna*. In urgent cases, a teaspoonful may be exhibited every half hour, until some change is produced in the symptoms. In less dangerous cases, the intervals of administration may be lengthened as circumstances require.

Aconite. Suitable in the first and second stages, when

there are burning and dry skin; red cheeks; full and rapid pulse; red and sensitive eyes; tongue natural or covered with a whitish slimy coat; lips and mouth dry; vomiting of mucus and bile; urine dark-red. Violent febrile reaction; sensation of intense heat; great thirst; acute pains in the temples, forehead, or on the side of the head; vertigo on rising, eyes weak and sensitive to light; pains and soreness in the back and limbs; nausea; general sense of debility; great heat and irritability of the stomach; short and anxious respiration. When the fever is on, great anguish, anxiety, and restlessness; for the most part nightly delirium.

Administration.—Dissolve in water as above. *Aconite* and *Belladonna* may sometimes be alternated with benefit in the first period of the disease.

In a majority of cases, a few doses of this remedy will be found indispensable, during the first reaction.

Nux vomica. Skin yellow; face pale or yellowish, especially around the nose and mouth; lower part of the sclerotica yellow; eyes inflamed, with redness of the conjunctiva; eyes surrounded with a dark circle and full of tears; tongue with a thick white or yellow fur, or dry, cracked, and brown, with red edges; pulse variable. Burning pains in the stomach; pressure or cramp-like pains in the epigastrium; vomiting of acid, bilious, or mucous matters; frequent and violent hiccough; eyes sensitive to light; vertigo, or pains in the head; tremors of the limbs, cramps in different parts; thirst for beer, brandy, or some stimulant; contraction of the abdominal muscles; loose discharges of slimy or bilious matters or blood; burning pains at the neck of the bladder, with difficulty in urinating; coldness, paralysis, and cramps in the legs; feet benumbed and cramped. Excessive anxiety, uneasiness, fear of death, despair, or loss of consciousness and delirium, with moaning or muttering.

Administration.—Same as *Belladonna*.

Mercurius. Yellow color of the skin; eyes red, blood-vessels of sclerotica injected; eyes sensitive to light; paralysis of one or more limbs; tongue with moist, thick, white fur, or dry and brown mucus; fæces variable; pulse irregular, or quick, strong, and intermittent, or weak and trembling. Excessive inclination to sleep, or restlessness from nervous irritation; sense of fatigue and debility; rapid loss of strength; dizziness, or violent pain in the head; violent convulsive vomiting of mucus and bilious matter; burning pain and tenderness of the stomach; constipation, or diarrhea with discharges of mucus, bile, or blood; coldness of the arms and legs, with cramps; excitability and sensibility of all the organs. Anguish and agitation; weakness of memory; apprehensions; discouragement; moroseness; raving.

ADMINISTRATION same as *Belladonna.*

Veratrum alb. Face of a yellowish or bluish color, cold and covered with cold perspiration; eyes dull, clouded, yellowish and watery; lips and tongue dry, brown and cracked; hiccough; coldness of the hands and feet; trembling and cramps of the feet, hands and legs; evacuations loose, blackish or yellowish; pulse slow and almost extinct, or small, quick, and intermittent. General prostration of strength; confusion of head, or vertigo; deafness; difficult deglutition; intense thirst; violent vomiting of green bile and mucus, or black bile and blood; burning in the stomach; great exhaustion; cramps in the stomach, abdomen, and limbs; diarrhea. Timid, despondent, restless, loss of sense; coma or violent delirium.

ADMINISTRATION same as in *Arsenic,* and with it in alternation.

Sulphur. Face pale, or yellowish; eyes red, or yellowish; aphthæ in the mouth; tongue dry, rough, and reddish, or with white or brownish coat; pulse hard, quick, and full; fæces whitish, greenish, or brownish, bloody or purulent. Dizziness, or sharp pains in the head; itching and burning pains in the eyes; roaring in the ears; nausea, with trembling and weakness; vomiting of bilious, acid, bloody, or blackish matter; pressure and pain in the stomach; pains in the back and loins. Melancholy, sad, timid, undecided, wandering.

Administration.—Dissolve in water as above; every four or six hours a teaspoonful.

Cantharides is sometimes indicated in the third stage with complete insensibility, cramps in the abdominal muscles and legs, suppression of urine, hemorrhages from the stomach and bowels, and cold sweat on the hands and feet. It may be employed in water, dissolved, every half hour a teaspoonful, until a decided impression is produced.

Carbo veg. and *Lachesis* have both proved curative in the third stage of yellow fever, and should always receive due attention in grave cases.

Application of Water.—See "Typhus."

Diet and Regimen.—Same as under "*Fevers.*"

Bilious Remittent Fever—Bilious or Gastric Fever.

(*Febris remittens, Enteropyra.*)

Diagnosis.—A more or less severe chill is followed by feverish heat, with dry skin, and rapid but soft pulse; the latter is frequently intermittent, mostly irregular. The patient has a feeling of oppression and swelling at the pit of the stomach; pressure on the stomach causes not much pain, but rather a disagreeable sensation by the gases in the stomach, which are belched up, smelling disagreeably, sometimes with vomiting of a tough, variously-colored mucus, with a bitter, putrid, or slimy taste. The patient has a foul tongue, with a yellowish or brownish coat; he complains of headache, particularly a pressing sensation over the eyes, of dizziness and unusual lassitude.

In the beginning of the disease, the bowels are constipated; in its progress, offensive discharges appear, of badly-digested food with mucus. The urine, generally, is turbid, resembling a mixture of butter with water (*urina jumentosa*).

There appear, sometimes, two varieties of this fever.

First variety, respecting the *stomach,* which sometimes is inflamed in several spots, exhibiting many symptoms of a real gastritis; such as vomiting after the least eating or drinking, continual eructation of gas and hiccough, beside great tenderness on pressing the region of the stomach.

Second variety, respecting the *febrile excitement,* which sometimes assumes the febrile type, particularly in persons of a plethoric constitution. In such cases the pulse becomes hard and full, with rush of blood to the head, the skin dry and hot, the tongue has a thin, whitish coat, the urine, at first dark brown, becomes turbid only on standing. The remission of these symptoms takes place in the morning, therefore, the name *remittent fever;* a complication with the *intermittent* is frequently observed, particularly in marshy regions.

CAUSES.—This fever mostly appears in the summer, when the atmosphere is moist or changeable; also, during long-continued hot weather. Persons of weak digestion, with irritable temperament, are predisposed to it; also, those of sedentary habits, and indulging in debauchery or eating to excess indigestible food. As exciting causes, we mention: overloading of the stomach, anger, fear, taking cold and exposures to inclement climates.

Duration and course are very indefinite; this disease may terminate in a few days or it may last for weeks. Under a judicious homœopathic treatment, its duration is very much shortened, as, by the specific action of the medicines on the disease, its termination does not depend on the appearance of a favorable crisis, whereby a great deal of time is saved. If, however, a crisis appears, it does not impede the homœopathic medication: if it is too excessive or debilitating, the proper remedies have to be applied. Such crises appear by vomiting of food or bile, and by diarrheas of bile, mucus and indigestible substances. It is very favorable during the course of the disease, if the skin becomes moist, the urine deposits a sediment, or fever blisters appear on the lips and nose.

This disease can change into the intermittent fever or typhus, if neglected or badly treated. In such cases we refer the reader to the chapters of these diseases.

TREATMENT.—As the premonitory symptoms of a bilious remittent fever indicate, generally, a derangement of the stomach, from errors in the diet, or exposures to the changes of the weather, it is necessary, above all, to counteract these effectually in the beginning. In this stage of the disease, commonly termed *biliousness*, there is no fever yet, which will soon appear, however, if the patient does not adhere to a strict diet and keep quiet. His diet must be of the lightest kind, gruels, light bread, black tea and cold water; complete rest on the bed or couch. In case of the stomach having been overloaded, take coffee without milk or sugar; if caused by the eating of fat meat, etc., take *Pulsatilla, China, Carbo vegetabilis;* and, if there still remains nausea and gagging, give *Antimonium crudum* (see "*Indigestion*"). If anger was the cause, give *Chamomile,* and, if accompanied by chilliness and headache, in alternation with *Bryonia* (see "Affections of the Mind"). If climatic influences, exposures to cold or damp weather caused the biliousness, give *Bryonia* and *Rhus*, particularly if pains in the head, arms, and limbs are present; administer as stated page 119; beside, consult the article on indigestion.

The principal remedies for the bilious remittent fever, are *Aconite, Pulsatilla, Bryonia, Nux vom., Ipecac., Tartar emet., Antimonium crudum, Chamomile, Colocynth, China, Phosphoric acid, Arsenic, Veratrum.* If the symptoms of the first variety predominate, consult the article on *gastritis*, if those of the second, see "*Congestion of the Head,*" and "*Inflammatory Fever.*"

SYMPTOMATIC DETAIL.—*Aconite.* High fever; rapid pulse, yellow coating on the tongue; bitter taste and eructations;

bitter, greenish or slimy vomiting; painful sensitiveness of the stomach; headache, worse when talking.

Pulsatilla. Foul tongue, with a whitish coat; foul, bitter taste, especially of bread; sour, or offensive belching; aversion to food, particularly warm; desire for acids; throwing up of food or mucus; flatulence; chilliness, with languor; ill-humor; inclined to a diarrhea.

Antimonium crudum. Dull headache, worse when going up stairs, loss of appetite, loathing, tongue coated or covered with blisters, thirst at night, nausea; eructations, painfulness of the stomach to the touch; flatulency. (*Bryonia* is suitable after it.)

Bryonia. Especially during summer in hot and damp weather, dry tongue, coated white or yellow, thirst, bitter taste, desire for acids, wine; bilious vomiting after drinking, dullness of the head with vertigo, worse after drinking, chilliness. (In alternation with *Rhus.*)

Chamomile. Bitter taste in the mouth, loss of appetite, nausea, vomiting of green, bitter, or sour liquid; tensions and pressure in the stomach, anguish and restlessness, tossing about; pain and fullness in the head, hot and red face; irritable temper. (Against the excessive use of Chamomile tea give *Cocculus* and *Pulsatilla.*)

Nux vomica. Bitter or foul taste in the mouth, painful pressure and tension in the pit of the stomach; constipation, with frequent but ineffectual urging to stool; rheumatic pains in the head and body, inability to think. (After it *Chamomile* suits frequently.)

Ipecacuanha. Loathing of food, with desire to vomit; violent, but ineffectual efforts to vomit; or easy vomiting, but with great force; violent pains in the stomach; aching in the forehead, or sensation as if all the bones of the skull were broken.

Arsenicum. Colic or burning pains in the stomach and abdomen; great sensitiveness at the pit of the stomach to touch;

burning pressure at a small spot in the stomach; great debility, wants to lie down; vomiting after drinking or motion; drinks often, but little at a time.

Mercury. Moist, white or yellowish coated tongue, painful sensitiveness of the pit of the stomach and abdomen, worse at night, with restlessness; drowsy in the day-time, sleepless at night. (Suits well after *Belladonna.*)

China. No appetite, loathing of food and drink; chilliness and shuddering after drinking; flatulence; diarrhea of undigested food; very weak from debilitating losses; in alternation with

Phosphoric acid, as directed in *Typhus fever.*

Colocynth. Vomiting or diarrhea after eating ever so little; spasmodic colic; cramp in the calves.

Tartar emetic. Constant nausea, with desire to vomit; gagging; slimy vomiting and diarrhea. (Suits well in alternation with *Bryonia.*)

Veratrum. Dry tongue, coated yellowish, bilious vomiting and diarrhea, debility, fainting after a stool; cutting pains in the abdomen.

Carbo vegetabilis. Acidity in the stomach with pains, when pressing on the pit; heaviness or dullness of the head with debility; offensive diarrhea with great prostration.

Sulphur. If the fever had its cause in abdominal plethora, which is frequently accompanied by hemorrhoidal affections.

Administration.—Give of a selected remedy every three or four hours a dose (four globules) until four or six doses are taken; then discontinue for twelve or fourteen hours, to await the result. It is very proper to give the medicine dissolved in water. If that can be done, dissolve twelve globules in half a teacupful of water, and give, every two or three hours, a teaspoonful; for four or six times.

Application of Water—see "Fevers;" beside, if constipation shall be removed, the effect of the proper homœopathic remedy can be supported by cold injections and drinking of cold water.

Diet and Regimen.—As in fevers generally, lemonade is very grateful to patients of this kind, must however be avoided, where there is severe diarrhea.

Intermittent Fever. Fever and Ague. Chills and Fever.

(*Febris intermittens.*)

The difference between *remittent* and *intermittent* fevers is very marked, and ought to be well understood.

Remittent is a fever in which the symptoms continue during the whole time of the patient's sickness, only varying, from time to time, in severity; but never leaving the patient entirely at any time.

Intermittent, however, is a fever, in which the symptoms, at certain times, cease, and the patient feels as if entirely free from them, or well. To this latter class belong the chills and fever, or fever and ague, which is caused either by a certain miasma, generated in marshy countries, or follows other diseases, acute as well as chronic; for instance, inflammation of the liver, indigestion, internal obstructions, etc.

Diagnosis.—The cold stage is preceded by languor, yawning, drowsy headache, numbness of toes and fingers, and blue nails. Then coldness of the extremities is felt, gradually increasing, until the patient sometimes begins to shake and tremble, his teeth to chatter, and delirium ensues.

During this time, the pulse is weak and oppressed; his thirst variable; the cold stage lasts from twenty minutes to three or four hours, and varies much in severity.

The hot stage shows all the symptoms characteristic of an inflammatory attack: hot, dry skin; thirst; full, quick pulse; congestion of the head, and sometimes, even delirium. Its intensity and duration are variable, the latter being from two to six or eight hours.

The sweating stage indicates an abatement of the fever, although, frequently, there are fever and perspiration at the same time.

TREATMENT.—Certain and general rules for the treatment of this disease cannot be given; it depends too much upon the individual, and exciting causes, to make up its general character. But we will try to be as practicable on the subject as possible.

Two or three attacks must have passed before we can know, for a certainty, that we have to do with an *intermittent*. These attacks will have been treated already, according to their appearance, either as bilious rheumatic, or gastric fevers, whereby we may have used remedies beneficial in fever and ague also. But if this shows itself clearly as such, adopt the following treatment: First, *Ipecac.*, four doses (six glob. each), given in regular intervals between two attacks of fever, during which no medicine should be given; but, after it is over, give one dose of *Nux vomica* (six glob.). If, then, the next attack is lighter, do not give any more medicine, as the disease will disappear, the attacks gradually growing lighter and lighter.

But if this general treatment does not succeed, select the specific remedy among the following, taking great care to find the one most similar to the symptoms of the disease. For its application, I will here give general directions suitable for every case.

ADMINISTRATION.—Having found the remedy, give three doses of it (six glob. each), commencing twelve hours before the next attack is expected, once in four hours a dose. During the attack, if the chilliness and fever are very severe, give, invariably, *Aconite*, in solution (eight globules in half a teacupful of water), every half hour or hour a teaspoonful, until the attack is over. If the next attack is lighter, give no more medicine; if not lighter, select for the next attack another more suitable remedy. In this way proceed for ten or fourteen days, trying to find the right *homœopathic* remedy, before adopting the method spoken of at the end of this article, which subdues the fever without, perhaps, eradicating it as safely as the homœopathic remedy would, if found.

We will give, in the following, the principal remedies useful in domestic practice, leaving more complicated forms of the disease for the treatment of a homœopathic physician, if one can be had.

Arsenic. For *great debility,* disposition to vomit, or *violent pains in the stomach;* great anguish in the precordial region; lameness of the extremities, or *violent* pains; *imperfect development* of chilliness and heat, or both; alternately sensations of internal chilliness with external heat; *drinking very often but little at a time.* The pains in the limbs or all over the body are almost insupportable, with anxiety and restlessness, oppression in the chest, nausea, bitter taste in the mouth. (Compare *China, Ipecac., Veratrum.*)

China. When, before the fever, there is nausea or thirst, voracious appetite, headache, palpitation of the heart, thirst *between* the cold and hot stages, or *after* the hot stage, or during the perspiration; cold and heat alternately; *no thirst* during the heat; great debility; *uneasy* sleep; *yellow complexion.* (Compare with *Arsenic* and *Lachesis.*) This remedy particularly is suitable for those intermittents, originating from marsh miasms.

Natrum mur. Violent headache during the chilliness and heat, with obscuration of sight, amounting almost to partial loss of consciousness; pains in the bones, yellowish complexion; fever-blisters on the lips and *ulcerated corners of the mouth;* thirst during the chills, more during the heat; sensitiveness at the pit of the stomach; bitter taste; no appetite, or slight chilliness with yawning, and stretching, without thirst, followed by high fever with thirst, then perspiration with drowsiness and sleepiness; particularly in cases where

Quinine had been given, to suppress the fever. (Compare with *Ignatia*, *Arsenic*.)

Ignatia. *Thirst only during the chill;* gastric symptoms, pain in the bowels during the chill, and eruptions on the lips, as in *Natrum mur.*; *external heat moderates the chill;* external heat with partial internal shuddering. (Compare with *Carbo veg.*, and *Natr. mur.*).

Carbo veg. *Thirst only during the chill;* rheumatic pains in teeth or limbs, before or during the attack; nausea; giddiness during the heat; chill comes on in the evening or at night; particularly appropriate in *damp or wet weather.*

Sabadilla. When the attacks return almost at the same hour, with chills of short duration; then thirst followed by heat, or where the paroxysm consists entirely of chills.

Ipecac. Much shivering with but little heat, or the contrary; *increase of the shivering by external warmth* (the opposite of *Ignat.*); oppression at the pit of the stomach; no thirst, or but little, during the chill; violent thirst during the heat; nausea and other gastric symptoms; clean or slightly coated tongue; nausea and vomiting; oppression of the chest before or during the paroxysm. (Compare *Nux vomica.*)

Nux vomica. External heat, with internal chilliness, or *vice versa;* desire to lie down, and to be constantly covered, even during the heat; rheumatic pains in the sides, abdomen, and limbs; during the heat, headache, buzzing in the ears, heat in head and face, with redness of the cheeks, thirst, and constipation. (Compare *Ipecac.*)

Pulsatilla. Gastric symptoms; chills, heat, and at the same time in the afternoon and evening (compare *Sabadilla*); no thirst during the whole paroxysm, or only during the hot stage; at intervals the patient feels very chilly. It is very suitable when a disordered stomach has caused a relapse, or after *Lachesis.* Beside, compare *Antimon. crud.*, *Bryonia*, *Chamomile.*

Lachesis. Chills after a meal or in the afternoon, with

pains in the limbs and back; oppression of the chest; *violent headache* during the hot stage, with delirium, burning thirst, restlessness, internal shuddering; *debility;* livid complexion during the intervals and when the fever returns easily after eating sour things; in which case it alternates advantageously with *Pulsatilla.*

Veratrum. External chill and cold sweat, particularly on the forehead, with internal heat and dark-red urine; delirium and red face, or chills with thirst and nausea; or, vomiting and diarrhea during the heat or in the beginning of the cold stage, with pains in the back and loins.

Sambucus, when the perspiration is very profuse, even during the intermission.

Antimonium crud. When the tongue is very much coated with nausea, and vomiting, little or no thirst, constipation, or diarrhea. (Compare *Pulsatilla.*)

Bryonia. For bilious symptoms, with much thirst, rheumatic stitches in the side during the heat.

Rhus. The paroxysms for this remedy consist of heat, preceded and followed by chills. If bilious rheumatic symptoms are present, alternate with *Bryonia.*

Capsicum. Chilliness *with* thirst, followed by heat *without* thirst, or thirst only during the hot stage; the chills are violent and last long; the heat is intensely burning; throat and mouth filled with mucus; cannot bear noise; diarrhea of acrid, slimy matter.

Sulphur. Intermittents, following suppressed cutaneous eruptions, or after the abuse of *quinine.*

Calcarea. Chills and heat alternate, sometimes external coldness, and internal heat, head and face hot, extremities cold, pains in the small of the back, diarrhea.

Opium. Intermittents of old persons and children, where drowsiness with loud snoring prevails, oppressed breathing with the mouth open; face looks bloated and dark-red; twitchings of the muscles of the extremities.

We will now give some general indications and the names of the medicines only. The symptoms may be examined in the Materia Medica, at the end of the book, and then the choice made accordingly.

For *marsh-intermittent fevers: China, Arsenic, Ipecac., Carbo vegetabilis.*

For *fevers prevailing in damp and cold seasons: Carbo veg., Rhus, Sulphur, China, Pulsatilla, Lachesis, Veratrum.*

For *mismanaged* fevers, by *large doses of Quinine: Pulsat., Arsenic, Natrum mur., Lachesis, Sulphur.*

For *daily fevers: Arsenic, Bryon., Carbo veg., China, Ignatia, Ipecac., Lachesis, Natrum mur., Nux vomica, Pulsatilla, Rhus, Veratrum.*

For *tertian,* or every-other-day fevers: *Arsenic, Carbo veg., China, Ipecac., Nux vomica, Pulsatilla, Rhus.*

For *quartan,* or every-fourth-day fever: *Arsenic, Pulsatilla, Veratrum.*

When the fever returns yearly, give *Lachesis, Carbo veg.,* or *Arsenic.*

Having tried to cure the *intermittent* fever with these remedies for a fortnight, without success, and being unable to procure a homœopathic physician, give the patient the following remedy:

Take four or six grains of *Quinine,* mix with eighteen or twenty grains of loaf sugar, and triturate thoroughly, in a clean mortar, for half an hour; make six powders of it, and give, twelve or eighteen hours previous to the next attack, one powder; and, afterward, every two hours one, until all are given. Give, then, a similarly prepared powder one hour before the next chill is expected to come on, for at least a week, and, afterward, continue to give such a powder every seventh day, in the evening, for thirteen weeks after the last chill. If the fever returns (which it seldom does), use *Pulsatilla, Arsenic,* and *Natrum mur.*

N. B. If the disease is complicated with *bilious rheumatic* symptoms, see this article in Index.

Application of Water in the cure of this disease is frequently of the greatest advantage, and ought to be preferred by homœopathists to any other expedient, on account of its efficacy and harmlessness. The wet sheet during the period of heat, the sitting-bath before going to bed every evening, except when in a fever-paroxysm, or during perspiration, and the wet bandage around the abdomen, are the principal modes of application. The proper homœopathic remedy must be given at the same time. It is frequently necessary to resort to the douche, particularly in obstinate cases, or where the reactive force of the system has to be aroused.

Diet and Regimen, as generally in fevers. (See "Common Fever," page 115.)

CHAPTER V.

AFFECTIONS OF THE MIND.

SUDDEN emotions are often followed by fatal consequences either immediately or soon after, and it is not well to neglect them, particularly in children and delicate women.

We will give, in the following tabular view, the most frequent emotions, with the principal remedies, whose symptoms are detailed below, and which must be compared with the patient's symptoms before a choice is made.

For the consequences of *fright and fear*: *Opium, Aconite, Belladonna, Ignatia, Pulsatilla, Mercury.*

Excessive joy: *Coffea, Opium, Pulsatilla, Aconite.*

Grief: *Ignatia, Phosphor. ac., Staphysag., Colocynth.*

Home sickness: *Phos. ac., Mercury, Capsicum, Staph.*

Unhappy love: *Hyoscyamus, Ignatia, Phosphor ac.*

Jealousy: *Hyoscyamus, Lachesis, Nux vomica.*

Mortification and insult: *Belladonna, Ignatia, Platina, Colocynth, Staphysag., Pulsatilla.*

Contradiction and chagrin: *Chamomile, Bryonia, Ignatia, Colocynth, Aconite, Nux vomica, Platina, Staphysag.*

If accompanied with *indignation*: *Colocynth, Staphysag.*

Violent anger: *Aconite, Nux vomica, Chamomile,* and *Bryonia, Phosphorus.*

SYMPTOMATIC DETAIL.—*Aconite.* Headache, with congestion to the head; constant fear, especially in children; or when *Opium* has not been given at once for fright.

Belladonna. Loss of consciousness, or constant anxiety,

with weeping, fear, *crying with malice,* particularly in children; also, when *Opium* and *Aconite* have been insufficient for fright.

Capsicum. For sleeplessness from home-sickness, with heat and redness of the cheeks.

Chamomile. For the following consequences of anger: bitter taste in the mouth, nausea, vomiting of bilious matter, *cutting colic, pressure in the stomach,* headache, fever, thirst, restlessness, asthma, *suffocating fits; in children,* convulsions or gastric derangement, after eating or drinking, shortly after an angry fit.

Bryonia. Chilliness and shuddering over the whole body; vehement anger; loss of appetite; nausea; vomiting of bile.

Coffea. Nervousness from great joy, with trembling and faintness, especially in females and children.

Colocynth. From chagrin or mortification — colic, cramps in the stomach, nausea, bitter vomiting, sleeplessness.

Hyoscyamus. From fear — stupefaction, and apathy, inability to swallow, convulsions, sudden starts or involuntary laughing during sleep, desire to escape; and, also,

From unhappy love—jealousy, restlessness, running about.

Ignatia. From fright, mortification, chagrin, grief, especially after losing a friend — irresistible grief, headache, vertigo, vomiting, gastric symptoms or even convulsions, especially in children, from fright or from unhappy love.

Mercury. From fright, mortification, or home-sickness — as great anguish, trembling, and restlessness; sudden starting from sleep; congestion of blood on the least motion; sleeplessness; cannot bear the warmth of the bed; nervousness; quarrelsome mood; complains of everybody, even one's own family; constant shivering; night sweats.

Nux vomica. From anger—particularly after having eaten or drank something, or after *Chamomile* or *Bryonia* has been given without effect.

Opium. From joy or fear, to be given immediately—loss

of consciousness; perspiration about the head, with coldness of the rest of the body; congestion to the head; involuntary *diarrhea;* snoring-like breathing; *fainting fits;* spasms; *epileptic fits,* with spasmodical rigidity of the whole body.

Phosphoric acid. From deep grief, unhappy love, home-sickness, or in any case where *Ignatia* is not sufficient, particularly when the patient is dull and listless; when the hair falls out, or turns gray; hectic fever, with profuse sweats; sleepy in the morning.

Platina. From anger and mortification — as indifference, sadness, and laughter; pride, with contempt for others; great anguish and dread of death.

Pulsatilla. From fear — diarrhea, with heat in the abdomen.

From anger — in persons of a bland disposition, or when *Chamomile* is not sufficient.

Staphysagria. From anger or indignation and ill-humor— the patient pushes violently away whatever is near him; restlessness; fear; also,

From deep grief, as sadness, with a disposition to take everything wrong — dread of the future; sleepy in day-time and sleepless at night; falling off of the hair; feeble and faint voice; hypochondriac mood.

ADMINISTRATION.—The selected remedy should be prepared and given as follows; Dissolve twelve globules of it in half a teacupful of water, and give, every half hour a teaspoonful, until three or four are given, or until better; if not better after three or four doses are taken, select another remedy, and give it in the same manner. As soon as the patient feels better, give the medicine at longer intervals.

APPLICATION OF WATER.—That in the various affections of the mind, when depending on material changes of the system, the water can be made a useful auxiliary, is evident; yet its application is only necessary, where the disease has been of long standing. In such cases it is possible to arouse by it the sleeping reaction of the system and prepare the way properly for the readier action of homœopathic medicines. Frequent bathing and washing are the principal modes of application.

Hypochondria. Hysteria.

These two diseases are not essentially, but sexually, different. Hypochondria is the name for it in a male person, Hysteria, in a female. Persons inclined to this disease have great disposition to spasms and nervous attacks; their idiosyncrasies and sympathies are very much developed, from which result a great variety of singular fancies and imaginary sufferings, changing frequently in expression and character; sadness and excessive joy, deep distress and buoyant hilarity follow each other in rapid succession. Their real disorders can be traced generally to obstructions in the abdomen and abnormal states of the sexual organs. Debilitating influences of any kind may produce them, particularly where constitutional predisposition is present; also, suppression of habitual secretions, as piles, fluor albus, etc. The female system is more liable to them, if an ungoverned and unsatisfied imagination is fed daily by reading novels, plays and trashy romances. This disease is by itself not fatal; but becomes very troublesome to the patient as well as others.

Treatment.—Part of the treatment must consist in encouraging the patient during the fits of distress and pain even if only imaginary; to the patient these sufferings are real, and it cannot be of benefit to him, to express doubts of their reality in his presence. A kind, patient, sympathizing attention, with occasional congratulations on his progressive recovery, etc., is more beneficial, and contributes much to gain his confidence.

During the hysteric fit or spasm, it is only necessary to admit fresh air, and sprinkle cold water in the face of the patient; let him smell from time to time on camphor, or hartshorn. Between the attacks, the patient's diet ought to be regulated according to the strictest homœopathic rules, allowing plenty of exercise in the open air, if it can be taken; diverting the mind from his own state of health; using hydropathic means, and giving those homœopathic remedies which suit his case.

The difference between a *congestive* and a *nervous* hypochondria and hysteria is very important, as it greatly facilitates the selection of the right remedy.

The *congestive* form is signalized mostly by red, swollen face, wild looks, full pulse, feverishness, and requires principally: *Aconite, Belladonna, Nux vomica, Bryonia, Opium, Calcarea, Natrum mur., Sulphur.* The *nervous* form exhibits a pale face, with distressed looks, general debility, weak pulse, chilliness, and requires mostly: *Aconite, Coffea, China, Igna., Puls., Chamo., Lach., Nux moschata, Phos., Platina, Vera.*

Symptomatic Detail and Administration of these remedies, see "*Affections of the Mind.*"

If the disease is based decidedly on obstructions in the abdomen, consult the following remedies particularly:

Nux vomica. Ill-humor; *aversion to life; disposition to vehemence;* disinclination to mental labor; unrefreshing sleep; *feels worse in the morning;* dullness of the head, with aching pains, or sensations as if a pin were sticking in the brain; aversion to the open air; *constant desire to lie down;* great exhaustion after walking; painful distension in the hypochondria and stomach; *constipation* of the bowels; disposition to, or presence of, the piles (hemorrhoids). *Sulphur* follows well after *Nux vomica.*

Sulphur. Lowness of spirits; solicitude about one's *affairs, health, salvation;* fixed ideas; anxious impatience; restlessness; vehement disposition; *bodily* and *mental indolence;* absence of mind; cannot think; exhaustion after mental labor; fullness and pressure in the stomach; *constipation;* feels very unhappy. *Calcarea carb.* follows well after *Sulphur.*

Calcarea carb. Lowness of spirits, with disposition to weep; anxiety, with congestion or palpitation of the heart; despair about one's health; apprehension of illness, misfortune, infectious diseases, insanity, etc.; dread of death; cannot think, or perform any mental labor. (*Natrum m.* follows well after *Calcarea carb.*)

Natrum mur. Lowness of spirits; weeping and lamenting about the future; *desire to be alone;* aversion to life; ill-humor; disposition to vehemence; cannot perform mental labor; headache, with want of appetite; indigestion after eating.

Administration.—Give of the selected remedy every third evening a dose (six glob.), until four or six doses are taken; then discontinue for the same length of time; giving afterward the next best remedy in the same manner; and so on, until better.

Application of Water. — Beside the modes of applying the water indicated on page 145, this disease requires sitting-baths, foot-baths, wet bandage around the abdomen, cold injections and the wet sheet; sometimes the douche is indicated when the symptoms of this disease resemble that of the following; in *melancholia* the douche is the principal application.

Melancholia. Mania.

A disturbance of the normal actions of the mind similar to the former, but more deeply seated, with general derangement of the system always requiring skillful medical aid.

If the patient is timid, unsociable, sad, listless, weak, we call it *melancholia;* if he is in the opposite state, and dwelling on a fixed idea, we call it *mania* and *frenzy*. The treatment of these disorders is so difficult and complicated, that it would be impossible to introduce it here with advantage. We only draw the attention of the reader to a few remedies, which may be given to commence a cure or satisfy immediate necessities, until competent help can be procured.

For deep *melancholy: Arsenicum, Aurum, Lachesis, Nux vom., Sulphur.*

For *silent melancholy: Ignatia, Cocculus, Lycopodium, Phosphor. acid, Pulsatilla, Veratrum.*

For *religious melancholy: Aurum, Belladonna, Lachesis, Pulsatilla, Sulphur.*

For *mania,* bending upon *self destruction;* to *hang* one's self, *Arsenicum;* to *drown* one's self: *Belladonna, Hyoscyamus, Pulsatilla, Secale;* to *shoot* one's self: *Antimon. crud., Carbo veg.*

For *restlessness, wandering about: Belladonna, Hyoscyamus, Stramonium.*

For *mania,* as if possessed by bad spirits: *Hyoscy.;* as if seeing ghosts: *Belladonna, Stramonium.*

For *frenzy, rage, cursing,* etc.: *Bellad., Hyoscyamus, Veratrum, Stramonium.*

Symptomatic Detail and Administration of these remedies same as under "*Affections of the Mind.*"

CHAPTER VI.

AFFECTIONS OF THE HEAD.

---

1. Congestion, or Determination of Blood to the Head.

(*Congestio ad caput.*)

Some persons have a predisposition to this disease; others acquire it by wrong habits, such as the use of spiritous liquors, leading a sedentary life, or by intense mental application. It becomes dangerous by long continuance, in which case the patient ought to put himself under the charge of a homœopathic physician.

For the single attacks, we will indicate the remedies below.

Diagnosis.—In such an attack, the beating of the arteries of the head is felt by the patient, the veins of the neck are swelled, the head feels full and heavy, and giddiness ensues, particularly when stooping, exercising, or walking in the sun, and when turning round suddenly. The head aches mostly above the eyes; increased by stooping, coughing; sleep is unrefreshing; drowsy.

Treatment.—In general, the patient ought to abstain from heating or ardent drinks, such as coffee, liquors and tea; drink cold water freely, and wash or bathe in it. Every evening take a cold foot-bath up to the ankles, rubbing the feet briskly after it. Never allow bleeding, as it would only increase the disposition afterward, without taking away the present attack sooner than the following remedies will do, if properly applied.

The principal circumstances, under which congestion to the head takes place, and their remedies, are:

From *great joy*: *Coffea, Opium.*

From *fright or fear*: *Opium.*

From *anger, violent*: *Chamomile, Bryonia, Nux vom.*

From *anger suppressed*: *Ignatia.*

From a *fall* or *blow*, causing *concussions*: *Arnica.*

From *loss of blood* or *fluids*: *China.*

From a *cold*: *Dulcamara, Bryonia, Rhus tox.*

From *constipation*: *Aloes, Opium, Nux vom., Bryonia.*

From *drinking liquors*: *Nux vom., Opium.*

From *sedentary habits*: *Aloes, Nux vom., Aconite.*

At the *critical period of girls, or*

From the *stoppage of menstruation*: *Pulsatilla, Aconite, Belladonna, Bryonia, Veratrum.*

From *dentition in children*: *Aconite, Coffea, Belladonna, Chamomile.*

Before giving one of the above remedies, examine the symptoms as detailed below.

Aconite is the first remedy to be given, if the head aches violently above the eyes, *as if it would burst,* particularly when stooping or coughing, or when it is caused by *fright or anger*, especially in children. (See "Affections of the Mind.")

Aloes. Periodical headache, alternating with pains in the small of the back; stitches in the left temple, worse when treading. Congestion of blood to the head from suppressed hemorrhoids and gout.

Belladonna. After *Aconite,* if necessary, or in alternation with it, if the congestive symptoms are more on one side of the head, and particularly the *right;* or if there is violent pressure in the forehead, increased by motion, stooping, noise, or the glare of light; darkness before the eyes; buzzing in the ears.

N. B. *Belladonna* and *Aconite* for young girls at the critical age. (See *Pulsatilla.*)

Opium. First remedy, if occasioned by fright (see "Affections of the Mind," under *Opium*), or in those serious cases of sudden congestion which occur in summer from a draught of cold water when heated, with the following symptoms: vertigo; buzzing in the ears; *stupor,* with sweat pouring off the head; pulse full and heavy, or quick and weak.

Also, in those cases which arise from extreme *constipation,* when the patient has no desire for stool (*Nux vom.* in constipation, with ineffectual effort to evacuate the bowels), with red and bloated face; dry mouth; wandering look; if, with acid regurgitations, nausea and vomiting, alternate with *Nux vom.;* the same, also, when from *debauch.*

Coffea. In cases of congestion caused by excessive joy, or in children when teething; sleeplessness, and agitation; sometimes in alternation with *Belladonna* or *Opium.*

Chamomile. Congestion caused by angry passion, particularly in children when teething; followed by *Bryonia* or *Nux vom.,* if necessary.

Ignatia. Congestion from *suppressed anger* or *grief.*

Arnica. By a fall on the head or other parts; congestions of the head take place either by actual concussion, or by fright and fear occasioned by a fall. In both cases, *Arnica,* externally applied (twelve drops of the tincture in half a teacupful of water), in wet bandages; and internally, in alternation with *Aconite.*

Also, in cases where there is heat in the head, with chilliness of the other parts; dull pressure in the brain, buzzing in the ears, and vertigo; obstruction of sight, especially when rising from lying down.

Nux vom. Congestion from sedentary habits; intense tudy, or drinking spiritous liquors; also from violent anger (see *Chamomile* and *Bryonia*), when there is nervousness, with painful feeling in the head when walking or moving, pressure in the temples; dim eyes, with desire to close them without being able to sleep; the symptoms worse in the morning, in the open air, or after a meal; bowels constipated, with ineffectual desire to evacuate.

N. B. In cases where *Nux vom.* does not give perfect relief, in persons fond of liquors, *Opium, Calcarea carb.*, and *Sulphur*, at intervals of four or six days, one dose (six glob.), are necessary. (See "Delirium Tremens.")

Pulsatilla. Congestion at the critical period of young girls, or in phlegmatic temperaments, when there is distressing pressure and pain on one side (particularly the *left*) of the head; relieved in the open air, or from binding the head; whining mood; anxiety; shivering; pale face, with vertigo.

Mercury. Congestion with sensation of fullness, or *as if the head were compressed by a band;* relieved by the pressure of the two hands around the head; *worse at night;* disposition to perspire—is often suitable after *Belladonna* and *Opium.*

Dulcamara. Congestion from the least cold; wet feet, particularly when there is continual buzzing in the ears, with dullness of hearing.

China. Congestion after loss of fluids, or blood-letting, or hemorrhage; when there is beating in the head, with palpitation of the heart, and dimness of sight; heavy breathing when lying with the head low; followed, in such cases, by *Calcarea carb.* and *Veratrum.*

Bryonia. Painful pressure in the temples, or sensation as if everything would fall out of the forehead when stooping, nose bleeds without relief; constipation. If in wet weather, alternate with *Rhus.* Administer every two or three hours a dose (four glob.), until three doses of each are given, or until better.

Rhus tox. Congestion with burning, throbbing pains, and fullness in the head; rheumatic pains in the limbs; worse after eating. (See *Bryonia.*)

ADMINISTRATION of the above remedies, the same as in *Affections of the Mind.*"

Application of Water.—This ought to form an important part in the treatment of this disease, at least, when caused by sedentary habits, intense study, or drinking spiritous liquors. Beside the proper homœopathic remedies, the patient ought to take, an hour before dinner every day, a cold sitting-bath, drink during the day from eight to twelve tumblers of cold water, and exercise a great deal in the open air; in the evening before going to bed it is well for him to take a cold foot-bath of ten minutes' duration, during which time the feet must be rubbed and after the bath dried off.

Diet and Regimen.—The diet ought to be light, farinaceous; no meat or broths, except in cases where loss of blood or fluids has preceded the congestion.

In the habitual form of congestion, early rising and daily exercise in the open air, bathing or sponging in cold water, are recommended.

2. Vertigo. Giddiness or Dizziness.

It arises either from disordered stomach, irritation of the brain and congestion to the head, or from suppressed eruptions, or ulcers; also from riding in a carriage.

In most cases it accompanies severe disorders of the brain and stomach, when it ought to be treated by an experienced homœopathic physician. Until such help can be had, the following remedies may be resorted to:

Treatment.—Vertigo from *disordered stomach: Nux vom., Arnica, Cham., Pulsat., Antimon. crud., China, Rhus, Coccu.*

Irritation of the brain, from excess of thinking, etc.: *Nux vomica, Arnica, Bellad., Chamomile, Hepar, Pulsatilla, Rhus.*

Suppressed ulcers and eruptions: Calcarea carb., Sulphur.

Riding in a carriage: Hepar sulph., Silicea, Cocculus, Petroleum.

Congestion of blood to the brain: Aconite, Aloes, Bryonia, Arnica, Belladonna, China, Lachesis, Mercury, Nux vomica, Opium, Pulsatilla, Sulphur.

Before giving one of the above remedies, read its detailed symptoms below.

Aconite. Vertigo on raising the head after lying down or stooping, attended with nausea, vomiting, dimness of sight, loss of consciousness.

Antimon. crud. Nausea and vomiting; aversion to food; disordered stomach; is followed well by *Pulsatilla.*

Arnica. Vertigo from over-eating, or during meals, with nausea, dimness of sight, red face; is followed well by *Nux vom., Chamomile, Rhus, Lachesis.*

In cases of this kind, frequently very dangerous, seek the advice of a homœopathic physician.

Nux vom. Vertigo *during* or *after* a meal, or when *walking in the open air; stooping* or *thinking;* worse in the *morning* or evening, *in bed,* when lying on the back, with sensation as if turning around or falling; fainting; loss of consciousness.

Opium. From fright, with trembling; stupor; dimness of sight; worse when rising from bed, and obliged to lie down again.

Pulsatilla. Vertigo when *looking upward,* or when sitting or stooping; worse in the evening, or after a meal; better in the open air.

Rhus. Vertigo when lying down in the evening, with fear of falling or dying.

Lachesis. Vertigo on *walking* in the morning, with absence of mind; intoxicated feeling; constipation; sensation as if the head were turning to the left side.

Mercury. Vertigo on arising in the morning, or in the evening, with nausea; dimness of sight; or when raising the head, with a desire to lie down again. (See *Bryonia.*)

Bryonia. Same as *Mercury,* and with feeling of intoxication and congestion when stooping and rising again.

Hepar sulph. Vertigo from riding in a carriage.

Cocculus. Same as *Hepar sulph.,* if this is not sufficient.

Petroleum. Same as *Cocculus,* if that is not sufficient.

Silicea. Same as *Petroleum,* if this is not sufficient, or the vertigo seems to rise from the back to the nape of the neck, and thence to the head; worse in the *morning* and *after emotion.*

Sulphur. Vertigo in the *morning,* or at *night, when ascending an eminence,* or after a meal; after suppressed ulcers and eruptions.

China. Vertigo, with fainting when raising the head. (See "Congestion to the Head.")

Calcarea carb. Same as *Sulphur,* and when with *trembling before breakfast; coldness of the head; congestion to the head.*

Chamomile. Vertigo in the morning or after eating, and drinking coffee, with *fainting turns.*

Administration. — Every two, three, or four hours, one dose (four glob.) until relieved, or another remedy is necessary. If in vertigo, caused by congestion to the head, see "Administration" in that article.

Application of Water, in this disease, is similar to that recommended in congestion of blood to the head; but the sitting bath for violent vertigo must be lukewarm, while cold-water bandages are applied to the head at the same time. The proper homœopathic remedies must be administered.

Diet and Regimen the same as in "Congestion to the Head."

3. Weakness of Memory.

This diseased state of the brain is principally caused by *debilitating loss of fluids,* such as bleeding, purging, sexual excesses, etc., for which give *China, Nux vom.,* and *Sulphur,* every week one or two doses (six glob.), in alternation, until better.

Sometimes it is caused by *excessive mental labor,* for which give *Nux vom.* and *Sulphur,* as above.

If caused by *external injuries*, a fall or blow, give *Arnica*. (See "Congestion to the Head.")

If by *congestion to the head*, give *Aconite*, *Belladonna*, *China*, *Mercury*, *Rhus*, and *Sulphur*. (See "Congestion to the Head.")

If by *excessive use of spiritous liquors*, give *Nux vomica*, *Calcarea carb.*, *Lachesis*, *Opium*, *Sulphur*, in the same manner as above, under "Debilitating Loss," etc.

ADMINISTRATION, DIET, AND REGIMEN as in "Congestion to the Head."

4. APOPLEXY. (*Apoplexia.*)

Short, thick-necked persons, of a full and fleshy growth, are predisposed to this disease; it is also hastened on by the too free use of spiritous liquors, by excesses of any kind, and suppression of the habitual perspiration of the feet. An attack of apoplexy is often preceded by heaviness and fullness of the head; buzzing in the ears; dim eyes; dullness of hearing; sleepiness; indistinct speech; numbness of limbs. If this state exists, particularly in old persons, or those predisposed to apoplexy, the greatest care should be taken in the diet, which ought to consist only of simple farinaceous and mucilaginous substances, and cool acidulated drinks; they ought not to exercise very much, particularly in the heat of the day, and should take the following remedies, as it is easier to *prevent* an attack than to cure it.

Opium. If in *old people* there is unusual stupor; buzzing in the ears; obtuseness of hearing; redness of the face; constipation; pulse slow and full. Give three times a day a dose (four glob.), until better.

Nux vomica. In people of a sedentary habit, or addicted to the use of ardent spirits, in alternation with *Opium* and *Lachesis*, particularly when, with the above premonitory symptoms, there is headache on the right side, with vertigo and a nervous bilious temperament.

ADMINISTRATION same as under *Opium.*

Lachesis. Same as *Nux vom.*; but particularly when the *left* side of the head suffers, and *lowness of spirits* is connected with it. Administration same as above.

Belladonna and *Aconite* under the same circumstances as stated under "Congestion to the Head."

Arnica. When symptoms of congestion to the head appear after a *meal.* If an apoplectic fit ensues, however, continue the same remedies as indicated above, only give them in solution (twelve globules to half a teacupful of water), every half hour a teaspoonful until better, or another remedy is indicated.

In such cases hasten immediately to procure a homœopathic physician. Avoid bleeding under any circumstances; the chances of killing the patient by such an act are too frequent.

Application of Water is of great advantage in this disease; beside the proper homœopathic remedies, apply cold water on the parts affected; use the wet sheet, even the douche.

Diet and Regimen as in "Congestion to the Head."

5. Inflammation of the Brain.

The brain and its two coverings (see Anatomical Part) are subject to inflammation separately, the characteristic symptoms of which show themselves, particularly in the beginning of a brain fever. We will, therefore, give them separately, as it is important and interesting, to be able to distinguish between the different localities of the disease.

Diagnosis. *First species,* called *meningitis,* if the *dura mater,* the skin next to the skull, is inflamed.

The *acute* meningitis attacks a person suddenly, exhibiting, *immediately,* stupor and drowsy symptoms; the patient cannot be raised easily, or keep his head erect; it inclines to fall on either side; he complains of no pain, except vertigo and dizziness; reels when walking; pupil contracted; sensitiveness to light, although the eyes are not red as yet; constipation; scanty, dark-red urine; fever, with a soft pulse.

N. B. Old people are most liable to this species of inflammation of the brain; also those who have indulged too much in the use of spiritous liquors, particularly after taking cold. It frequently precedes an apopletic fit.

Second species. Called *arachnoiditis,* if the covering next to the brain is inflamed. This species does not commence with stupor, and not without pain, like the first species, but with violent pains over the entire head; increased by paroxysms of congestion, with violent beating of the arteries of the neck and temples; sleeplessness; low muttering; pulse quick; if stupor ensues suddenly, the patient dies soon after.

Third species. Encephalitis vera, or inflammation of the substance of the brain, in its various parts.

It commences with violent congestion and pulsation of the arteries on the neck and head; face red and bloated; eyes bloodshot and brilliant; intense heat of the head, and violent delirium.

The patient tosses about, screams, and evinces great muscular strength and sensitiveness to light; pupil contracted; cannot hear well. The deeper the interior of the brain is affected, the more the senses are stupefied, so that, in some cases, the patient can, finally, neither see nor hear; dry skin; violent thirst; hard, full pulse; fever accordingly; frequent vomitings or retchings.

Treatment.—It is easily to be conceived that, in such a violent disease, no layman would trust his own judgment, except in cases of absolute necessity; and, on this latter account, we give the following treatment of the above three species of brain fever, which is the same as regards the *internal* remedies, and differs only in the *external applications,* as will be seen below.

External Applications.—*First species*—cold water bandages.

Second species—warm water bandages.

Third species—cold-water bandages, or pounded ice.

INTERNAL TREATMENT.—*First species*— *Opium*, *Hyoscyamus*, *Bryonia*.

Second species—*Aconite*, *Belladonna*, *Hyoscyamus*.

Third species—*Aconite*, *Belladonna*, *Stramonium*, *Bryonia*, *Hyoscyamus*.

Before giving the medicine selected, read the symptoms presented below.

Aconite is generally given first, when there is inflammatory fever, delirium, violent burning pains through the whole brain, particularly in the forehead; red face and eyes; hot and dry skin. Six hours after give *Belladonna* or continue the use of *Aconite* in alternation with *Belladonna*, until better.

Belladonna. This remedy is almost a specific in inflammation of the brain, particularly when there is *great heat of the head*, red and bloated face, *violent pulsation of the arteries* on the neck and temples; *burying the head in the pillow;* sensitiveness to the *slightest noise* and *light;* burning and shooting pains in the head; *bloodshot* and *brilliant* eyes, with a wild expression; contracted or dilated pupils; *violent* and *furious* delirium; raving; loss of consciousness; sometimes low mutterings, convulsions, vomiting, violent thirst. Administer alone or in alternation with *Aconite* (see above), or with *Stramonium* and *Hyoscyamus* (see below).

Hyoscyamus. Stupor, loss of consciousness, delirium; sudden starting; talks about his affairs; inarticulate speech; singing, muttering, smiling, picking the bed clothes; skin dry; red face; desire to escape; involuntary stool and urine.

Stramonium. Red face; staring look; *frightful visions;* sleep natural, but with twitching, tossing about, and absence of mind when awaking; desire to escape, and screams.

Bryonia. Constant stupor, with delirium; sudden starting from sleep, screams, cold sweat on the forehead; burning and shooting pains in the head, or stitches through it.

Opium. Stupor, with heavy breathing; eyes half open; confusion and giddiness after waking; complete listlessness and dullness of sense; also, no desire for anything, or complaining of anything.

ADMINISTRATION.—Dissolve twelve globules of the selected remedy in half a teacupful of water, and give either alone or in alternation with another remedy, similarly prepared in another teacup, every hour or two hours a teaspoonful, until better or another remedy is needed. Each remedy must have its separate teaspoon, with which it is given to the patient. If signs of amendment appear, discontinue all medicines.

DIET AND REGIMEN as in "Common Fever."

Inflammation of the brain in children. As the brain of children is very tender, its diseases must necessarily be more dangerous and frequent, and we give, therefore, in the following, a more special and somewhat modified treatment for inflammations of the brain in children:

If a *child's head is very hot, feet cold,* skin dry and hot, it *sleeps with eyes half open,* has scanty urine, with or without vomiting or diarrhea, let the cause of the disease be what it may, in such a case give at once *Belladonna* and *Hellebor.*, in solution (twelve globules in half a teacupful of water, each remedy in a separate cup), every two hours a teaspoonful, alternately, until better, or until the symptoms require a change of remedy, generally *Sulphur* or *Mercury.* (See Materia Medica, at end of book.)

If the child gets worse, or exhibits at the beginning the following symptoms, beside those above-mentioned: motionless eyes, with insensible pupil; loss of consciousness; moaning; icy coldness, with bluish color of the skin; pulse nearly imperceptible; respiration interrupted; give *Belladonna* and *Zincum* in alternation; to be prepared and given in the same manner as *Belladonna* and *Hellebore,* above.

The above suggestion is *important,* as cases of inflammation of the brain occur so often in children, when, as is said, the disease goes to the head. For instance in teething; in common cold, with fever; in scarlet fever (see this article); or in other eruptions, when suppressed; also, worm fevers.

If such a state should continue in a child for some time, *dropsy of the brain* (see "Hydrocephalus") would speedily ensue; the above treatment will surely prevent this, if applied in time.

N. B. If, at any time during the treatment of inflammation of the brain, the patient is very restless and sleepless, we may give, with great advantage and without injury to the effect of the other medicines (which are discontinued during that time), *Coffea* cc. and *Belladonna* cc., alternately, every hour a dose (four glob.), until better. This may be done often in the night.

6. Sunstroke.

Is a species of inflammation of the brain; the principal remedy is *Glonoine*, 2d atten., every five minutes a dose.

If not better in half an hour, give *Camphor*, in alternation with it, at intervals of five or ten minutes, if he is sweating profusely while unconscious, and breathing heavily.

Belladonna, after *Camphor* has been given, in alternation with

Lachesis, every half hour, in solution (twelve globules of each in separate teacups half full of water), a teaspoonful at a time.

Externally, wash the head and face occasionally with brandy, and give, internally, small quantities of brandy until the patient revives. Put neither cold water nor ice upon the head.

7. Headache.

This disease, so frequent and troublesome, requires to be treated with particular minuteness; the more so, as its treatment falls almost entirely within the legitimate sphere of domestic practice, except where headaches are the concomitant symptoms of severe fevers, as in the typhus, etc., or the forerunner of dangerous attacks, as in apoplexy, etc., in which cases the respective articles must be consulted.

Administration of Medicine in Headache. — For this purpose we divide all headaches into *habitual* and *accidental*. This requires two modes of administering the medicine: one for the cure of an attack of headache, be it accidental, or one of the habitual attacks; and the other, for the eradication of the habitual headache, or the predisposition to it.

First. Administration of medicine *for an attack*.—Having selected a remedy (from those stated below), dissolve of it six globules in three tablespoonfuls of water, and take, according to the severity of the headache, from half an hour to two, three, or six hours, a teaspoonful, until three are taken, when its benefits must be apparent. If beneficial, continue with the same, only at much longer intervals, as long as necessary. If not beneficial, select carefully another remedy, and prepare and take in the same manner.

Secondly. Administration of medicine for *eradicating the disposition* to certain kinds of headache; for instance, sick headache.—Having selected a remedy, take of it, every third or sixth evening, a dose (four glob.), until four or six doses are taken; when the next best remedy has to be taken in the same manner, or until better.

Application of Water, in the various forms of headache, must be modified according to its different causes. If constipation shall be removed quickly, apply cold injections, if the pains are very severe, sitting-baths of short duration must be used, or cold foot-baths; these means dare not be used during menstruation. Beside, we refer the reader to the chapters, in which the prescriptions for the causes of headache are given.

a. Headache from Congestion of Blood to the Head.

Aconite. Violent throbbing; heaviness; fullness in the forehead and temples, with a sensation as if the head would burst; burning pain through the whole brain; red, bloated face, and red eyes; sensitiveness to light and noise; worse on moving, talking, drinking, rising up; full and quick pulse. After it, or in alternation with it, *Belladonna* may be given, if necessary. (See "Congestion of Blood to the Head.")

Belladonna. *Violent aching pain, as if the head would split,* or as if the brain would protrude through the forehead; heat in the head and coldness of the feet; *undulating feeling, as of water in the forehead;* violent throbbing of the arteries of the neck and temples; delirium, either with red, bloated face, bloodshot eyes, great *sensitiveness to light, noise, and touch,* or vertigo and deeply-seated, violent, pressing pains, with pale face, drowsy unconsciousness (compare, in such a case, article on "Apoplexy"); worse on moving the eyes, or raising or moving the head. In alternation with *Aconite* or *Rhus,* if the symptoms agree. (See *Aconite* and *Rhus.*)

Bryonia. Distending pressure from within, particularly through the forehead, on stooping or moving, with violent beating or single *stitches* in the head; *desire to lie down;* constipation of the bowels; bleeding at the nose. Before it, *Belladonna* frequently suits; after it *Rhus.* (See these remedies.)

Rhus. Fullness of the head, with burning and throbbing pain; oppressive weight in the back part of the head, with a sensation as if a fluid was rolling inside; a feeling of *looseness,* particularly in *wet weather.* In alternation with *Bellad.* or *Bryonia.*

Pulsatilla. Oppressive, dull pains on one side of the head, commencing in front at the root of the nose, and going back, or *vice versa;* better in the *open air,* or by *compressing the head,* or lying down; worse toward evening, or when sitting or *looking upward;* pale face, agitated mind, *inclined to weep.* It suits *females* and persons of a *mild* character, and *lymphatic* temperament.

Nux vomica. The opposite of the former. Pains; *worse*

in the *morning* and in the *open air;* heaviness of the head, especially when *moving the eyes* or *thinking;* a *sensation as if the skull would split; contusive pain in the brain,* worse when stooping or in motion; *constipation,* with rush of blood to the head; *irritable, rash,* or *lively* temperament, full habit, and for persons of *sedentary* habits, or who use *coffee* and *ardent spirits* freely. (Compare *Bryonia, Belladonna,* and *Chamomile.*)

Mercury. Fullness of the head, as if it would fly apart, or *was tied up* with a bandage; better by *pressing* the head with *the hands,* but worse at night, in the *warmth of the bed,* and not relieved by profuse sweating.

Opium. Constipation with rush of blood to the head; violent tearing, pressing pains through the whole brain, and heaviness with beating in the head; unsteady look. (See "Congestion to the Head.")

b. Headache from Catarrh and Cold in the Head.

The principal remedies are *Nux vomica, Mercury, Sulphur, Aconite, Chamomile.* (See, for other remedies, "Catarrh.")

Nux vomica.—Heaviness in the forehead; obstructions or running of the nose; feverish heat of the head, cheeks, and body, alternately with chilliness, constipation. After it *Mercury* often suits.

Mercury, is particularly useful in those headaches accompanying the epidemic catarrh (*influenza*), when there are *pressing* pains in the forehead, over the root of the nose; frequent sneezing and running at the nose, with redness and excoriation; also, with painful itching in the nose; fever, with chilliness, pains in the limbs, and thirst. It alternates well with *Nux vomica* or *Sulphur.*

Sulphur. After *Mercury* has relieved, but not entirely cured the cold, and when there is still felt fullness, pressure and heaviness in the forehead, stitches, and painful jerking;

especially on the *left side*, with heat and rush of blood to the head; constipation.

Aconite. *Pressing, dull feeling* and *heat* in the forehead; worse at night; better in the open air; fever, intermixed with chills; running at the nose and eyes.

Chamomile. Intolerable *tearing* and *jerking* on one side of the head, down to the jaws, with sore throat, hoarseness, and bitter, foul taste in the mouth. Is frequently suitable after *Aconite*.

c. *Headache from Rheumatism.*

The principal remedies are *Chamomile, Colocynth, Ipecac., Pulsatilla, Bryonia, Mercury, China, Nux vomica.*

Chamomile. Drawing, tearing pains on one side of the head, down to the jaws; very *sensitive to touch;* hot sweat about the head; *one* cheek *red*, with *paleness* of the other; and if the pain almost drives to *despair*. Suits well after *Coffea:* after it *Bryonia, Pulsatilla*, and *China*, are suitable.

Colocynth. Violent tearing, drawing, cramping, or aching pains, with nausea and vomiting; worse when stooping or lying on the back; pains appear in the afternoon, with restlessness.

Ipecac. Drawing in the forehead; worse or excited by touch; headache, with nausea; sensation through the skull, extending to the tongue, as if the brain were *bruised;* pains better after vomiting; relieved by heat.

Nux vomica. Tensive *drawing* pains on one side of the head, with a bruised sensation in the head; worse when stooping or in the *open air*, with nausea and sour vomiting; constipation.

Pulsatilla. *Darting, rending*, jerking pains on one side only, particularly in the temples; pain as if the *brain were lacerated*. (See "Nervous Headache.")

Bryonia. *Rending* and *shooting* pain, from the neck up to the sides of the head, with shivering or fever; worse by *motion* and *at night*, or during changeable weather. In alternation with *Rhus*.

Mercury. *Burning*, *shooting*, *throbbing*, and *rending* pains on one side principally, down to the teeth and neck, and in the ears; worse at night, and in the *warmth of the bed*, with perspiration which does *not* relieve.

China. Aching pains at night, with sleeplessness, jerking, tearing; boring on top of the head, with a bruised feeling of the brain; worse in the open air, by touch, motion, draughts of air and wind; sensitiveness, even of the *roots* of the hair, to *touch*.

d. *Headache from Constipation and Gastric Derangement.*

1. *Constipation*, which causes congestive headache, is generally cured by *Bryonia*, *Nux vom.*, or *Opium*, according to its concomitant symptoms (see these three remedies, under "Headache from Congestion to the Head," p. 163), or by *Pulsatilla* and *Mercury*. (See their symptoms under the same heading.)

But, if the constipation has a *chronic character*, give

Silicea. When there are *beating* pains in the head, mostly from congestion, from the nape of the neck to the top of the head; pressing in the head, *as if it would split*, with sleeplessness at night, and worse in the morning when awaking, or when reading, writing, or thinking; constipation, with ineffectual urging. Suits, frequently, after *Lycopodium*, or

Lachesis and *Lycopodium*, in alternation, when there is, *cutting as with knives in the top of the head*, or *hammering* on stooping, with congestion to the head; disposition to faint, and great restlessness; whining mood; yellowish complexion.

Sepia. Headache on *shaking* or *moving* the head, or walking, with tendency of blood to the head, heaviness, and confusion, with nausea and vomiting; worse in the morning and on looking at bright sunlight.

Sulphur. If the former remedies do not cure, or when the

headache is more on one side (the *left*), with heat and congestion; roaring in the head; worse by thinking, in the open air, or walking, or when it appears every morning, or night, or every week.

2. *Headache from Gastric Derangement*, is generally accompanied by a *furred tongue, loss of appetite, fullness* in the forehead, as if it would split, with beating pain; worse when stooping. It is frequently connected with bad taste in the mouth, and nausea or vomiting, and *sour risings (acid stomach) caused* by *indigestion.* (See these articles.) The principal remedies are,

Antimonium. When the pain is worse on going up stairs, and better in the open air. With nausea, loathing, and aversion to food, *Bryonia, Pulsatilla, Nux vomica.* (See "Headache from Congestion" and "Indigestion.")

e. Headache from External Causes.

There are many external circumstances that produce headache; we will state the most frequent of them, with their remedies, whose detailed symptoms must be consulted under the headings mentioned within the brackets, and at the end of the book, in the "Materia Medica."

a. Headache from *drinking coffee—Nux vomica, Chamomile, Ignatia.*

b. From *over-heating—Aconite, Belladonna, Bryonia.* (See "Congestion to the Head.")

c. From drinking *ardent spirits—Nux vomica, Arsenic, Lachesis.*

d. From *loss of sleep, long watching—Nux vomica, Cocculus, Pulsatilla, Lachesis, Carbo veg.*

e. From abuse of tobacco—*Hepar sulph., Nux vomica, Antimon. crud.*

f. From excess of *mental* or *bodily labor—Nux vomica, Sulphur, Lachesis, Lycopodium, Silicea.*

g. From *grief—Ignatia, Staphy.* (See "Mental Diseases.")

h. From *anger* or *chagrin*—*Chamomile, Nux vomica.* (See the same.)

i. From *bad changeable weather*—*Bryonia, Rhus, Carbo veg.* (See "Headache from Cold.")

j. From *bathing*—*Pulsatilla, Antimon. crud., Calcarea carb.*

k. From *suppressed eruptions*—*Antimon. crud., Sulphur.* (See "Skin Diseases.")

l. From *mechanical injuries, blows, etc.*—*Arnica, Bellad., Aconite.* (See "External Injuries.")

N. B. In regard to the administration of the above medicines, we refer the reader, in all cases of headache, to what is said about it in the beginning of that article, p. 163.

Sick Headache.

This form of headache, so well known under the above name, is of a chronic nature, appearing periodically, and depending mostly upon gastric, rheumatic disorders in persons of a psoric constitution, and may be eradicated by a systematic homœopathic treatment. Although this requires the skill of medical attendance, we will try to bring within the reach of every intelligent person sufficient knowledge for the commencement of a treatment, which, if successful, will encourage him to seek further medical advice.

First, we will give the treatment of the attack itself:

Ipecac. and *Apis mellif.*, in almost all cases which commence with nausea, after which a bruised feeling of the whole head manifests itself, followed by vomiting or retching.

Administration.—Of this and the following remedies, as directed in the beginning of the article, page 163. If not better within an hour, select one of the following remedies:

Belladonna. If with headache there is great sensitiveness to light, worse in the warmth of the bed, on lying down or in a draught, and from noise, such as shutting the door, etc. (See "Congestion to the Head.")

15

Thuja. *A boring* pain over the eye; relieved by pressure; in alternation with *Belladonna.*

Spigelia. If there is great sensitiveness to *noise,* with the pains worse on the *left* side, and insupportable beating in the temples, the pain sometimes descending into the face and teeth, worse by stooping or motion and in the open air. The headache appears generally at a *regular* time in the morning, growing worse with the ascending sun (*sun pain*). In this case, in alternation with *Belladonna.*

Sanguinaria. If there is great sensitiveness to the *walking* of others in the room, with fullness of the head, as if it would burst, worse on the *right* side, with a feeling as if the eyes were pressed outward, chilliness, nausea, inclination to lie down.

(Compare *Bryonia* in "Congestion to the Head.")

Aconite. (See this remedy in "Congestion to the Head.") When the patient has a great *sensitiveness to all kinds of odors,* the pain mostly on the *left* side. In this case in alternation with *Sulphur,* or *Ignatia.* (See "Nervous Headache.")

Aloes. If the patient complains of stitches in the left temple; the headache appears periodically, alternating with pains in the small of the back. (See "Congestion to the Head.")

Sepia. If there is a great dislike to be *touched,* and sensitiveness to thunder-storms and the cold air. (Compare with *China* in "Headache from Rheumatism." If the patient is easily vexed, pain mostly above the right eye and worse by shaking or moving the head.

Beside, consult the articles on "Congestion to the Head," "Headache from Rheumatism," and "Neuralgia in the Head."

Second, to eradicate the disposition to sick headache, take *Sepia, Silicea,* and *Sulphur,* each remedy for six weeks, commencing with *Sepia.* During the six weeks take of that remedy, the first three weeks, every week, two doses (six glob.)

in the evening, on going to bed ; for the last three weeks, every week one dose (six glob.). If during that time attacks of sick headache occur, treat them as directed above and resume the other treatment again after they are over.

Nervous Headache. Neuralgia in the Head.
(*Megrim.*)

In this kind of headache, to which nervous persons and females are mostly subject, the head is generally cool, the face pale, with a suffering expression ; in females great quantities of colorless urine are discharged ; if vomiting sets in, it only relieves for a short time ; the pain is mostly concentrated in one spot, with the characteristic feeling, as if a *nail were driven through the head* (*clavus hystericus*); the patient is generally very nervous, fickle-minded, dejected, hysterical, or hypochondriacal.

Treatment.—Beside the medicines mentioned under "Sick Headache," which are suitable in this kind of headache, also (see this article), there are the following :

Coffea. *Pain as if a nail was driven into the head*, or as if the brain were torn or bruised ; *pain seems to be intolerable ;* also, noise and music ; the patient is very restless, screams, weeps, feels chilly and has an aversion to open air and drinking coffee, though being, at other times, fond of it. The headache generally arises from cold, close thinking, or vexation.

Ignatia. Aching pain above the nose, relieved by bending forward ; sensation as if a nail had been driven into the head ; with nausea, dimness of sight, and yet dread of light ; pale face, copious and watery urine ; *pain is momentarily relieved by a change of position ;* tendency to start ; fitful mood ; taciturn and sad.

Pulsatilla. Tearing pains, worse toward evening, with pale face, whining mood, loss of appetite, *no thirst*, chilliness sometimes with palpitation of the heart ; pains are worse during rest, when *sitting*, better in the *open air*, and when the head is bandaged tight; particularly suitable for *mild phlegmatic* persons.

Aconite. (See "Sick Headache.") When it arises from cold, with catarrh, buzzing in the ears and pains in the abdomen; also, when there is a sensation as if a ball was rising up into the head, as if of cool air.

Belladonna. (See "Sick Headache.") When there are wavering shocks, and a sensation of fluctuation or undulation, as of water. This pain sometimes commences very *gently*, but increases rapidly on one side (mostly the *right*) to piercing pains, which produce agonizing lamentations and temporary delirium, dimness of sight, buzzing in the ears.

Thuja. A *boring* pain over the eye; suits well after *Belladonna* and *Apis mellifica.*

Platina. Suits often after *Belladonna*, particularly in females, when there is roaring in the head as of water, with coldness in the ears, eyes, and one side of the face; also illusions of sight, viz: objects appearing smaller than they really are; violent cramp-like pains over the root of the nose, with heat and redness of the face, restlessness, and whining mood.

Hepar sulph. Suits after *Belladonna* or *Mercury*, if there is pain as from a nail in the brain, with violent nightly pains, as if the forehead would be pulled apart, and when painful tumors appear on the head.

Mercury. After *Belladonna*, if the pain shoots down into the teeth, neck, and left ear; worse at night, with perspiration, which does not relieve. The pain is better by pressing the head with both hands.

Chamomile. Suits often for children and *persons unable to bear the least pain*, and when there are acute, shooting pains in the temples, or a rending, drawing pain on one side extending to the jaw, especially when one cheek is red, the other pale, the eyes painful, sore throat, and bitter taste.

Colocynth. Violent, excruciating, tearing, drawing pains

on one side, or cramp-like, compressive sensation, aching, with nausea; worse when stooping or lying on the back, with great restlessness; perspiration smells like urine; copious watery urine during the pains, or scanty, offensive discharges of urine between the paroxysms.

Arsenic. Pains in the head, sometimes very severe, almost maddening, with nausea, buzzing in the ears, weeping and moaning, tenderness of the scalp; cold applications relieve the pain for the time; suits frequently after *Pulsatilla;* when better in the open air, worse within doors.

Veratrum. Maddening pains on one side with great weakness, fainting when rising, cold perspiration, chilliness, diarrhea, tenderness of the scalp; suits well after or before *Arsenic.* If these two remedies will not relieve, give

China. Suitable for persons sensitive to pain, feverish, dissatisfied dispositions, talkative and restless at night; the pains are aching, preventing sleep, or are piercing, jerking in the forehead, with a bruised feeling in the brain; worse by *touch,* reflection, conversation, open air, motion, draughts of air; the *scalp* very sensitive to the *touch.*

Sepia. (See "Sick Headache.") When the pain in the temples renders them very sensitive to the touch; quietness and darkness relieve; also, a good sleep.

Sulphur and *Silicea.* For the chronic treatment, as directed in "Sick Headache," 169.

ADMINISTRATION.—The above-mentioned remedies must be given according to directions in "Sick Headache."

APPLICATION OF WATER, see page 163.

FALLING OFF OF THE HAIR. (*Allopecia.*)

This frequently happens after severe fevers, when *Hepar sulph.*, *Silicea,* and *Lycopodium* suit; or after *debilitating losses,* such as depletion, excesses, profuse sweats, etc., when we may give *China* and *Mercury;* or, if it happens to *women when nursing, Calcarea carb.* and *Sulphur.* If *long-continued grief* is the cause of it, give *Phosphoric acid* and *Staphysag.* If caused by frequent attacks of nervous headache, give *Hepar sulph.* and *Nitric acid.* If caused by having taken too much calomel, give *Hepar* and *Carbo veg.*

ADMINISTRATION.—As it takes a long time to see the effects of a remedy in this disease, do not change it quickly for another, but take every week one dose (six glob.) of a remedy for four weeks, and then discontinue two weeks before taking another medicine. If by that time the loss of the hair seems less, do not change the medicine.

Externally, use the same remedy by washing with a solution of twelve globules in half a teacupful of water every other night.

If the *hair is dry* and *splits easily*, cut it often, every month or six weeks a little; use nothing but pure bear's oil; all other preparations and pomatums are of little use, and often very injurious.

For the *dandruff, scales of the scalp*, take *Calcarea carb.*, *Graphites* and *Staphysag.*; if with *itching*, take *Graphites*, *Lycopodium*, and *Sulphur*.

Administer same as above.

CHAPTER VII.

AFFECTIONS OF THE EYES.

General Remarks.

The diseases of the eye ought to claim our most careful attention, as this important organ is, from its position and complicated, delicate structure, subject to a great variety of diseases, which, heretofore, have been very badly treated under the allopathic system.

All external applications, in the form of strong eye-waters and salves, are injurious, and even if, as in scrofulous sore eyes, for instance, these salves seem to have effected a cure, it is only by driving the disease from the external parts to some internal organ, which is, at the time, the weakest—in most cases to the lungs. If external remedies are wanted, pure water is preferable in all cases of inflammation, applied either cold or warm, according to the feelings of the patient. In cases of external injuries to the eye, the arnica lotion (ten drops of *Arnica* tincture to half a teacupful of cold water) must be used externally.

But, when erysipelas affects the eyes, nothing wet ought to be applied, but warm bags filled with bran. (See "Erysipelas.")

When the inflammation of the eyes and face is caused by the poison of the sumach, or other weeds, apply nothing outwardly, but give the internal remedies recommended for that disease. (See "Poisoning by Sumach," page 71.)

1. Inflammation of the Eyelid and its Margins.

a. *Inflammation and Swelling of the Eyelid.*

Aconite. In all cases where the inflammation and the pain is great, attended with fever and restlessness, or where the lids are *swollen, hard,* and *red,* with *heat* and sensation of *burning* and *dryness,* or when there is a copious secretion of mucus in the eyes and nose, with dread of light, fever, and thirst; after it *Belladonna, Sulphur,* or *Hepar sulph.,* are often necessary. (See these.)

Belladonna. If *Aconite* is not sufficient; or when there is a feeling of burning and itching in the red and swollen eyelids, which stick together, and bleed easily when opened; also, when the edges are turned to the outside, and feel as if paralyzed (see *Hepar sulph.*).

Hepar sulphuris. If there is a sensation of *ulceration* or *contusion* in the *red* and *swollen* lids on *touching* them, with sensitiveness to light, and spasmodic contractions of the lids in the morning. In alternation with *Aconite, Bellad.,* or *Mercury,* as the symptoms indicate (see these remedies), every three or six hours a dose (four globules), until better.

Sulphur. Frequently in alternation with *Aconite,* when the swelling and redness are very bad, with pressing, burning pains in the eye and lids (as if from sand in the eyes), great secretion of mucus, and sensitiveness to light. After it *Calcarea carb.* is frequently necessary.

Mercury. If there is a hard swelling, with cutting pain, and difficulty of opening the lids, as if from contraction, ulcers and scabs on the edges, worse in the night, and in the warmth of the bed, with restlessness and perspiration, or if there is a *burning itching* in the eyes, worse in the open air, with great dread of the light of the fire. After, or in alternation with it, give *Hepar sulph.,* every six hours a dose (four glob.) until better.

Euphrasia. In cases where the eyelids are red and swelled, their margins ulcerated, with itching in the day-time, sticking together in the morning, constant catarrh, headache, heat in the head and dread of light, with *profuse secretion of mucus and tears*. In alternation with *Nux vom.*, if the eyeball is very red, and there is burning with the itching; if the patient is very irritable, and feels *worse* in the open air; but in alternation with *Pulsatilla*, if he is of a mild character, and feels *better* in the open air.

Arsenic. Inflammation of the inside of the lids, with inability to open the eyes, and *violent burning pain*.

Spigelia. In inflammation and *ulcerations* of the lids, with biting soreness, difficulty of raising the lids (as if from stiffness), with burning in the eyes and pain in the head, worse on the least motion.

Calcarea carb. Frequently after *Sulph.*, when there are *cutting*, burning pains, especially when *reading*, with red, hard and great swelling, and copious secretion of mucus, and the lids sticking together in the morning.

Hyoscyamus and *Chamomile* in alternation, when the eyelids are closed spasmodically, with a sensation of heaviness or pressure.

ADMINISTRATION.—Give every two, four or six hours a dose (four globules) of the selected remedy, either alone or in alternation with another, until the patient is relieved, or another remedy is necessary; discontinue the medicine altogether, as soon as the patient is improving.

APPLICATION OF WATER, either cold or warm to the eyes, is strongly recommended; if constipation is present, use cold water injections, and drink cold water freely.

b. Inflammation of the Margins of the Lids.

The principal remedies in this disease, which frequently appears without affecting the whole lid, are *Bellad.*, *Euphrasia*, *Pulsat.*, *Nux vom.*, *Mercury*, *Hepar sulph.*, and *Chamomile*.

(See the detailed symptoms of these remedies in the preceding article: "*a.* Inflammation of the Eyelids.")

2. Inflammation of the Eyeball. (*Ophthalmia.*)

In most cases where the eyeballs are inflamed, the lids will also be affected, and the remedies stated under "Inflammation of the Eyelids," will be beneficial. This is particularly the case, when *Aconite, Bellad.*, and *Euphrasia* are indicated, which are the most important remedies in diseases of the eyes, and to which we refer the reader, in the preceding article. But frequently the eyeballs alone are implicated, especially when cold, together with a scrofulous or rheumatic predisposition, is the cause.

The first remedy in this disease, particularly when it appears suddenly, is *Aconite.* When the eyes are *very red,* with dark redness of the vessels, and intolerable burning, stinging, or aching pains (worse on moving the eyes), dread of light, copious flow of tears, yet with dryness of the eyelids and fever.

Belladonna. When the white of the eye is very much inflamed, sensitive to light, either copious flow of burning hot tears, or great dryness of the eyes, which ache all around, or deep inside, with stitches proceeding from the eyes to the head (worse on moving the eyes), and a severe cold in the head, or a *violent headache,* with stupor and vertigo, sparks of black spots before the eyes, and a short dry cough, it suits mostly after *Aconite;* but frequently, too, after *Hepar sulph.*, and *Mercury.*

Euphrasia. Same as *Bellad.*, and when this is insufficient; or when the pain in and above the eyes, in the head, is more *pressing,* and the cough not dry, but loose; also, with profuse running at the nose; worse in the evening.

Nux vomica. When the eyes are bloodshot, smarting as if from sand, with swelling and softening of the eye, irritable temper, coated tongue, redness of the corners of the lids, with stiffness and itching, acrid tears, dread of light in the morning, headache every night, and stoppage of the nose.

Ignatia. If the pain is more like pressure in the eyes, which are not much inflamed, but with copious flow of tears and nasal discharge, great sensitiveness to light, mild, quiet, disposition.

Pulsatilla is often effective, after *Aconite* has subdued the worst inflammation, and severe pains remain (tearing, stitching, and cutting), in *rheumatic* inflammation of the eyes, where there is sensitiveness to light; worse in the afternoon and evening; the patient is fretful and inclined to weep.

Bryonia. After *Pulsat.*, when the redness still remains, the lids are swollen, with pain in the head when the eyes are opened; worse at night.

Rhus. After *Bryonia*, or in alternation with it, in damp, wet weather, or when the eye continues to burn and stitch, with the running of water, or the eyelids are swollen as if from erysipelas.

Spigelia. Aching, stitching, or boring pains, penetrating into the head, and returning regularly at the same time of day, with a sensation as if the eyeballs were too large. The pain is at times insupportable.

Sulphur (See "Inflammation of the Eyelid") is also necessary, after *Mercury* and *Pulsatilla.*

ADMINISTRATION the same as in the foregoing article.

APPLICATION OF WATER. (See p. 177.)

DIET AND REGIMEN, in all diseases of the eye must be light, as in fevers generally (see these). Rest and quiet in the room are necessary. The room itself should be dry, airy, and darkened.

3. CHRONIC INFLAMMATION OF THE EYES.

The treatment of these inflammations varies according to their causes, which are either hereditary or acquired.

a. From Gout and Rheumatism.

For the severest symptoms use *Aconite, Bellad.*, and *Spigelia*, as stated in the preceding article; also,

Colocynthis. When there is violent burning and cutting, extending far back into the head and nose, with great anguish and restlessness; or violent pressure in the forehead; worse when stooping, or lying on the back; severe drawing pain in the head, with vomiting.

Hepar sulph. If *Bellad.*, or *Spigelia*, is insufficient; or when there is redness of the eyes and eyelids, with soreness *when touched;* sensitiveness to light, especially in the evening; sight at times dim and obscured, at others clear; pressure in the eyeball, as if it would *start out of the head.*

ADMINISTRATION, the same as under "Inflammation of the Eyelids."

APPLICATION OF WATER in this and the following diseases of the eyes, can be made either for the purpose of palliating the present condition or of eradicating them entirely. If the first is our object, we refer the reader to page 177, where these means are detailed; if we want to eradicate the disease by the use of water as a principal means, we recommend the reader to have recourse to a water-cure establishment, where a systematic use of water will be found highly beneficial in these diseases.

b. From Scrofula. (Scrofulous Sore Eyes.)

Scrofula frequently affects the eyes, after an inflammation of the lids or eyeball has set in, from causes above stated, by which complication such cases are rendered much worse, and more difficult to cure; for dimness of sight and ulcers on the ball of the eye often remain; they require medical attention, as the consequences of neglect, or family treatment, would be too serious; and the necessity for the eradication of scrofula is, of itself, obvious.

In the beginning of such an attack, give *Aconite* and *Belladonna*, as stated under "Inflammation of the Eyelids" and "Eyeball." Also, all the other remedies mentioned there, if they are required by the symptoms. Beside these,

Dulcamara is of use, when cold is the cause of the sore eyes, and when they are made worse by reading, with dimness of sight, and a sensation as if sparks of fire were flying out of the eyes; pain over the eyes; worse when at rest; better when walking.

ADMINISTRATION the same as above.

For ulcers on the eyeballs, remaining after the inflammation has subsided, give *Euphrasia*, *Hepar sulph.*, and *Silicea*, each remedy during one week; two or three times every evening a dose (four glob.). When *Silicea* is given, apply externally a wash of twelve globules of *Silicea* in half a teacupful of pure cold water. Make the application several times a day.

For *specks*, give *Euphrasia*, *Hepar sulph.*, *Silicea*, *Calcarea carb.*, *Nitric acid*, in the same manner as stated under "*Ulcers on the Eyeball.*"

DIET AND REGIMEN.—See "Inflammation of the Eyeball."

c. *From Syphilis or Venereal Disease.*

The eyes may be implicated in this disease, and become inflamed, particularly when a gonorrhea is suppressed and transferred, as it were, to the eyes, or when syphilis has penetrated the whole system. In the latter case, a homœopathic physician must be consulted. In Inflammation of the eyes and lids from *suppressed gonorrhea*, administer at first *Aconite*, as stated under "Inflammation of the Eyes;" after it *Pulsatilla*, in the same manner; then wait two or three days, and give, if necessary, *Nitric acid*, *Mercury*, and *Sulphur*; commencing with *Nitric acid*, and taking four doses the first week; four doses of the next remedy, the second week; and so on, until better.

In the real Syphilitic Eye-affections: Nitric acid, Mercury, and *Thuja,* are the principal remedies—to be given as above.

DIET AND REGIMEN.—See "Inflammation of the Eye-ball," and "Syphilis."

d. *From abuse of Mercury.*

This drug, given in allopathic doses, frequently produces severe affections of the eye; for which must be given, *Hepar sulph., Nitric acid, Pulsat.,* and *Sulphur,* in the same manner as stated above, under "Syphilitic Eye-Affections." Diet, also, the same.

4. STY ON THE EYELID.

A sty is a small boil on the eyelid, produced by the swelling of the Meibomian glands, which are imbedded all along the margins of the lid.

The specific remedy in the commencement of this complaint is

Pulsatilla. A dose (four glob.) twice a day, until four doses are taken; then discontinue two days; and if not better, or if suppuration appears, take *Mercury* in the same manner, in alternation with *Hepar sulph.*

If no suppuration, but induration takes place, or hard spots remain, and if the sties appear often, give *Staphysag.*, a dose (four glob.) two or three times, during one week; and afterward, for two or three weeks, give each week two doses of *Calca. carb.* (each dose four glob.), until better; and if not, *Sulphur,* for the same length of time, and in the same manner.

Externally, apply nothing; but bathe occasionally in warm water.

DIET AND REGIMEN.—The diet light; no animal food; and regimen cool.

5. WEEPING OR WATERY EYES.

If this complaint arises, as is mostly the case, from an obstruction of the lachrymal duct, or a swelling of its entrance, in the internal corner of the eye, a homœopathic physician should be consulted. In the meantime, use the following remedies:

Bellad., *Pulsat.*, *Calca. carb.*, *Sili.*, *Petrol.*, *Sulph.*; the first two remedies alternately, every day a dose (four glob.) of each, until the acute symptoms subside; the other remedies each for four or six weeks, every week two doses (six glob. each), until better.

But if the watery eyes arise from a general weakness of the organ, *Euphrasia* and *Spigelia* in alternation, ever two or three days a dose (six glob.), will generally be found beneficial. Let this treatment be followed, at the end of two weeks, by two doses of *Sulphur*, on two successive nights (each dose six glob.).

Diet.—The usual homœopathic diet must be observed during the whole time.

6. Cataract. (*Glaucoma.*)

This disease, which consists of the gradual darkening of the lens in the eye (thus preventing the light from reaching the optic nerve), is, in its commencement, curable by medicines, if carefully selected and applied. As this, however, ought to be done by a homœopathic physician, we will here merely notice a few remedies, which may be taken in the beginning, until a physician can be consulted.

By this means, an operation for the cataract may frequently be avoided.

Pulsatilla, *Sulphur*, *Silicea*, *Conium*, *Phosphorus*.

Administration.—Give each remedy for four or six weeks, every three days one dose (six glob.), in the evening, until better, or until the next remedy has to be taken

Diet and Regimen.—Light, without animal food; otherwise, the usual homœopathic diet.

7. Weakness of Sight. (*Amblyopia.*)

Blindness (sudden and incipient)—Amaurosis.

Short-sighted and far-sighted persons have not, strictly speaking, *weak* eyes; this latter is a defect in the optic nerve itself, which is weakened or paralyzed, in a greater or less degree. If this nerve is not much paralyzed, so that only dimness of sight exists, we call it *amblyopia,* or *weakness of sight;* if the nerve is more or entirely paralyzed, it is incipient or real blindness—*amaurosis.*

This disease can be cured; but it must be taken in time, and a homœopathic physician ought to be counsulted *immediately,* as delay in this case is very dangerous.

In the meantime take, for *simple weakness of sight, Pulsatilla, Sulphur, Bellad., Calcarea carb., Phosphorus,* and *Ruta.*

Administration the same as stated under "Cataract."

If *Ruta* shall be used, drop two drops of the tincture in half a teacupful of water, and wash the eyes three times a day with it; particularly when the weakness of sight resulted from excessive reading, sewing, etc., everything appearing dusky and foggy before the eyes.

For *incipient blindness,* give the same remedies as for simple weakness of sight,

Attacks of sudden blindness; if caused by congestion to the head, and accompanied with pain in the head and convulsions, give *Bellad.* and *Hyoscyamus* in solution (twelve glob. in half a teacupful of water), every fifteen minutes a teaspoonful, until better (see "Congestion of blood to the Head"); but for sudden blindness, without an apparent cause, give first *Aconite;* then *Mercury;* every two or three hours a dose (four glob.), alternately, until better.

For *night-blindness; Belladonna.*

For *day-blindness,* where the patient can only see in the evening; give *Sulphur,* and afterward *Silicea.*

Diet the same as in "Cataract.'

8. Short-Sightedness. (*Myopia.*)

This affliction, if not of too long duration, may generally be mitigated or cured by *Pulsatilla;* or, if caused by abuse of calomel, give *Carbo veg.* and *Hepar sulph.;* if from debilitating causes and typhus fevers, *Phosphoric acid.*

These remedies to be administered in the same manner as stated under "Cataract."

Diet and Regimen, also, the same.

9. Far-Sightedness.

This frequently occurs after excessive use of ardent spirits; in which case *Nux vom.* must be given; every day a dose (four glob.) for a week; followed by *Sulphur*, in alternation with *Lachesis;* every week two doses of each, for four or six weeks, or until better; followed by *Silicea* and *Phosphorus* in lean persons, or *Calcarea* in fleshy persons. If not relieved, consult a physician.

10. Squinting. (*Strabismus.*)

A frequent cause of squinting, in young children, is that from the position of their cradle, they constantly have the light on the same side. To obviate this, alter the position of the cradle so that the light will be directly in front.

If, however, squinting continues, notwithstanding, and the heads of the children are hot, give *Belladonna* and *Bryonia,* in alternation, every four or six days a dose (two glob.) until six doses of each are taken, or the child is better. If not better, consult a homœopathic physician.

11. Falling of the Eyelids. (*Paralysis.*)

If the upper or lower eyelid falls down, and cannot be raised easily, give *Spigelia, Belladonna, Sepia, Veratrum, Opium, Cocculus, Nitric acid.*

Administer the same as stated under "Cataract."

ing its effect, and, if not better, give one of the following remedies, according to the symptoms:

Camphor. If the chilliness still continues, or there is great difficulty of breathing and failing of strength; let the patient either smell champhor or drop three drops of spirits of camphor in half a tumbler of water, and give every fifteen or thirty minutes a teaspoonful, until better.

Mercury. Particularly in the commencement, when the head symptoms prevail, such as sneezing and running of the nose, with rheumatic pains in the head and body, red watery eyes, or when a loose cough, with profuse perspiration without relief, sets in; also, when there is a slimy diarrhea, with straining like dysentery. Give it in the same manner as *Arsenic*, above. This remedy is considered almost a specific in this disease. (Compare also, "Materia Medica," at the end of the book.)

Bryonia. In alternation with *Aconite*, every two or three hours a dose (four glob.), if inflammatory symptoms appear; fever; dry, hot skin, with a hard shaking cough, and stitches in the chest.

Belladonna and *Aconite*, in the same manner, if the cough is dry and spasmodic, with severe headache and dryness in the mouth and throat.

Hepar, if the cold was better, but is worse again, or when the patient had previously taken much calomel.

Euphrasia, when with a discharge of white mucus from the nose, the eyes are sore and run water profusely.

Phosphorus and *Tartar emet.*, in alternation, in the same manner, if the lungs feel oppressed, weak, and sore; and when coughing or breathing there is rattling in the chest.

Causticum. If the feeling of *excoriation* in the chest is prevailing, with a dry cough, so violent that the urine escapes involuntarily; give twice a day a dose (four glob.).

Pulsatilla. After *Mercury*, or in alternation with it, every three or four hours a dose, if the cough is loose, and the nose discharges thick, yellow mucus; soreness of the chest in the morning, after expectoration; foul tongue; disagreeable or insipid taste in the mouth; no thirst.

Silicea, in chronic catarrh, which returns frequently, when it is either running or causes obstruction.

Sudden suppression of the influenza sometimes produces *headache*, for which give

Aconite, Pulsat., China; or

Difficulty of breathing, for which *Ipecac.*, and *Bryonia*, are suitable, followed by a dose of *Sulphur*, if necessary.

Administration.—Every three or four days a dose (four glob.), until better or another remedy is necessary. (Consult also the article on "Coughs.")

Application of Water. (See page 203.)

Diet and Regimen.—No meat or coffee; for drink, water or lemonade, if there is no diarrhea; gruels and toast-water. Keep the face from the direct influence of the fire in the grate or stove; it is preferable to remain in bed, where a gentle warmth may be maintained.

5. Cough.

As cough is in most cases, only a symptom of some other disease, such as pneumonia, bronchitis, influenza, hooping-cough, consumption, etc., we must refer the reader to their respective chapters. Sometimes, however, a cough appears isolated from any marked disease, and is either caused by cold (*catarrhal cough*), or sympathy, or derangement of other organs (*nervous, spasmodic,* and *gastric cough*); so that we have to mention here their appropriate treatment.

a. Catarrhal cough, caused by a severe cold on the lungs, is, in the beginning of the day, harsh and painful; afterward it becomes loose, with heavy expectoration, relieving the chest from pain and oppression.

Treatment.—If such a cold is combined with pains in the

head and limbs, chilliness, and thirst (commonly called *bilious*), give *Bryonia*, and *Rhus tox.*, alternately, every two or three hours a dose (four glob.), until better, or until three doses of each are taken; then wait twelve or sixteen hours before the next remedy is taken, which will suit the remaining symptoms of the cough. (See "Symptomatic detail.")

When the *cough* is *dry*, without expectoration: *Aconite, Chamomile, Bryonia, Rhus tox., Belladonna, Hyoscyamus, Capsicum, Ignatia, Nux vom., Phosphorus, Hepar.*

When the *cough* is *loose: Pulsat., Mercury, Tartar emet., Phosphorus, Dulcamara, Stannum, Lycopodium, Sulphur.*

b. Nervous and *spasmodic* cough, caused by nervous irritation or excitement, either original, or transferred to the lungs from other organs; for instance, pain in the womb (*neuralgia*) may cease suddenly, and, by being transferred to the lungs, creates here the *hysterical* cough. (See article "Hysteria," especially.) All the nervous coughs are dry; but they may affect the stomach, and cause *vomiting* or *retching;* sometimes *spasms* in the lungs may take place; *fits of suffocation*, which are generally of not so much danger as they appear to be.

TREATMENT.—For *nervous* and *spasmodic cough: Bellad., Hyoscyamus, Ipecac., Bryonia, Drosera, Hepar, Cina, Sulphur.*

If accompanied by *vomiting, retching: Ipecac., Mercury, Bryonia, Tartar emetic, Pulsat., Sepia.*

If by fits of suffocation: *Ipecac., Tartar emetic, Opium, Chamomile, Bryonia, Drosera, Hepar, Lachesis, Sulphur, Arsenic, China.*

Cough, caused by *sympathy* from other diseases, such as *worms, dentition* (*teething*), *dyspepsia; growing too fast* causes in young persons such coughs. Look for these in their respective chapters.

N. B. After having found the kind of cough in the above, select the best remedy from those designated for such kind of cough, comparing the symptoms.

SYMPTOMATIC DETAIL.—*Aconite*. *Violent, short* cough; sometimes with pains and anxious oppressions in the chest.

Chamomile. Dry cough, from constant tickling in the throat and chest; worse after talking *in the night;* with fever and coughing during sleep; particularly in children, when they cough after crying, or a fit of anger or passion, or a tickling cough, which ceases after the patient gets warm in the bed; also when in the morning tough, bitter mucus is thrown up. (Compare "Croupy Cough," "Cold in the Head," and "Hoarseness.")

Bryonia. Dry cough, from irritation in the throat, or with pain in the chest; worse in the open air; sometimes from taking cold in damp, frosty weather; with rheumatic pains in the head and limbs; also chilliness, followed by fever and thirst (in alternation with *Rhus tox.*); or a loose cough, with yellowish expectoration, or spasmodic cough after eating or drinking. (For children, see "Croupy Cough.")

Rhus tox. Short, dry cough, from a tickling in the chest; worse in the evening, or before midnight; with weakness in the breast, and shortness of breath; restlessness at night; dry tongue (see *Bryonia*); worse in the air, better when exercising, or in the warmth; or cough, with a taste of blood in the mouth; bloody saliva runs from the mouth *during the sleep*.

Belladonna. Short, dry cough, particularly at night; worse when moving; with dryness and tickling in the throat, and redness of the face, *dry spasmodic cough*, with retching, *mostly after midnight; dry cough* day and night, with soreness of the abdominal muscles, or in the region of the hip, as of falling of the womb; or when the attacks end with sneezing, as if the person had taken a heavy cold. (For children, see "Croupy Cough.")

Hyoscyamus. Suits well when *Bellad.* has afforded only partial relief, or when the cough at night is temporarily mitigated by sitting up in bed; much rattling in the throat and tickling or dry hacking cough, with weak respiration; worse by muscular action or motion; the patient can hardly walk up stairs. (See "Consumption Beginning or Galloping.")

Capsicum. Particularly in persons of *phlegmatical* temperament; easily *chilled after drinking cold water;* cough *worse toward evening and night;* with pains in various parts of the body; bursting headache; painful pressure, and aching in the throat and ears; cough, with offensive breath and disagreeable taste in the mouth.

Ignatia. Dry cough, with running at the nose day and night, in the same degree; or short, hacking cough, as if from a stricture in the throat, or the tickling of a feather; aggravated by the continuation of the cough; particularly in persons who are easily affected by grief, or when the cough is worse after *eating,* or on *lying down at night,* or on *rising in the morning.*

Nux vomica is one of the most useful remedies for various kinds of cough from cold. (See "Influenza," "Cold in the Head," etc.) *Tickling cough; worse early in the morning;* sometimes with *catarrhal hoarseness,* and scraping around the palate; tough mucus in the throat and lungs, with an itching, tickling sensation in the throat, and chilliness; cough worse by movement, reading, or meditation after meals; and followed sometimes by retching or vomiting; or *fatiguing cough,* with pains in the head, as if it would burst; or pains in the pit of the stomach, as if from a *blow* or *bruise;* worse in the night, or after lying down; cough dry during the after part of the day and night, with oppression on the chest, as if from a weight; expectoration toward morning. Suits well for persons of an energetic, sanguine, choleric temperament, and for those who drink much coffee and ardent spirits.

Carbo vegetabilis. Cough, with *hoarseness,* worse toward evening or in the morning, and by speaking; nervous, spasmodic cough, exciting vomiting in paroxysms throughout the day. The cough is attended with *burning* pain and a sensation of *scraping* or excoriation in the chest; particularly during damp, cold weather. (In alternation with *Phosphorus.*)

Phosphorus. Dry cough, from tickling in the throat, but more in the chest; worse when laughing, *talking*, and drinking, hoarseness, and pains in the chest, particularly on the *left* side, as if from *excoriation; lying on the left side excites the cough.* (In alternation with *Carbo veg.*, or *Hepar sulph.*)

Hepar sulph. In alternation with *Phosphorus,* in dry, hoarse cough; worse after talking; or excited when *any* part of the body becomes *cool,* particularly at night.

Tartar emetic. Loose cough, *with much rattling* on the chest; quick breathing, almost amounting to suffocation; hot and moist hands, with perspiration on the forehead; bluish lips (in alternation with *Phosphorus,* see "Inflammation of the Lungs"); or cough, with *vomiting of food* after eating; *deep, hollow cough; expectoration of mucus in the night.*

Dulcamara. Loose cough, after taking cold; spitting of light-red blood; hooping cough, excited by drawing a deep breath; worse in a room, or when lying still; better when moving and out of doors.

Stannum. Hard, dry cough in the *evening;* excited by laughing, talking, and singing; also, a loose cough, with much expectoration of mucous or sweetish matter, with feeling of soreness of the chest after it (see "Consumption"); lying on the *right* side excites the dry cough.

Lycopodium. Cough worse in the night, or after drinking; or a tickling cough, excited by drawing a *deep breath,* with a saltish expectoration, and stitches in the *left* side of the chest (see "Consumption"); dryness of the tongue without thirst.

Sulphur. Dry cough, worse in the *evening* and *during the night,* or when lying down; loose cough with expectoration of thick mucus, and feeling of soreness in the chest (particularly suitable after *Mercury*); cough, with pain and stitches in the chest or the head; also, a sensation of spasmodic constriction in the chest, as if caused by the vapors of brimstone.

Ipecac. Nervous or spasmodic cough, sometimes with nausea, retching, and vomiting; worse at night or when walking in the cold air; accompanied by oppression in breathing, almost amounting to suffocation, as if *from the accumulation of mucus* (*congestion to the lungs*), particularly in children; when the face looks livid and dark, and the body becomes rigid and stiff. (See "Hooping-Cough.")

Drosera. *Dry, spasmodic cough,* with *retching;* worse immediately after *lying down,* in the *night;* chronic *cough,* and *hoarseness* after *measles; dryness,* and a *rough, scraping* sensation, deep in the throat, which causes coughing. (See "Bronchitis," and "Hooping-Cough.")

Cina. *Dry, spasmodic cough,* with shortness of breath, pale face and moaning, also in the night, with restlessness and crying. (See "Worms," and "Hooping-Cough.")

Pulsatilla. *Severe shaking, dry* cough mostly in the *morning,* with *retching* and *inclination to vomit;* or *loose* cough, with much expectoration of a *bitter, yellow* mucus.

Mercury. Cough, with hoarseness (see "Influenza"), or excited by tickling in the throat; shaking, dry cough, mostly at *night,* or loose cough, with expectoration *streaked with blood,* and an inclination to *perspire easily,* but *without* relief. In children the cough is frequently attended by bleeding of the nose, sickness at the stomach, hoarseness and diarrhea.

China. Severe cough, from ulceration of the lungs (see "Galloping Consumption"), after hemorrhage, or other losses of blood; or *asthmatic* cough in the night, with acute pain in the chest and the shoulder-blades.

Arsenic. When *China* only ameliorates, without curing; or when there is *dry cough* after *drinking;* or cough, with bloody expectoration in the night, with a *burning* sensation over the whole body; asthmatical cough (see "Asthma").

Opium. Cough when swallowing or *breathing,* with *anxious, heavy,* and *intermitting* respiration, worse during repose; full, red face (see "Congestion of the Lungs").

Sepia. Dry cough in the evening in bed, frequently with sickness at the stomach and bitter vomiting; or loose cough, with *much saltish* expectoration, particularly in the *morning* and *evening* (see "Consumption").

Lachesis. *Short, dry, suffocating* cough, as if from something sticking in the throat, with ineffectual efforts to expectorate.

Administration. — Of a remedy, having been carefully selected, dissolve twelve globules in half a teacupful of water, and let the patient take every two, three, or six hours a teaspoonful (children half a teaspoonful), until three or four doses have been taken; then wait from four to twelve hours, according to the severity of the case; and if not better, select and give the next best remedy in the same manner. This will suit for recent attacks. In coughs of a longer standing, give the remedy for two days, evening and morning a dose (four glob.); then discontinue two or three days; if then not better, take another remedy in the same manner. To very small children, give the medicine in globules altogether, if they cannot take it dissolved in water; one or two globules at a time is a dose for them.

Application of Water. — If the cough is very dry and exhausting, put a warm water compress over the whole chest, renewing it from time to time, until the cough becomes looser and the patient relieved. If possible, let the patient drink plenty of cold water and wash his breast and neck frequently with it, rubbing well afterward with a dry towel.

Diet and Regimen.—If the cough is accompanied by fever or biliousness, abstain from meat and butter; if not, these may be used: otherwise, keep the diet prescribed in chronic diseases. If persons are habitually liable to take cold, they ought to harden themselves against the changes in the atmosphere, by the systematic use of cold water, externally, and internally, as spoken of in the latter part of the book (see "Hydropathy"); persons, however, with tubercular affections must not use it. Another great dietetic rule is, that persons liable to colds on the lungs ought to abstain from *all* spiritous liquors.

The bathing of children in cold water, when they have cold on the lungs, may be suspended for the time (except when allowed by a physician especially); as in many cases it might not be admissible at all.

A patient with a cough should not occupy a damp room, facing to the north; but a dry, airy chamber, exposed to the midday sun, and susceptible of easy ventilation and even temperature. If the cough at any time is very dry and painful, use, as a loosening drink, an infusion of the roots of althea and liquorice, in equal parts, as freely as the patient finds it necessary, cold or warm. In chronic coughs, where the expectoration is tinged with blood, no warm drinks are allowed. In fall and winter, until summer, a plaster of Burgundy pitch on the breast is recommended to those who have weak breasts; but, after taking it off in the summer, they must wash and rub the breast well.

Hooping-Cough. (*Tussis Convulsiva.*)

This is one of those diseases which exclusively befall children, from the infant on the breast up to twelve or fourteen years. It appears mostly as an epidemic, and is as such, infectious. In some seasons its attacks are milder than in others; sometimes it commences immediately with hooping; at other times, it is preceded by all the symptoms of an inflammation of the lungs, with great tendency to convulsive and spasmodic affections. The real hooping seldom commences in the earliest stage.

Diagnosis.—We recognize, generally, two stages for this disease:

The *first*, or *febrile stage*, showing all the symptoms of a heavy cold; running at the nose; watery, heavy eyes; sneezing; irritating and painful cough, with feverishness and difficult respiration. It is in this stage that congestions to the head and lungs often occur, particularly when children are teething at the time, which, of course, adds materially to the danger of the case. The old practice is almost powerless in such cases, while homœopathy offers a safe and successful treatment.

The *second*, or *nervous spasmodic stage*, begins as soon as the feverishness diminishes, and the hooping commences; the latter increases by degress, until the paroxysms become, at least in severe cases, really appalling.

The little patients dread the attack, and run, as it were, to the mother for help, or hold fast to something, when they feel the approach of it. In severe paroxysms, the face swells and becomes livid, while quantities of mucus are forced from the mouth, and frequently blood escapes from the mouth and nose; respiration seems to cease for a minute, when a deep inspiration ensues, which ends the attack for the time, and the patient recovers quickly; being, in the intervals, almost always perfectly well, except, perhaps, a little fretful and weak.

Duration.—If this disease is not treated at all, or only by allopathic medicines, its duration is left to its own natural limits, and not shortened in the least; in such cases, the first stage may last from three to eight, or even twenty-one days, and the second stage, from the beginning to its height, from five to six weeks; from thence to its total disappearance, the same length of time. Frequently, the cough reappears in those patients in the fall or winter, who had it in the preceding summer.

But under the proper homœopathic treatment, its duration is very much shortened; sometimes the disease is cut off in its progress within five or six days. Very seldom has a person the hooping-cough twice in his lifetime, except as above stated.

TREATMENT.—*In the first stage,* where the children apparently have a cold, select from those remedies recommended in the articles on "Cough," and "Croupy Cough," by the use of which the cough frequently entirely disappears. These remedies are mostly *Chamomile, Belladonna, Bryonia,* etc.

Aconite. If the cough does not cease in a few days, but becomes very dry and whistling; the child has fever and complains of a burning pain in the windpipe. Administer as in Croup, until better, or some of the following remedies are indicated.

Dulcamara. If the cough is loose and moist, with copious expectoration of a thin mucus with hoarseness, apparently brought on by exposure to wet or dampness, evening and morning a dose (three or four glob.) for two days.

Pulsatilla. In the same manner, if there is a *loose cough* with vomiting of mucus or food; also, a slimy diarrhea.

Ipecac. and *Nux vomica,* alternately, if the cough is dry, accompanied by great anguish, strangling, and bluish face; worse after midnight, until morning; *with vomiting* and bleeding at the nose. Give alternately every hour or two hours a dose (three glob.), until better.

Tartar emetic and *Phosphorus,* in alternation, in the same manner, is frequently necessary in this period, if there is rattling in the lungs, short breathing, great debility, drowsiness, and thirst; also, retching, with diarrhea.

Carbo veg., is the principal remedy, when the cough exhibits the first signs of hooping; particularly, when it is worse in the *evening,* the patient complaining at the same time of sore throat when swallowing; shooting pains in head and chest; especially useful, when the weather is damp and cold. Give it the same as *Dulcamara,* above.

In the second stage, when the hooping or spasms during coughing have really commenced, the principal medicines are:

Drosera, Veratrum, Cuprum, Tartar emetic, Phosphorus, Cina, Bryonia, Belladonna, Mercury, Iodium, Opium, Hepar sulph., Arnica, Sulphur, Hellebor.

Drosera. After the *Carbo veg.*, when the paroxysms become more violent, with real hooping, vomiting of food and mucus, without or with fever, which is characterized by chilliness, heat with thirst, hot perspiration in the night; the patient feels better when moving about.

Veratrum. After *Drosera*, or in alternation with it, for similar symptoms, only accompanied with great weakness; small and quick pulse; slow fever, with cold perspiration on the forehead; child is unable to hold up its head; miliary eruption (prickly heat) over the whole body; apathy and drowsiness, from weakness; child dislikes to move or speak.

Cina. If the child, during the hooping-cough, exhibits symptoms of worms—as picking at the nose, sudden pains or gripings in the bowels, or itching at the anus—or if it becomes *stiff* during a paroxysm of cough, after which a gurling noise is sometimes heard, descending from the throat into the stomach. This remedy can be given in alternation with *Mercury* (see "*Mercury*"), if there is bleeding from the nose and mouth at the same time.

Cuprum. If the paroxysms appear *very often* during twenty-four hours, rendering the little patients *rigid* and *unconscious;* if with drowsiness and rattling of mucus in the chest between the paroxysms, in alternation with *Tartar emetic* (see "*Tartar emetic*:" compare, also, "Congestion to the Head"). This remedy is particularly useful, when convulsions appear instead of the cough, and cease when the paroxysms return; as if the paroxysm of the lungs had been temporarily transferred to the brain. (See "Convulsions.")

Tartar emetic and *Phosphorus.* See page 260.

Belladonna. Before or after *Cuprum*, when the brain becomes affected; patient cannot bear the light, noise, or motion; head seems to ache; burning fever; thirst; restlessness; delirium; convulsions (see "Inflammation of the Brain"); in such cases, in alternation with *Hellebor.*: paroxysms terminate in sneezing.

Hellebor. At any time during the hooping-cough, when symptoms of congestion to the head appear, particularly when the patient sleeps with the eyes half open (see *Belladonna*, above); it is of great service when children are teething, or otherwise weakly and delicate.

Bryonia. Sometimes in alternation with *Hellebor.*, when *Belladonna* was insufficient, for similar symptoms; or when the paroxysms of suffocating cough appear more in the evening or at night; mostly, however, after eating or drinking, which is vomited up.

Mercury. The principal remedy, when the child *bleeds profusely* at the nose and mouth when vomiting, with copious sweat at night, and great nervousness; also, if there are worm symptoms (see "*Cina*").

Sulphur. At any period, if the paroxysms are accompanied by vomiting, which will not yield to other remedies.

Iodium. If the patient pines away, or has a chronic, watery diarrhea, of lightish color.

Opium. If the best indicated remedies seem not to have the desired effect, or if there is stupor (see "Congestion to the head"), with hot perspiration; *irregular breathing*, with great anguish; constipation.

Hepar sulph. When the cough is better, but yet hollow, hoarse, and dry, with retching and *crying* after a paroxysm.

Arnica. When the child cries much after coughing, or coughs after crying (in alternation with *Cina*$^{c.c.}$ or *Hepar*).

ADMINISTRATION.—Whenever no reference is given to other chapters, give the remedies as follows: Dissolve twelve globules in half a teacupful of water, and give for two days a teaspoonful, morning, noon, and night; then wait two or three days for the effect; if the cough is slightly improved, wait still longer; because the hooping-cough needs, beside the right medicine, a little time, to disappear by degrees; but, if no better, give the next remedy, in the same manner.

Application of Water.—The washing of the breast with cold water, and the frequent drinking of it, is strongly recommended.

Diet and Regimen.—In cases with fever, see the diet in "Croupy Cough;" where there is no fever, give the usual diet without coffee and spices. A great deal of fresh air is good for the young patients, if they have no feverish symptoms. The same holds good in relation to their usual bathing, which must be discontinued, if fever is present.

Inflammation of the Lungs. (*Pneumonia.*)

This disease generally commences with chills, followed by fever, with difficulty of breathing, and a short dry cough; pulse soft in the beginning, afterward hard, but always very quick; dull pains in the chest at every deep respiration, with great oppression; expectoration of a tough, lumpy mucus, afterward mixed with blood; the patient generally prefers to lie on his back; is not inclined to speak, or when speaking pauses after every articulation; is sometimes sullen, and wishes to be quiet; in some cases, the face turns to a bluish *purple*, with red cheeks; tongue dry, parched; great thirst; skin dry, hot. As soon as the skin becomes moist and natural, the oppression in breathing diminishes, and a thick mucus is coughed up abundantly; the danger is over, and the patient needs only good nursing and rest in bed during convalescence. If this is not the case, however, the inflammation runs either into the nervous or typhoid stage (see "Typhoid Fever"), or into *hepatization* of the lungs (the air-cells are filled with lymphatic matter); both very dangerous and critical situations for the patient.

Causes of Pneumonia are, mostly, exposures to cold, north or northeast winds; particularly, when at the time one is over-excited by fast running, etc.; also, suppression of hemorıhages or habitual secretions; inhalation of obnoxious gases; irritating treatment of catarrh (I have seen inflammation of the lungs follow the use of hoarhound candy, in a simple cold, and hooping-cough). Pneumonia appears in its highest inflammatory degree in the north, while toward the south it gradually decreases in violence, but not in danger; because here the bilious complication occurs more frequently (*bilious pneumonia*), where bleeding is *particularly injurious.*

TREATMENT.—This disease requires quick and energetic action; and the first remedy to be given, under almost all circumstances, is

Aconite. In the chill, as well as the highest fever, in the commencement (either alone, in water dissolved, twelve globules to half a teacupful), every half hour a teaspoonful, until the fever is broken, and the pain and oppression in the chest are ameliorated; or in alternation with

Bryonia, when oppression and pain in the chest are very severe (resembling pleurisy—see that article); worse by every movement or cough; expectoration bloody, of a brick-dust-color; also, pains in the extremities; tongue is coated, often dry, with great thirst; constipation.

Administer the same as *Aconite,* only every hour or two hours a teaspoonful.

If after these two most important remedies the disease still seems unchecked, give, in six or eight hours afterward, if not better,

Phosphorus, in alternation with *Tartar emetic,* dissolved in water, the same as *Aconite* and *Bryonia,* every hour, or two hours, a teaspoonful, until three or four teaspoonfuls of each are taken; wait for the effect of these remedies, from eight to twelve hours, as frequently their effects are not seen immediately. If necessary, repeat both the above prescriptions, or choose among the following remedies, if the patient, in place of being better, has run into the *typhoid* or *hepatized* stage of the pneumonia.

The *typhoid* stage of pneumonia commences when the patient is restless, particularly at night; throws himself about and becomes quite delirious, or lies motionless on his back in a stupor; breathing quick and irregular; snoring with his eyes half closed, and rattling of mucus in his lungs; tongue dry, pulse quick and thread-like; skin dry, or covered with clammy sweat (See "Typhus Fever").

TREATMENT.—In the beginning of this state give

China. Particularly if the patient, in the early part of the disease, under allopathic advice, had been bled, or lost blood by other means, such as hemorrhage, or a fall or blow (in the latter case, in alternation with *Arnica*); or when the patient complains mostly of a *pressure* in the chest, stitches in the *breast* and *sides*, together with palpitation of the heart when breathing or coughing; beside, great weakness, fine, quick pulse and yellowish coated tongue. Administer two or three times, every two or three hours a dose (four glob.); then wait from four to six hours, after which recourse may be had to *Bryonia* and *Rhus tox.*, as prescribed in "Typhus Fever" (see this article). If the disease still progresses, it will be necessary to give

Opium (see this remedy in "Typhus Fever"); or

Arnica, under similar symptoms, but without delirium; or

Hyoscyamus (See "Typhus Fever"), if the cough is spasmodic or very irritating.

Belladonna (see "Typhus Fever"), when the oppression is very great.

Veratrum. If the pulse is very small and weak; extremities cold; delirium; vomiting and diarrhea; sinking; no sleep whatever.

Camphor and *Coffea,* in alternate doses, in a similar state, particularly if the patient is covered with cold perspiration.

Phosphoric acid. If after the patient has been relieved by the above remedies, there is yet diarrhea present. (See "Typhus Fever.")

Sulphur may be given once or twice, if the amelioration brought about by previous remedies seems not to be permanent; then return to those medicines again, which previously were the most efficacious.

Administration the same as in "Typhus Fever."

Hepatization, or the *second* stage in pneumonia, when infiltration of the lungs with coagulated lymph takes place, is indicated by greater difficulty of breathing, and a dull sound by percussion of those parts of the breast where the pain was the severest.

Treatment.—*Sulphur* has first to be given (twelve glob. dissolved in half a teacupful of water, every two or three hours a teaspoonful) four times; then wait from eight to twelve hours, and, if not better, give

Lachesis, *Lycopodium*, *Phosphorus*, one after the other, in the same manner as *Sulphur*, until better.

Arsenic and *China*, in alternation, in the same manner, when fetid expectoration, of a dirty, green color appears.

Application of Water.—In the different stages of this disease relieves greatly and accelerates the specific effect of the proper remedies. The wet bandage, frequently changed, is generally sufficient to afford relief in the inflammatory stage, mitigating the fever and preventing its return. During the typhoid stage or when hepatization has taken place, the wet sheet will accelerate the cure under the proper remedies.

Diet and Regimen.—As in fevers generally; but particularly as in "Typhus."

After-Diseases.—If pneumonia threatens to become *chronic*, or consumption ensues, see this article; when the patient expectorates clear matter, *China*, *Mercury*, *Sulphur*, *Stannum*, *Lachesis*, *Hepar*, *Lycopodium*, are the principal medicines to be given, as stated in "Consumption."

Pneumonia in infants and *children* up to two or three years of age is very frequent; in fact, every cold on their lungs affects them more or less in an inflammatory manner, and ought not to be neglected for a moment.

Beside heat, fever, thirst, dry mouth, there is quick, *oppressive breathing*, with *short cough, after* which *the child always cries:* these latter symptoms are a *sure sign* of inflammation of the lungs in children, and unless they are relieved or disappear (particularly the respiration is slower and regular), we must not feel secure in regard to the safety of the young patient.

TREATMENT.—The principal remedy is

Aconite. In solution or dry: half a teaspoonful, or two glob., every two or three hours, three or four times, or until better; after which, if necessary, give

Bryonia. In the same manner, if the cough is very bad; or

Belladonna. In the same manner, if the head is very hot at the time. If these remedies do not relieve in from twelve to twenty-four hours, give

Tartar emetic and *Phosphorus,* in alternation (ten glob. of each, dissolved in two teacups, each half full of water), every hour, alternately, half a teaspoonful, for twelve or twenty-four hours, until better; discontinue for the same length of time, and repeat afterward, if necessary; if, during that time, the child is very sleepless and restless, give

Coffea ^{cc}, and *Belladonna* ^{cc}, in alternation, a dose (three glob.) every hour, until better. Continue with this treatment for three or four days, and in the most severe cases it will prove successful.

If convulsions, or congestions to the head occur, see these articles, and treat accordingly.

APPLICATION OF WATER, see page 266.

DIET AND REGIMEN.—Keep the patient as quiet as possible; in a darkened chamber, if the head suffers; not too warm; if the child does not take the breast, give cold water freely, if thirsty; of solid food, crackers soaked in milk or water; neither broth nor meat; gruels are good.

Pneumonia in Old People. (*Pneumonia notha.*)

This disease shows itself in old people as follows: They become at once prostrated, having symptoms of a common cold, with a cough, chills, and fever; the cough is loose, and the expectoration white, yellow, slimy, and streaked with blood; the respiration quick and labored; pain in the breast, when drawing a long breath, mostly on a small spot; fever is not high; pulse soft but quick; cheeks slightly flushed; skin generally moist at night, without relief; during the day, the patient feels tolerably comfortable; the voice, however, is weak, almost in a whisper. As these symptoms do not *seem* to indicate any danger, the disease is frequently left to itself, but very often with the most fatal results; because paralysis of the lungs soon ensues, and death is inevitable.

TREATMENT.—*Aconite.* Every three hours a dose (six glob.) will be first necessary, three or four times, during the fever, after which give

Mercury. In the same manner; wait twelve hours, and then, if not better, in alternation with

Belladonna. Particularly when the cough becomes short and dry, and the breathing difficult and suffocating; if not better, give

Sulphur once or twice; afterward repeat *Mercury* and *Belladonna.*

Veratrum and *Arsenic.* If they sink very low; cold extremities, etc. (See "Typhoid Pneumonia.")

Tartar emet. and *Phosphorus.* If, with constant rattling in the lungs, paralysis threatens; alternately every half hour a dose (three or four glob.).

Compare, also, the remedies under "Pneumonia."

APPLICATION OF WATER; wet bandages around breast and stomach, and drinking moderate quantities of cold water, are recommended; also to excite perspiration in a slight degree between wet sheets.

Diet and Regimen.—The same as in "Pneumonia," only more nourishing as soon as the inflammatory symptoms have left in the least; the yolk of an egg with sugar; broth of beef with rice, etc. After-diseases, see "Consumption."

There is another disease, called *galloping consumption*, in which the inflammation of the lungs forms the most important part. This species of pneumonia occurs mostly in young people of florid complexion, at the time of development, and needs a separate article. (See "Galloping Consumption.")

It is evident, from the nature of pneumonia and the dignity of the organ affected, that a good homœopathic physician ought to be consulted, if he can be procured; but if this cannot be done, rely on the above rules and prescriptions.

Remarks on Pneumonia.

This disease may frequently be complicated with other diseases, such as inflammation of the pleura, heart, and brain; also, with bilious, rheumatic, or gastric symptoms; the treatment, however, does not vary from the above; beside, consult the respective articles.

Pleurisy. (*Pleuritis.*)

a. Real Pleurisy. (*Pleuritis serosa.*)
b. False Pleurisy. (*Pleuritis muscularis.*)

a. Real Pleurisy.

If the sac around the lungs (called pleura) becomes inflamed, we call it *real pleurisy;* this can be the case with or without inflammation of the lungs. If complicated with pneumonia or bronchitis, these articles must be consulted together with this chapter.

Diagnosis.—In real pleurisy the pain is preceded mostly by a chill and fever, as in pneumonia, but it does not produce so much general oppression in breathing as pneumonia; however, in pleurisy the pain is more severe on a fixed spot (mostly in one of the sides of the chest), from which it radiates; increased often to intolerance by deep inspiration or hard pressure between the ribs, where the pain is located; the breathing is, on this account, short, and the lying on the affected side impossible; if the back part of the pleura toward the spine is inflamed, the pains increase by moving the spine, and running up into the neck impede frequently the swallowing of food, with inclination to vomit, or produce real vomiting.

Fever is never wanting, but not so evident as in pneumonia; neither is the cough so distressing, but more a short and dry one, very seldom, with much expectoration of mucus.

This disease terminates frequently in the formation of lymphatic effusion, which result may be known by the following change of symptoms, different from the above real pleuritic ones: respiration becomes more anxious and short; the patient cannot now lie on the well side either, or, if he does, he feels in danger of suffocation, because the water presses over toward the well lung; by turning, which is very difficult, he feels something moving within the chest, like water; the fever becomes hectic; the urine is offensive, and has a sediment.

This description will be sufficient to distinguish pleurisy from pneumonia; but there is another form of pleurisy, the so-called

b. False Pleurisy. (*Stitch in the Side.*)

Which resembles the true or real pleurisy very much, yet is different in origin and location, as well as in termination.

DIAGNOSIS.—This false or spurious pleurisy, is not an inflammatory, but a rheumatic affection of the intercostal muscles, and occurs mostly in persons subject to rheumatism; it is preceded generally by pains in the neck, shoulders, and throat, as if from cold, without much of a chill, fever, or thirst; the pain in the side is worse by *exhaling;* in real pleurisy, worse by *inhaling; slight* pressure on the affected side increases the pain in real pleurisy, while only *hard* pressure with the fingers between the ribs increases it in false pleurisy, which has a *slight* cough only; in real pleurisy the cough is *dry* and *painful.*

TREATMENT. *a. Of Real Pleurisy.*—*Aconite* and *Bryonia.* First of all, in the same manner as described in "Pneumonia," for so long a time as the pain is very intense; if not better in thirty-six or forty hours, give

Sulphur. Twelve globules dissolved in half a teacupful of water, every two or three hours a teaspoonful, until four or six are taken, particularly if the fever continues with the painful oppression on the chest, yet the skin has become a little moist; this is the principal remedy, also, when effusion of plastic lymph is feared, or has taken place; it is well enough to give the patient even a dose (six glob.) of *Sulphur,* if *Aconite* or *Bryonia,* or both, have restored him so far as to be able to be out of bed. If *Aconite* ameliorates the pains, do not be in haste to give *Bryonia* immediately, but wait until the disease increases again; do the same in regard to *Bryonia.* In general, do not give another remedy as long as the former has shown a decided beneficial effect.

If the patient is sleepless and restless at night, give at any time *Coffea*$^{cc.}$, and *Belladonna*$^{cc.}$, in alternation, every hour a dose (four glob.), until better.

If the patient complains of lying hard on his side, in consequence of which he changes his position often; has cold hands and feet, yet feels hot inwardly; or if a short, dry cough troubles him very much, particularly by increasing the stitching pain in his side, give *Arnica* once or twice, every two hours a dose (four glob.).

If the real pleurisy is complicated with pneumonia (*pleuro-*

pneumonia), give the remedies described under "Pneumonia," such as, *Belladonna, Rhus tox., Lachesis, Sulphur, Phosphorus, Lycopodium, China, Sepia,** according to the symptoms indicating their use.

N. B. As these pleuro-pneumonias are frequently of a *bilious* character, the remedies for *bilious* or *bilious rheumatic* fever must be consulted.

TREATMENT. *b. Of False Pleurisy* (*Stitch in the side*).—If there is any fever, give first once or twice a dose (four glob.) of *Aconite*, every hour and a half one dose; after which administer the principal remedy:

Arnica. Every two hours a dose (six glob.), and in alternation with *Apis mellifica* or

Pulsatilla. If the patient is not better in two hours; but if he is relieved, scarcely anything more is needed, but rest and perspiration in bed. In two or three days afterward one dose of *Sulphur* (four glob.) may be given to complete the cure.

Nux vomica. Stitch in the side, with painful sensibility of the external parts of the chest on pressing between the ribs; worse on taking deep inspiration or by any movement.

If at any time the patient becomes feverish, with pains in limbs, side, and head, give *Bryonia* and *Rhus tox.* (See "Rheumatic Bilious Fever.")

APPLICATION OF WATER.—See page 266.

DIET AND REGIMEN.—As in fever generally. In false pleurisy frequently a mustard draught, or some other heating substance—for instance, a bag of heated salt—will relieve, and may be used with advantage.

* *Sepia* once cured an old man of a most violent attack of *pleuro-pneumonia* on the left side, caused by a metastasis of an inflammation of the liver, which had been subdued, but not cured, a few days previous, by excessive allopathic blood-letting; *China* had preceded the *Sepia*, without decided effect.

Diseases of the Heart.

a. *Inflammation of the Heart.* (*Carditis.*)

It is well that inflammation of the heart does not occur frequently, as its course is very rapid and dangerous, and its diagnosis difficult.

Diagnosis.—The prominent symptoms are *violent* pains, mostly *burning* or *cutting*, in the region of the heart and toward the pit of the stomach; great oppression in breathing, which shows itself in the distorted and anxious features of the patient; the pulsation of the heart is *violent* and *irregular*, while the pulse on the wrist is small, frequent, and trembling; the patient prefers lying *quietly on the back;* sometimes there is delirium, difficulty of swallowing, fainting spells, vomiting, starting in the sleep.

Causes.—This disease is caused mostly by taking cold in drinking cold water when the body is heated; also, by wounds, blows, etc.; the most frequent cause, however, is acute rheumatism, particularly in the knees. See "Rheumatism of the Heart."

It must be well understood that not every palpitation of the heart is inflammation of the heart; the latter has always an agonizing feeling of oppression and pain.

Treatment and Administration.—In every case give first *Aconite*, as directed in "Pneumonia;" afterward *Bryon.*, *Nux Vomica*, *Cocculus*, *Arsenic*, *Pulsatilla*, and *Cannabis sativa*, at intervals of from two to four or six hours, until better; each remedy, when used, may be dissolved in water (twelve globules to half a teacupful), and every half hour a teaspoonful given; but, if possible, procure the advice of a homœopathic physician *immediately*.

Application of Water.—Wet compresses on the chest in the region of the heart will be beneficial, but they must be frequently changed; the water which the patient drinks may be very cold. If the pains are very severe, and the extremities become cold, a warm foot-bath may be applied.

b. *Palpitation of the Heart.* (*Palpitatio cordis.*)

Young people in their growing years, as well as old persons of high age, are troubled with this disease; the former from development and congestion, the latter from contraction, ossification, and want of blood. Between these two extremes of age, persons sometimes are taken with it by violent emotion of the mind, by the use of ardent spirits, or by constitutional predisposition, particularly when inclined to be affected by rheumatism, which latter mostly causes the chronic palpitation of the heart. In pregnancy this disease is frequent, as, also, in persons of a plethoric habit, and at the time of change of life, or during floodings, in consequence of loss of blood.

If it is dependent on organic disorders of the heart, as polypus, ossification, etc.—as, also, in the chronic form—we advise strongly to apply in time to a homœopathic physician, as frequently a permanent cure may be effected.

TREATMENT.—If caused by *fright: Opium* or *Coffea.*

By *sudden joy: Coffea.*

By *fear* or *anguish: Veratrum.*

By *disappointment: Aconite, Chamomile, Ignatia, Nux vom.*

By *congestion of blood,* or *plethora, Aconite, Belladonna, Coffea, Ferrum, Lachesis, Aurum, Phosphorus, Opium, Sulphur.*

By *loss of blood,* or *other debilitating losses: China, Phosphoric acid, Nux vomica, Veratrum.*

If it is present in *nervous persons, hysterical females,* etc.; *Coffea, Ignatia, Chamomile, Cocculus, Nux vomica, Lachesis, Pulsatilla, Veratrum.*

In *young, growing people: Aconite, Pulsat.*

In *old, decrepid people: Arsenic, Lachesis,* particularly when with temporary dimness of sight.

After the suppression of an eruption: *Arsenic, Lachesis, Sulphur.*

For ameliorating the frequent attacks in *chronic palpitation* of the heart, the most suitable medicines are, *Pulsat.*, *Arsenic*, *Lachesis*, *Aconite*, *Sulphur*, *Phosphorus*, *Aurum*.

Administration.—Dissolve of the selected remedy twelve globules in half a teacupful of water, and take from one to twelve hours a teaspoonful, according to the severity of the case; or, if traveling, take of the medicine a dose (four glob.) from one to six or twelve hours; if not better after from one to twelve hours, select another remedy.

Application of Water varies according to the character of this disease. If it is caused by plethora, cold bandages around the chest will be indicated, at the same time that the feet may be put in warm water. If caused by loss of blood or other debilitating influences, a cold ablution will invigorate the system and support the effect of the proper remedies. In almost all cases of palpitation of the heart, a lukewarm foot-bath in the evening will be found beneficial.

Diet and Regimen.—Diet as usual in chronic diseases.—Sleep as quiet as possible during the administration of the medicine; be careful always to have dry, warm feet; avoid getting wet by exposure to rains, etc. Young people must abstain from eating much in the evening, but drink freely of cold water.

c. *Rheumatism of the Heart.* (*Rheumatismus cordis.*)

Diagnosis.—In this disease the palpitation of the heart is only *one* of the symptoms; the principal symptom is a sensation of weight in the region of the heart, with occasional stitches through it; beside, tearing pains in the external muscles of the chest and in those of the left upper-arm, either constantly or only periodically. With the palpitation of the heart and its violent action, the character of the pulse on the wrist does not harmonize; the latter is invariably weak, small, and contracted.

Causes.—This disease appears mostly in young persons of both sexes at the age of development, at which time it is dangerous; if neglected or badly treated, the heart will inflame or increase in size. It is also frequently caused by the translation of acute or inflammatory rheumatism (*see this article*) to the heart; the treatment in this case remains the same; it is favorable, if the rheumatic symptoms reappear in the extremities.

TREATMENT.—The principal remedies are: *Aconite, Arnica, Bellad., Bryon., Spigelia, Pulsat., Arsenicum, Lachesis.*

Aconite. Palpitation of the heart, with great anguish, feverish heat, particularly in the face; the heart beats rapidly, while the pulse is slow and intermittent. Stitches and oppressive aching in the region of the heart, as if from a heavy load; the patient cannot breathe well in an erect position.

Arnica. Stitches in the heart from the left to the right side, with fainting fits, quivering of the heart, with a pain as if it was squeezed together.

Belladonna. Palpitation of the heart with intermitting pulse; great anguish about the heart; tremor of the heart with anguish and pain; oppression of the chest. (After *Aconite,* or before *Lachesis.*)

Spigelia. Tumultuous pulsation of the heart with suffocative sensation and spasms of the chest, increasing in a sitting posture and bending the chest forward; tremulous motion of the heart. (In alternation with *Pulsatilla.*)

Pulsatilla. Palpitation of the heart with great anguish, clouded sight and impeded respiration, particularly when lying on the left side; anxiety, pressure, and burning sensation in the heart.

Bryonia. Respiration impeded by stitches in the chest with palpitation of the heart and violent oppression (after *Aconite,* where acute rheumatism of the extremities had been transferred to the heart).

Arsenicum. Violent palpitation of the heart with great anguish and restlessness; great heat and burning of the chest, with cold extremities; in such cases, in alternation with *Veratrum;* or with *Lachesis,* when the pulse becomes weaker and the pulsation irregular.

Lachesis. Irregularity of the pulsation; great anguish about the heart with heaviness on the chest, in rheumatism; very weak.

Administration.—Dissolve twelve globules of the selected remedy in half a teacupful of water, and give every half hour or hour a teaspoonful until relief is obtained; and if this is not the case within one or two hours, select another remedy and give it in the same manner. Externally apply a mustard poultice on the breast, put the feet in hot water and cover the patient well.

Application of Water.—See page 274.

Diet and Regimen, as in fevers. Apply to a homœopathic physician as soon as possible.

Congestion of the Chest. (*Plethora pectoris.*)

Congestion or *determination of blood* to the chest is a frequent complaint in young people, during the time of the development of their systems, and in persons of a phthisical habit. It ought never to be treated by bloodletting, even if this means relieves for the time, as it does not remove the disposition or the bad consequences, in the system, but has a tendency, if once resorted to for palliation, to augment the difficulties for a final cure, rendering the lungs weaker by each successive attack. The homœopathic remedies, on the contrary, relieve in a different manner, and in a much shorter time.

Diagnosis.—Great fullness, weight, and pressure in the chest; more or less palpitation of the heart, with oppression, short and sighing breathing; cold hands and feet, and anxious look; sometimes a hacking, short cough.

Treatment.—*Aconite.* Particularly in plethoric females during menstruation; *violent oppression,* with palpitation of the heart; shortness of breath; dry cough; heat and thirst.

Belladonna. If *Aconite* does not suffice, and if the head is congested at the same time. See "Congestion to the Head."

Nux vomica. Heat and burning in the chest, more at night, with sleeplessness and agitation; or fullness and throbbing in the chest, with palpitation; worse in the open air; clothes feel too tight around the chest.

China. In consequence of debilitating losses, as of blood, etc.; violent oppression, with great anguish; loss of sight; palpitation of the heart; cannot breathe with the head low.

Phosphorus. Violent oppression, with heaviness, fullness, and tension in the chest; palpitation of the heart, which is felt in the throat.

Mercury. After *Aconite,* if there is anxious oppression for breath, with a desire to take a long breath; heat and burning in the chest; cough, with expectoration of mucus streaked with blood.

Pulsatilla and *Bryonia.* In alternation, before menstruation, or when this has stopped suddenly; also, when the piles have been suppressed; or when there is ebullition of blood in the chest, with external heat.

Spongia. When movement increases the anguish, and produces danger of suffocation, nausea, fainting, and prostration; particularly in persons subject to sick-headache, or other nervous affections of the head, which frequently attack the chest in this manner.

Sulphur. After *Nux vomica* or *Pulsatilla,* if necessary.

ADMINISTRATION, DIET, and REGIMEN, same as in "Palpitation of the Heart."

APPLICATION OF WATER.—See page 274.

HEMORRHAGE OF THE LUNGS. (*Hæmoptysis, Pneumorrhagia.*)

Spitting or *coughing* up of *blood* is generally considered by persons such a dangerous, and, for the life of the patient, fatal symptom, that they lose, when it occurs, all presence of mind, frequently incapacitating them for the right action in the case; yet not all the hemorrhages of the lungs are alike in their character; some are dangerous, it is true, but most of them yield readily to the proper remedies, and some even cease of themselves. It will be necessary to distinguish well between them, and act accordingly, not in too great haste, but in the right manner; in this way, time is saved. Moreover, we will see hereafter that the most dangerous kinds of bleedings from the lungs leave ample time to provide means, while the milder forms take more by surprise, thereby causing more fear than injury, with the exception of one form, the so-called "Apoplexy of the Lungs," which is easily distinguished by marked symptoms. Be careful to examine whether the blood coughed or hawked up is from the lungs, or merely from the nose or palate.

DIAGNOSIS. — Without going into the distinction as to the different places in the lungs and windpipe from whence the blood may issue, as this would be without practical advantage, we will give now the qualitative difference of hæmoptysis, which has the highest practical bearing. We distinguish two varieties:

1. The *active* or *idiopathic* hæmoptysis, caused by congestion of the lungs, or mechanical injury; this is the most frequent and least dangerous.

2. The *passive* or *symptomatic* hæmoptysis, caused by the ulcerative process in consumption, which gradually consumes the substance of the lungs (*if not arrested*), and causes the rupture of larger blood-vessels; although this is the most dangerous form, as it is caused by a destructive and sometimes incurable disease, yet it does not occur frequently, and even then its appearance may be expected and measures taken accordingly.

First. *Active hemorrhage of the lungs* depends always on congestion of blood to the lungs, which is sometimes constitutional, at other times caused by external circumstances, such as quick running, violent exercise of any kind, lifting, etc., the frequent inhaling of injurious dust, such as from lime, gypsum, or plaster of Paris, tobacco, flour, or metal filings, or of obnoxious gases, such as from nitric and sulphuric acid.

Beside these causes, it sometimes appears epidemically, mostly at the time of the equinoxes, on account of the rapid changes in the temperature of the atmosphere; the abuse of spiritous liquors is a frequent cause of hemorrhage of the lungs; also, suppression of discharges of blood from other organs, as stoppage of the menses, sudden disappearance of the piles, etc.; excessive growing and consequent weakness of the chest predisposes to it, as in general young or middle-aged persons are more liable to it. It occurs in attacks, accompanied with more or less fever, frequently of an intermittent type, worse toward night.

This form of hemorrhage of the lungs presents itself in the most various degrees, from the least spitting of blood to a violent effusion; the highest degree, which really endangers life immediately, is the *apoplectic hemorrhage* (apoplexia pulmon.) of the lungs, where all the symptoms of an apoplectic fit are present; the patient loses his consciousness, looks as if he was suffocated, eyes protrude out of their sockets, bloody mucus issues from the mouth.

Treatment. — The first thing necessary in severe cases is to let the patient keep as quiet as possible, in a half-sitting, half-lying posture; he must remain perfectly quiet, without speaking or being spoken to, except when it is indispensably necessary; if no homœopathic medicine is at hand, give every five or ten minutes a teaspoonful of table-salt in water, but cautiously, that it may not make him cough; or, if *sulphuric acid* is convenient to be had, drop five or ten drops into a tumbler full of water, and give a teaspoonful every five or ten minutes, until the severest bleeding ceases. If homœopathic medicine is at hand, give directly,

Aconite. Twelve globules dissolved in half a teacupful of water, every ten or twenty minutes a teaspoonful, until the severest bleeding ceases; afterward administer it at longer intervals, from three to six hours. This remedy suits always at first, but particularly when there is ebullition of blood in the chest, with a fullness and a burning pain; palpitation of the heart; anxious looks, with paleness of the face; profuse expectoration of blood at intervals, provoked by a slight cough. Try this remedy at least for two hours; if not better, give

Ipecac. When there yet remains a taste of blood in the mouth; frequent, short cough; expectoration of mucus streaked with blood; *nausea* and weakness; or,

Arsenic. When there is yet palpitation of the heart, with great anguish, dry heat, and desire to leave the bed; it is particularly applicable for drunkards after *Hyoscyamus* has been given.

Opium. Often in the most serious cases, especially in persons addicted to spiritous liquors; or when there is expectoration of thick, frothy blood; cough worse after swallowing; oppression and anguish; weak voice, drowsiness and anxious starts; cold extremities, and heat in the chest.

Nux vomica. Suits well after *Opium*, *Ipecac.*, or *Arsenic;* particularly when there is cough, affecting the head, caused by tickling in the chest; or when the hemorrhage was caused by a fit of passion, by taking cold, or suppression of piles. *Sulphur* suits well after it.

China. If the patient has already lost much blood; or when the cough is violent, hollow, dry, and painful, with taste of blood in the mouth; shivering and flushes of heat; weakness, faintness, cloudiness of sight, roaring in the head.

Ferrum. After *China*, if this has in severe cases relieved, yet there is great fatigue after talking; slight cough, with expectoration of scanty, bright red blood, with pain between the shoulder-blades; difficulty of breathing.

Hyoscyamus. Dry cough at night, with expectoration of blood; frequent waking with a start; particularly in drunkards, after *Opium* and *Nux vomica,* and followed by *Arsenic.*

Dulcamara. Tickling cough, from cold; the hemorrhage was preceded for some time by a loose cough.

Carbo veg. Hemorrhage, with violent *burning* pain in the chest, in persons susceptible to changes of weather, or who have taken much calomel.

Pulsatilla. In obstinate cases, when *black* and *coagulated* blood is expectorated, more in the morning or night, particularly in timid persons, or in females when caused by suppression of the menses.

Arnica. In slight hemorrhages of *black* and coagulated blood, with stitching, burning pains and heat in the chest, palpitation of the heart, difficulty of breathing; or caused by *mechanical injuries, fall, blow, lifting,* leaning against a table by studying, sewing; or when the expectoration is clear, frothy, mixed with pure lumps of matter; hacking cough, from tickling under the breast-bone; pains in the limbs, as if they had been beaten. It is often administered in alternation with *Aconite.*

Belladonna. Cough from tickling in the throat, with hemorrhage; sensation of fullness, as if from blood in the chest, with pressing or shooting pains, worse when moving; is especially suitable for hemorrhages of the lungs in females of full habit, at the change of life, and then in alternation with *Aconite.*

In very serious cases, *Aconite, China, Ipecac.,* and *Opium* will be found most efficacious.

For the bad consequences of pulmonary hemorrhage, such as weakness, cough, etc., give *Carbo veg.* and *China.* If possible, procure the advice of a physician immediately.

Administration of the above remedies, in very severe cases, the same as in *Aconite,* stated above; in less severe cases, or mere spitting of blood, give every six or twelve hours a dose (four glob.) until better, or until another remedy is necessary.

Application of Water in the form of wet compresses on the chest is recommended; sometimes a cold foot-bath will be necessary, the feet being rubbed constantly while in the bath.

Diet and Regimen.—The patient must be kept cool; his drinks, for two weeks, at least, must be cool, not spiritous or exciting, but more slimy, such as rice and barley water, water with raspberry syrup, lemonade, etc. If the feet are cold, put them in warm water, mixed with ashes or mustard.

In *apoplectic* hemorrhage of the lungs, give *Aconite* immediately, same as above; if not better in twenty or thirty minutes, *Opium* and then *Ipecac.;* afterward, if necessary, *Belladonna* or *Lachesis,* in the same manner. Put the feet in hot water, with mustard; also the hands, if they are cold. Send immediately for medical aid.

Second. *Passive* hemorrhage of the lungs, or rupture of a blood-vessel in tubercular consumption, requires principally *Aconite, China, Pulsatilla, Arsenic, Lycopodium,* to be given in the same manner as described under active hemorrhage. See, also, "Pulmonary Consumption."

Diet and Regimen the same as above.

Asthma.

As this disease is well known in regard to its symptoms, we will only mention here that distinction in its character which has a practical bearing. There are two kinds of asthma, as regards the cough and expectoration of mucus in an attack; it is either a *dry* or *humid.* The former is more sudden and violent in its attacks; has only slight cough and expectoration, but great difficulty of breathing. The attack of the latter, or humid asthma, proceeds slowly—has a severe cough, with gradually increasing and afterward copious expectoration of mucus, which relieves greatly. Asthma in itself, is not a dangerous, but a very distressing disease, sometimes hereditary, but oftener acquired; its different causes will be enumerated below, with their respective remedies attached. In general it is curable, although it takes a comparatively longer time than most other chronic diseases require, particularly when it is constitutional. A radical cure must only be undertaken by a skillful homœopathic physician. We subjoin below the treatment for the attack itself, to alleviate temporarily, advising the patient, at the same time, not to omit any favorable opportunity by which he may be allowed to place himself under the care of a physician, for the final cure of the disease.

TREATMENT.—When caused by *congestion of blood* to the chest (see this article): *Aconite, Bellad., Nux vom., Phosphorus, Pulsat., Spongia, Sulph.*

By *derangement of the menstruation: Bellad., Cocculus, Bryon., Pulsat., Veratrum, Sulph.*

By *vapors of Sulph.* (brimstone): *Pulsat.*

By *vapors of Arsenic* or *Copper: Ipecac., Hepar, Mercury.*

By a *chill: Aconite, Ipecac., Bryon., Bellad.*

By *a fit of passion: Nux vom., Chamomile.*

By *fright: Opium, Ignatia, Aconite, Bellad., Veratrum.*

By *sudden joy: Coffea, Aconite.*

By a *suppressed catarrh,* or *cold in the head: Ipecac., Nux vom., Arsenic, Apis mellifica.*

By *dust* from *stone* or *flour: Calcarea, Silicea, Sulph.*

By *suppression of piles: Nux vom., Sulph., Arsenic.*

By *flatulency: China, Chamomile, Nux vom., Sulph.*

If it is present in *children: Aconite, Bellad., Ipecac., Chamomile, Bryon., Tartar emet., Sambucus.*

In *hysterical women: Coffea, Ignatia, Pulsat., Ipecac., Chamomile, Bellad.*

In *aged persons: Arsenic, Lachesis, Opium.*

When it is *constitutional: Ipecac., Arsenic, Sulph.*

When *dry,* or without much expectoration (similar to *cramps* in the chest): *Cocculus, Cuprum, Bellad., Nux vom. Sambucus.*

When *humid* or *moist*, with considerable expectoration of mucus: *Ipecac.*, *Arsenic*, *China*, *Pulsat.*, *Sulph.*

In the above tabular view, we have arranged the different kinds of asthma, as regards their origin and appearance; so that, in search for a remedy, the number of remedies to be looked for is reduced to very few. Their distinguishing symptoms are given in detail below, and their administration at the end of the article. The principal and first remedy in most all attacks is *Ipecac.*, after the administration of which one may proceed with more calmness to find out the next best remedy, by comparing carefully its symptoms with those of the case present.

SYMPTOMATIC DETAIL.—*Ipecac.* Difficulty of breathing; *nocturnal paroxysms of suffocation, spasmodic constriction of the throat, rattling in the chest, from an accumulation of mucus;* short, dry cough, *great anguish*, cries, agitation, fear of death; alternately either redness and heat, or paleness, coldness, and ghastliness of the face; sometimes nausea, with cold perspiration on the forehead; breathing at the same time *anxiously* and *rapidly*, with moaning and rattling. After it follows well *Arsenic*, *Bryonia*, or *Apis mellifica*.

Arsenic. In all cases of acute or chronic asthma, with an accumulation of thick phlegm; difficult breathing after a meal; oppression of the chest and want of breath, rendered almost intolerable by any motion, such as walking, going up stairs, laughing, etc.; constriction of the chest and throat; *suffocating fits*, more at *night;* panting, wheezing, as if *dying* with *cold perspiration;* these paroxysms grow lighter on the appearance of a cough, with expectoration of mucus, or of viscid saliva; the attacks render the patient *very weak;* burning pain in the chest. Suits well after *Ipecac.*, and before *Sulphur*, or *Apis mellifica*.

Nux vomica. Asthma, resembling that of *Arsenic*, only the spasmodic constriction is felt worse *in the lower part of the chest*, where even loose clothes seem to be too tight; *short*, dry *cough*, sometimes with a little blood; congestion of the chest (*see this article*); asthma, better by *lying on the back;* occasionally turning, or sitting up; suits well for persons addicted to the use of spiritous liquors, or after *Arsenic*, or before *Sulphur*.

Pulsatilla. Asthma in children, after suppression of a miliary eruption; in weak, timid females, after cessation of menstruation, or after having taken cold; *choking, as from the vapors of Sulphur; paroxysm of suffocation, with deadly anguish, palpitation of the heart*, and spasmodic constriction of the throat or chest; worse at night, or when lying horizontally, or when moving; better in the open air; expectoration, with much mucus, streaked with blood, which sometimes is coagulated; with a feeling of fullness and pressure of the chest.

China. Under similar symptoms as *Pulsatilla*, after which it suits well, if there is, with the asthma, *great weakness*, and *easy perspiration in sleep*.

Sambucus. Asthma, similar to *China*, but more in children (see "Asthma in children"); when there is *much perspiration;* suits well after *Ipecac.*

Sulphur. Almost in any acute or chronic attack of asthma, if several other remedies were insufficient. After *Sulphur*, if necessary, select carefully another remedy. It suits principally when there are paroxysms of asthma, almost *suffocating*, mostly at *night*, with *fullness* and *weariness*, *burning*, or *spasms* in the chest; expectoration of white mucus, detached with difficulty, sometimes bloody; constriction and pain in the breast-bone; bluish redness of the face; short respiration, and inability to speak.

Phosphorus. Asthma worse in the evening or during *movement;* attack of *suffocation* in the night, as if from paralysis of the lungs (in alternation with *Tartar emetic*); congestion of blood to the chest, with stitches, and fullness or sensation of heat to the throat, and palpitation of the heart (in alternation with *Belladonna*) phthisical habit.

Tartar emetic. Asthma in *old persons* and *children* particularly when there are *choking, retching,* and paroxysms of *suffocation* in the evening, with *rattling* in the chest, and wheezing (in alternation with *Phosphorus,* see "Inflammation of the Lungs").

Aconite. Asthma in sensitive persons, young, and of plethoric habit, easily excited by mental emotions. In children, especially, when they cough *at night spasmodically,* as if they would *suffocate;* or with congestion to the head, with vertigo; cough with expectoration of blood.

Belladonna. Asthma in children (see "Croupy Cough"), or in *plethoric women* at the critical period; congestion to the lungs, with stitches under the breast-bone, and fullness in the chest; *dry cough at night;* anxious moaning; respiration, sometimes *deep,* at other times *short* and *rapid;* constriction of the throat, as if to suffocate, with loss of consciousness and relaxation of all the muscles.

Bryonia. Asthma, worse by *motion* and in the *night,* with pain in the chest; breathing like that under *Belladonna;* suits well after *Ipecacuanha,* or when it arises from suppressed eruptions.

Coffea. Asthmatical breathing from sudden joy; short, dry cough.

Opium. Suffocating cough, with bluish-red face; deep, rattling, respiration, especially when fright was the cause.

Chamomile. Asthma in children, after taking cold (see "Croupy Cough"), or when the hypochondriacal region is swollen, painful to the touch; crying, and drawing up of the thighs; asthma caused *by passion.*

Cocculus. Asthma of hysterical women, especially when they complain of constriction of the throat and chest, with oppression; worse at night; congestion of the lungs in nervous persons (in alternation with *Belladonna*).

Ignatia. Asthma after fright or indignation, especially in women; choking and constriction in the pit of the neck, as if from the vapors of *Sulphur; want of air in walking*, and *cough when resting;* short spasmodic cough.

Spongia. Want of breath, and paroxysms of suffocation after every movement, with fatigue; rush of blood to the head and chest; heat in the face; respiration wheezing, deep, or slow, as if from weakness (*nervous asthma* in persons who are habitually addicted to neuralgic affections).

Cuprum. In hysterical women, after fright or anger, or before or during the menses; *spasms* and *oppression* in the chest; worse on speaking or going up stairs; short, spasmodic cough.

Veratrum. Paroxysm of suffocation when rising up, during movement, especially before the menses; coldness of the face and extremities; faint pulse and cold perspiration. Suits well after *Ipecac.*, *Arsenic*, or *China.*

Lachesis. Slow and wheezing, or short respiration; worse after eating; paroxysms of *suffocation when lying down*, especially in persons suffering from water on the chest. (Suits well after *Arsenic.*)

Calcarea carb. In chronic asthma, with *frequent dry cough;* worse *at night;* or caused by the habitual inhalation of dust.

Silicea. In chronic asthma, caused by the inhalation of stone-dust; oppression worse when lying on the back, when running, or coughing.

Administration.—Dissolve twelve glob. of the selected remedy in half a teacupful of water, and give, in severe cases, every half hour; in less severe cases, every two or three hours, and in chronic cases, twice a day a teaspoonful, until three or four are given. If better, discontinue until the symptoms are worse again; if not better, prepare and give the next remedy in the same manner. In very small children, give one or two glob. of the medicine at the same intervals, dry, on the tongue.

Application of Water.—The wet bandage around breast and abdomen during the night will be beneficial; to prevent an attack the patient must wash frequently in cold water, and exercise afterward in the open air; constipation is relieved by cold injections and drinking freely of cold water.

DIET AND REGIMEN.—Persons suffering from chronic asthma, ought to abstain from coffee, meat, and greasy substances almost altogether, and live mostly on farinaceous diet, such as gruels, etc.

Sometimes, in very severe attacks, the burning of a piece of paper, soaked in a solution of saltpeter, and filling the chamber of the patient with its smoke, will relieve; or smoking tobacco, or gympsum-weed (stramonium).

Asthma of Millar.

See "Children-Diseases."

DROPSY IN THE CHEST. (*Hydrothorax.*)

This disease appears mostly in consequence of previous diseases, either acute or chronic, and is too dangerous in its course and results to be managed by domestic treatment alone. Skillful medical aid is indispensable; yet we will briefly notice its symptoms, and some few remedies which mitigate its immediate distresses.

DIAGNOSIS.—We distinguish an acute and chronic dropsy of the chest; the principal distinguishing feature of both kinds is, the difficulty of breathing, when moving, particularly going up stairs, or lying with the head low; swelling of the feet in the evening, and of the eyelids in the morning; thirst for water, yet scanty urine.

The *acute dropsy* of the chest occurs mostly in young people after eruptive fevers, such as scarlet fever, measles (see *these diseases*), or after the suppression of other eruptions by salves, ointments, etc.

The *chronic dropsy* of the chest occurs mostly in old age, or in persons addicted to the habitual use of ardent spirits.

TREATMENT.—To alleviate the difficulty of breathing, and render the patient more comfortable, give *Arsenic* (twelve

25

glob. dissolved in half a teacupful of water), every hour a teaspoonful, until the judicious advice of a homœopathic physician can be obtained. Beside *Apis mellifica, Bryonia, Carbo veg., Laches., Merc., Spige., Acon., Sulph.*, are beneficial *Digit.*, in decoction, and *Aspar.* are strongly recommended.

Application of Water.—The wet sheet, with its consequent perspiration, will support the action of the proper remedies very much.

Pulmonary Consumption. (*Phthisis Pulmonalis.*)

We distinguish several forms of this disease, the most frightful destroyer of human life and happiness; but, as its treatment would be too complicated for a work of this kind, we would advise our readers to apply, in time, to a homœopathic physician; as consumption, in its beginning, is in most cases curable.

Diagnosis. — If some of the following symptoms appear, we advise to seek medical aid: constant hacking cough, either dry, or with an expectoration of a frothy mucus; shortness of breath, pain in the chest, derangement of the stomach, hectic fever, chilliness followed by flashes of heat, burning in the hands and soles of the feet, night-sweats; circumscribed redness of the cheeks during the fever, but pale cheeks at other times. The so-called *tubercular* consumption consists in the softening of the small tubercles, which are in the lungs frequently for years, without disturbing health, when they remain in their compact state; their softening, however, produces irritation and ulceration of the lungs. In the beginning, this process can be repressed, and the patient saved.

The *galloping* consumption is peculiar to young persons, in their growing years, or after debilitating diseases, and requires the most careful attention of a physician. It is very rapid, and is rightly called *galloping;* as it is most acute, sometimes even infectious, on that account. *Aconite, Hyoscyamus*, are remedies, frequently useful in this species of consumption, to allay the high fever and restlessness, and particularly for the dry, short, irritating cough and shortness of breath, with great weakness in the night.

Under *scrofulous* consumption, we understand an ulceration of the lungs, caused by the transfer of scrofulous affections from other parts of the system, such as swellings of the glands of the neck, etc., and all other more specific diseases, such as syphilis, cancer, etc.; also, when eruptive fevers fall with their fatal decision on the lungs, and there produce ulceration.

Application of Water in this disease is to be made very cautiously and ought not to be instituted except under the advice of a competent physician; in the so-called tubercular consumption the use of water is not beneficial; and as it is very difficult for laymen to decide between the different forms of consumption, we must advise them not to trust their own judgment but seek proper medical advice at once.

As this subject is so extensive and important to all, we refer our readers to a separate work, entitled "Consumption treated homœopathically," by A. C. Becker, M. D.

Contusion of the Chest by a Fall or Blow.

When the chest, externally or internally, is injured by a fall or blow, apply tincture of *Arnica* externally, as directed under "*Sprains*," and internally give *Aconite*, and *Arnica*, alternately, in solution, as directed under "Hemorrhage of the Lungs," until the patient is better; if, after two or three days, the fever still continues, with an ulcerative pain in the chest, give *Pulsatilla;* and in alternation with *Mercury*, if there is a heavy, thick, yellow mucus expectorated; the latter remedy, however, in exchange with *China*, if night-sweats occur, and derangement of the stomach, bad appetite still continues, with sleeplessness and fever.

Diet and Regimen.—The same as under "External Injuries."

CHAPTER XIV.

AFFECTIONS OF THE STOMACH AND BOWELS.

Want of Appetite. (*Anorexia.*)

Most diseases, particularly those of the bowels and those of an inflammatory character, produce loss of appetite, which, in such cases, is more beneficial than otherwise; as it prevents the suffering system from being burdened with nourishment, at a time when the organs for its digestion and use are out of order. This applies to most of the acute, and to a great many of the chronic diseases. When these have disappeared by the use of proper remedies, the appetite returns of itself. But sometimes persons complain of loss of appetite without any apparent cause; in which case, it mostly proceeds from a derangement of the nerves of the stomach. For such patients, it is of no permanent advantage to use stimulating drinks or food, such as bitters, mustard, or coffee. These things only create an artificial appetite, never removing the cause of the disease. The best remedy, which is applicable in almost all cases of loss of appetite, is *cold water*, externally in ablutions and bathing, and internally freely drank at any time in the day and evening; in large quantities, before, during, and after meals, etc., with the precaution, not to be overheated at the time. Beside this dietetic remedy, as it were, the following remedies are recommended: to be used according to directions given in "Dyspepsia." — These remedies are *Nux vomica, Chamomile, China, Antimon., Ipecac Bryonia, Lachesis, Hepar, Arnica, Sulphur*

2. Morbid Appetite. (*Bulimy.*)

A morbid, craving, or voracious appetite, manifests itself in consequence of another disease present in the system, such as worm affections, dyspepsia, etc.; or it frequently is the necessary result of severe loss of strength, after violent, debilitating diseases. In every case it consists in a weakness and derangement of the nerves of the stomach, and is treated in the respective diseases of which it is generally a concomitant symptom.

We will here only indicate some of these affections, with the remedies attached, which arrangement will be particularly useful. For their application and administration, see the respective chapters of these diseases.

If there exists a craving for food in

Worm affections: Hyoscya., Cina, Merc., Silicea, Spigelia.

Pregnant women: Nux vomica, Sepia, Petroleum, Natrum muriaticum.

Convalescence after *violent diseases,* or *loss of fluids: China, Veratrum.*

Dyspepsia, where unnatural hunger is present: *China, Veratrum, Nux vom., Sulphur, Bryonia, Ignatia, Mercury, Pulsatilla, Lachesis, Lycopodium.*

In satisfying an unnatural appetite, care ought to be taken not to overload the stomach. Frequent, but moderate meals, are preferable.

3. Dyspepsia, or Weak Stomach.

Diagnosis.—Dyspepsia is generally characterized by weakness of digestion, with loss of appetite, slight or irregular appetite, painful and disordered stomach, flatulency, sour risings, ill humor, drowsiness after a meal, sometimes vomiting of acid, or mucus, secreted in great quantities in the digestive organs.

Causes.—The causes of this disease are as numerous as the symptoms vary, under which it shows itself in different constitutions and periods of life. A principal cause lies in the irregularity of the diet: eating too much, too rich, or too indigestible food; using stimulating drinks, tea, coffee, liquors, to an excess, and at an unreasonable time; eating too quickly, or fasting too long between meals; studying or laboring mentally too intensely, or after a full meal; this is particularly the case in our country, where merchants are in the habit of confining themselves to their arduous business too closely after full dinners, when a few hours' complete rest, bodily and mentally, would be of the greatest benefit to them; lastly the immoderate use of tobacco, especially in the way of chewing, the use of such deleterious medicines as calomel, etc., by which weak stomach, or dyspepsia, is produced.

TREATMENT.—Avoiding the above-named causes of this disease is the first indispensable requisite in its successful cure; at the same time, the following remedies will be of the greatest benefit, to be applied according to the symptoms.

The principal remedies for recent dyspepsia are *Nux vom.*, and *Pulsatilla;* for chronic dyspepsia, *Hepar, Calcarea, Sulphur.* (See their symptoms below.)

To facilitate the choice of the remedies, we classify the disease according to its appearance and causes, with the remedies attached to each kind; before selecting a remedy, consult its details below.

If dyspepsia is present in *children: Ipecac., Bryonia, Calcarea, Nux vom., Sulphur.*

In *old persons: Antimonium, Nux vomica, China, Carbo vegetabilis.*

In *hypochondriacal persons: Nux vom., Sulphur.*

In *hysterical females: Ignatia, Pulsat., Sepia.*

If the *dyspepsia is caused* by *sedentary* habits: *Nux vomica, Sulphur, Sepia.*

By *prolonged watching: Nux vom., Arnica, Pulsat., Verat., Carbo veg.*

By *excessive study: Nux vomica, Sulphur, Lachesis, Pulsat., Calcarea.*

By *debilitating losses,* such as bleeding, purging, vomiting, etc.: *China, Carbo veg., Lachesis, Nux vom., Sulph., Calcarea.*

By *sexual excesses: Phosphoric acid, Nux vomica, Mercury, Staphysag.*

By the abuse of ardent spirits: *Nux vomica, Sulphur, Lachesis, Arsenic, Carbo veg.*

Of coffee: *Nux vom., Ignatia.*

Of tea: *Thuja.*

Of tobacco: *Nux vom., Hepar, Cocculus, Staphysag.*

By *over-eating: China, Pulsatilla, Antimon.*

By *distressing emotion,* such as *grief, anger,* etc.: *Chamomile, Nux vom., Phosphoric acid, China, Staphysag.*

By *mechanical injuries,* blow, fall on the stomach, etc.: *Arnica, Bryonia, Rhus tox., Sulphur.*

If *the dyspepsia is worse* after *partaking of almost anything: Nux vom., Sulphur, Lachesis, Carbo veg., China.*

After drinking *cold water: Arsenic, China, Pulsatilla, Veratrum.*

After drinking *beer: Arsenic, Calcarea, Rhus tox., Sepia, Sulphur.*

After drinking *milk: Bryon., Nux vom., Calcarea, Sulphur.*

After using *bread: Nux vom., Sulphur, Pulsatilla, Bryonia, Mercury.*

After using *acids: Nux vomica, Sepia, Sulphur, Arsenic, Lachesis.*

After partaking of meat: *China, Sulphur.*

After partaking of *fat substances: Pulsat., Sulphur, China, Carbo veg.*

If the dyspepsia is combined with *diarrhea: Pulsat., China, Phosphoric acid, Carbo veg., Veratrum, Arsenic, Mercury.*

With *constipation: Nux vom., Sulphur, Bryonia, Lachesis.*

With *sour stomach: Pulsatilla, Sepia, Phosphoric acid, Nux vom., Calcarea.*

With *headache:* See this article.

With *piles: Nux vomica, Sulphur, Sepia.*

SYMPTOMATIC DETAIL.—*Nux vomica.* In most cases of dyspepsia at the commencement, particularly in persons with a tendency to piles (see this article) and habitual costiveness; or when dissipation and late hours, the abuse of ardent spirits, or exposure to cold, was the immediate cause of this disease; this remedy is especially indicated for *sour* or *bitter taste in the mouth,* and if *food,* particularly *bread,* tastes sour, bitter, or insipid; patient has not much appetite, but a *craving for beer,* wine, or spirits, or he has great hunger, but a little satisfies him; after eating he is troubled with *nausea, eructation, vomiting of food, vertigo,* hypochondriacal humor, or, after a meal, lassitude, sleepiness, drowsiness, distension, fullness, and tension in the stomach, tender to the touch; around the waist a *sensation of tightness of the clothes;* sour risings and belchings; *water-brash;* sour stomach; makes the patient unfit for intellectual labor; with constipation, and *frequent heat* and *redness* of the *face, restlessness,* and *irascibility.* After it, *Sulphur* suits well.

Sulphur. Is in cases of long standing the principal remedy after *Nux vomica,* or when there is no *appetite* for *meat* and bread, but a *craving* for *acids* or wine; *milk, acids,* and *sweet substances* disagree; after a meal, difficulty of *breathing, nausea, pain in the stomach, belching* or *vomiting of food, shivering, acidity,* and *water-brash,* with flatulency and constipation; sad, morose humor, with irascibility. After it, *Calcarea carb.* is often suitable.

Pulsatilla. In recent cases of dyspepsia, particularly those caused by *over-eating,* or the use of *fat* or *pork,* or any greasy substance, causing flatulency and indigestion (in such cases in alternation with *China*); no *thirst; bitter* or *sour* eructations; the taste of the food comes up again, *water-brash, sadness, melancholy,* inclined to *loose* bowels. *China* or *Sulphur* suits well after it.

China. Dyspepsia from loss of blood or other humors, or caused by exposure to miasms in marshy countries, near canals, etc. (see "Fever and Ague"); particularly if there is *indifference to food* and *drink*, as if *from satiety;* craving wines or acids; food tastes *acid* or *bitter;* after a meal uneasiness, *drowsiness*, *fullness*, *distension;* patient wants to lie down, sensitive to draughts of wind, ill-natured and dislikes everything. After it suits *Bryonia*, *Rhus tox.*, *Carbo veg.*

Bryonia. Dyspepsia especially in *summer* or *damp weather;* or when there is *headache*, *chilliness*, *pains in the limbs*, arms, and *small of the back*, *aversion to food;* eructation of wind, pressure and pain in the stomach after a meal; cannot bear tight clothes; *vomiting of food*, constipation, with restlessness and irascibility. In alternation with *Rhus* or *China.*

Rhus tox. Always in alternation with *Bryonia* (see "Bilious Rheumatic Fever"), especially when there is great restlessness, thirst, and dry tongue during the night.

Carbo veg. Bitter taste in the mouth, aversion to food, milk, or fat, with acidity in the mouth; *frequent flatulency* and belching up, tasting the fat and food which had been eaten; *nausea in the morning*, water-brash during the night; heart-burn; hiccough during motion; pains under the short ribs, particularly on the left side, in the form of stitches, with pressing and fullness; cannot bear the clothes around him tight; worse in damp weather; *offensive diarrhea.*

Ipecac. Almost the same as *Carbo veg.*, but especially suitable for children after indigestion, when they have vomiting of food, drink, mucus or bile; retching, vomiting, with coldness of the face and extremities; sinking at the stomach. (See "Cholera Morbus.")

Veratrum. After *Ipecac.*, if this should be insufficient, or there is still diarrhea, attended with griping in the bowels; great thirst.

Antimon. crud. After *Ipecac.*, if this has not removed the nausea and vomiting, with a sensation of great fullness in the stomach, and much flatulency.

Ignatia and *Staphysag.* See "Diseases of the Mind."

Hepar. One of the most useful remedies in this disease, where a person has taken much calomel, and is easily taken with indigestion, with a longing for stimulating things, wine, or acids; nausea in the morning, with eructation or vomiting of sour, bilious, or mucous substances; hard, light-colored, difficult evacuations, or else whitish diarrhea. (In this case alternate with *Nux vomica;* otherwise with *Mercury* or *Lachesis.*)

Calcarea. Sensation of coldness in the head, with inclination to sick-headache; *acid stomach; water-brash; fullness and swelling in the region of the stomach,* with great *tenderness to touch;* evacuations similar to those of *Hepar,* but the diarrhea in children has a sour smell. Follows well after *Sulphur.*

Sepia. In persons subject to habitual sick-headache, who frequently suffer from dyspepsia when their heads feel comfortable; aversion to food, or else great craving; taste sour, and after a *meal* acidity in the mouth, and swelling of the abdomen, or else pressure, as if from a stone in the stomach, with much belching, mostly sour or painful; inclined to constipation; suits well for nervous, hysterical persons, or those who are subject to congestion of the head or bowels.

Arnica. Frequent eructations, sometimes with a taste of rotten eggs; great sensitiveness and nervous excitement; tongue dry, thick, yellowish coated; putrid, sour taste, hypochondriacal humor; inclined to diarrhea.

Phosphoric acid. Great mental and physical debility, caused by *grief, unrequited love,* or loss of bodily strength by losing too much and too constantly animal liquid. In diarrhea, alternate with

China. After every meal pressure in the stomach, as if

from a load; perception of the taste of food, particularly of *bread*, long after it is taken.

Lachesis. Irregular appetite; repugnance to bread, with craving for wine and *milk; frequent nausea* and *eructation, vomiting of food;* uneasiness, indolence, heaviness, fullness and pains in the stomach after every meal; *constipation*.—Suits well before or after *Mercury*.

Mercury. Putrid, sweetish or bitter taste in the morning; repugnance to *solid food* and *meat*, with craving for cooling things; inclined to diarrhea, with straining, or to perspiration; has much saliva in the mouth.

Cocculus. Sensation of emptiness and hollowness in the stomach; sour taste, with aversion to acids; dryness of the throat; nausea, even to fainting; constipation.

Phosphorus. *Vomiting after a meal;* burning in the stomach; acidity and sour taste in the mouth.

Thuja. Weakness of the stomach after the abuse of tea; rancid or bitter eructation, and throwing up of that which has been eaten.

Administration.—In severe and painful cases of dyspepsia take of the selected remedy from one to six hours a dose (four glob.) until better; but in chronic cases take only every evening or every other evening a dose (six glob.) until four doses are taken; then discontinue four days, and, if not better, take the next medicine in the same manner.

Application of Water.—Is in the various forms of this disease of the greatest benefit, beside the use of the proper remedies. In most cases the wet bandage around the abdomen, with cold ablutions morning and night, drinking of cold water and exercise in the open air, will be sufficient to support the action of the medicine sufficiently to secure success. In very severe and inveterate cases it is necessary to resort to an hydropathic institution, where the patient can receive the proper treatment.

Diet and Regimen.—Beside avoiding those excesses in the diet and regimen which we have mentioned in the "Diagnosis," as so many causes of this disease, it must be borne in mind that everything even allowed under other circumstances must not be indulged in, as soon as it disagrees with the patient. Keep busy and cheerful; avoid fatigue and exposure; the application of cold water, in a systematical way, externally and internally, is highly recommended. (See "Hydropathy.") Exercise freely in the open air; travel and mingle in cheerful society.

4. Water-brash. Heart-burn. (*Pyrosis.*)
(*Indigestion. Flatulency. Sour stomach.*)

These ailments are mostly comprehended under the name of dyspepsia, of which they form some of the most distressing symptoms; but where they occur more isolated their remedies may be found in the following tabular view; reference to the details of these medicines may be had in the article "Dyspepsia."

Treatment.—For *water-brash: Nux vom., Arsenic, Carbo veg., Sepia, Calcarea carb., Phosphorus, Lycopodium, Sulphur.*

For *heart-burn: Nux vom., Pulsatilla, China, Phosphoric acid, Sepia, Sulphur.*

For *vomiting or throwing up,*

a. Of *food, Arnica, Bryon., Carbo veg., Nux vom., Phosphorus, Pulsat., Sulphur.*

b. Of *indigested* food (*indigestion*): *China, Bryon., Pulsat., Ignatia, Lachesis, Phosphorus.* (See end of this article.)

c. Of *acid: Nux vom., Chamomile, Calcarea carb., China, Phosphorus, Sulphur.*

For *flatulency,* or *frequent rising of wind: Arnica, Nux vomica, Pulsatilla, Bryonia, Rhus tox., Sulphur, Carbo veg., Veratrum.*

a. After eating *flatulent food: China.*

b. After eating *pork* or *fat meat: Pulsat., China.*

c. After *drinking: Nux vom.*

d. Colic from flatulency: See "Colic."

In regard to *indigestion* and its consequences, we will particularly remark here, that if it is caused by an *overloaded stomach,* a cup of *coffee,* without milk or sugar, will remedy most of its bad consequences; the remaining symptoms require *Pulsat., Nux vom., Ipecac.*

Indigestion from *fat food, pork, pastry,* etc., requires *Pulsat., China, Carbo veg., Ipecac.*

That which is caused by *ice-cream, fruit,* or other things which chill the stomach, requires *Pulsatilla, Carbo veg., Arsenic.*

If caused by the abuse of *wine: Nux vom., Lachesis, Carbo veg., Pulsat., Antimon. crud.*

By *acid wines: Antimon., Pulsat.*

By *sulphurated wines: Pulsat.*

By *vinegar, sour beer,* and *other acids: Aconite, Carbo veg., Arsenic, Hepar.*

If *tainted meat* or *fish* causes indigestion, give first a little *pulverized charcoal* in brandy; afterward *China,* or *Pulsat.*

If *salt food* causes indigestion: *Carbo veg.*

Indigestion frequently produces the following disorders, which require the remedies attached to them:

Fever: Acon., Bryon., Antimon. (See "Gastric Fevers.")

Eruptions, like *nettle-rash: Ipecac., Pulsatilla, Bryon.* (See "Nettle-rash.")

Diarrhea: Pulsatilla, Coffea, Ipecac., Nux vomica. (See "Diarrhea.")

Colic: Pulsat., Nux vom. (See "Colic.")

Flatulency: China, Pulsat., Carbo veg. (See "Flatulency," above.)

In regard to *heart-burn* or *sour stomach,* we would remark that it will often be relieved by taking of a mixture of one drop of *Sulphuric acid* in a teacupful of water, every hour or two hours a teaspoonful; or by drinking lemon-water in moderate quantities. This is particularly recommended to pregnant women, who frequently suffer from acidity of the stomach from constitutional causes.

ADMINISTRATION, APPLICATION OF WATER, DIET AND REGIMEN, the same as in "Dyspepsia."

5. BILIOUSNESS. GASTRIC DERANGEMENT.

Biliousness, or bilious complaints, as a popular term, comprises different disorders of the digestive organs, which mostly have nothing to do with the bile or liver, but with the stomach alone. For practical purposes we divide these diseases:

Into *gastric affections*, where the stomach alone is implicated; and,

Into *gastric bilious affections*, where the derangement of the liver reflects its morbid consequences on the stomach.

These attacks occur without much fever.

1. *Gastric affections* (*gastroataxia*). This is a general name for all those disorders of the stomach, which we have already treated in the articles on "Dyspepsia," "Indigestion," "Heartburn," "Water-brash," and "Flatulency," to which we refer the reader.

2. *Gastric bilious affections* (*gastrodynia biliosa*). This disease is characterized by an *oppression* and *swelling* in the pit of the stomach, with inclination to vomit, and eructation of wind, of an offensive smell, like rotten eggs or meat; no appetite, and particularly a dislike for meat; thirst great, especially for acids; tongue thickly yellowish coated; either constipation or looseness of the bowels, of dark (black) offensive operations, with a great deal of wind. With these really bilious symptoms are combined a yellowish color in the face, around the nose and mouth; headache in the evening, with a full pulse and a feeling of heat without much fever.

CAUSES.—Persons removing from the north to the south

are subject to this disease very often, which sometimes runs into bilious fever. Otherwise, it is caused more by the imprudent use of too much meat and alcoholic drinks in warm climates; also, by mental derangement, such as anger, grief, etc. It is, frequently, the forerunner of bilious fever.

Treatment.—Similar to "Bilious remittent Fever," in its early stage. See page 135.

Application of Water.—See page 135.

Diet and Regimen.—Oatmeal gruel, with sugar and lemon-juice; lemonade, in small but often-repeated quantities; oranges; dry or milk toast; cold water. Meat, meat-soups, and eggs, are strictly forbidden. When recovering, a few oysters are allowed. If the bowels are very loose, the acids must not be used too freely, but very cautiously, if at all.

Cold baths are beneficial, particularly mornings and evenings. Exercise can be taken on hills, or dry places.

Nausea. Vomiting.

Nausea and vomiting seldom occur as solitary symptoms, except when caused by errors in the diet; in which case, the ejection of the noxious substances by vomiting is most beneficial, and ought rather to be fostered, by drinking freely of lukewarm water, than checked by medicine. But when nausea or vomiting is caused by, or connected with, other diseases, their respective chapters must be consulted; where, generally, these two, as prominent symptoms, are mentioned and prescribed for.

We will, however, furnish the reader here with a list of the most frequent diseases in which nausea and vomiting exist, and attach the principal medicines thereto.

The principal remedies, useful in most cases of nausea and vomiting, are: *Antimon. crud.*, *Ipecac.*, *Nux vomica*, *Arsenic*, *Veratrum*, *Tartar emetic*, *Bryonia*, *Pulsatilla*, *Arnica*, *Cuprum*, *Sulphur*.

Before time can be had, to select with care the proper homœopathic remedy in a case of vomiting, it is of no disadvantage, to give at once:

Ipecacuanha, if the tongue is *clear;* or

Antimonium crud., if the tongue is much coated, white or yellow.

Then proceed calmly to study the patient's case and select the proper remedy from the following symptoms.

If nausea and vomiting is present:

In *pregnant females: Nux vom., Ipecac., Arsenic, Veratrum.* (See "Diseases of Females.")

In *drunkards: Nux vom.., Arsenic, Opium, Lachesis, Sulphur.*

In consequence of *riding* in a carriage, *sailing*, etc., *Cocculus, Petroleum, Arsenic, Ferrum, Secale, Belladonna.* (See "Sea-Sickness.")

In consequence *of worms: Cina, Aconite, Ipecac., Nux vom., Mercury, Sulphur, Lachesis, Carbo veg.* (See "Worm Disease.")

In consequence of *overloaded stomach: Pulsat., Ipecac., Antimon., Nux vomica, Arsenic, Bryonia, Rhus tox., Sulphur.* (See "Indigestion.")

After *drinking: Arsenic, Ferrum, China, Bryon., Chamomile, Aconite, Arnica, Silicea.*

After *eating: Pulsat., Nux vom., Bryon., Arsenic, Ferrum, Sulphur.* (See "Dyspepsia.")

In the *morning: Nux vom., Arsenic, Drosera, Veratrum, Hepar., Lycopod., Silicea.*

In the *evening* or *at night: China, Arsenic, Nux vom., Ferrum, Silicea, Sulphur.*

After a *fall on the head: Arnica*, internally and externally (See "External Injuries.")

In connection *with a cough:* See "Hooping-Cough."

In connection with *headache:* See "Sick Headache."

In connection with *diarrhea:* See "Cholera."

Or, in regard to *ejected substances*,

If *blood* is vomited (*hæmatemesis*): *Aconite, Arnica, Ipecac., Nux vomica, Ferrum, Hyoscyamus, Bryonia, China.* (See "Inflammation of the Spleen," "Cessation of Menses," and "Hemorrhoids"). Generally, medical aid is immediately required, when blood is vomited. If the blood is very *dark*, *Black vomit* (*melaena*), with discharge of similar blood by the stool: *Veratrum, Arsenic, China, Ipecac.* (See "Diarrhea, Typhus.")

If *fæcal* matter is ejected: *Opium, Nux vom.* (See "Constipation," and "Ileus.")

If *bile* is vomited, of greenish look and bitter taste: *Chamomile, Ipecac., Nux vom., Pulsat., Antimon., Cuprum, Veratrum.* (See "Biliousness," etc.)

If *mucus* of a sour taste or smell; *China, Calcarea carb., Nux vom., Pulsat., Sulphur.* (See "Dyspepsia.")

If *watery substances*: *Bryon., Ipecac., Belladonna, Pulsat., Sulphur.* (See "Water-Brash," etc.)

Administration. — Give the medicine either dry, every hour or two hours, from three to six glob.; or, dissolved in water (twelve glob. in half a teacupful), every half hour a teaspoonful, until better, or until three or four doses of a medicine are taken, when another remedy must be selected, if the patient is not better.

Application of Water.—See the different diseases, of which nausea and vomiting are symptoms; beside, if it is desirable to have the stomach emptied of its contents, as in the case of an overloaded stomach, poisoning, etc., let the patient drink lukewarm water until this object is accomplished. If the vomiting or nausea is disconnected from other diseases, the action of the proper remedies will be supported by the use of the wet bandage and the sitting-baths; in case of attending constipation, by cold injections and drinking of cold water; habitual coldness of the feet is regulated by cold foot-baths.

DIET AND REGIMEN. — In feverish attacks, see "Fever." In all others, see their respective chapters.

SEA-SICKNESS.

This distressing complaint depends greatly on constitutional peculiarities, to which the remedy must be adapted. As the cause (the motion of the vessel) continues, it is necessary to repeat the medicine frequently. It will be of service to be careful in the diet just before embarkation; especially to avoid rich, fat food.

TREATMENT.—The principal remedies are:

Cocculus. In giddiness, headache, nausea; the patient feels better when lying down.

Nux vomica. The same. The patient feels better when *not* in the open air.

Pulsatilla. The patient feels better *in the* open air, on deck.

Colchicum. After *Pulsatilla,* or when the smell of food or the scent of the vessel sickens.

Tabacum. If *Pulsatilla* or *Colchicum* are insufficient, or when the patient sickens at the *slightest movement* of head or body, with *deadly paleness of the face.*

Petroleum. In cases of great debility.

Arsenic. If the patient becomes *very weak,* and there is violent retching.

Ipecac. If there is frequent vomiting, without feeling weak.

Hyoscy. at commencement of nausea, and dizziness of head.

For *constipation,* during a voyage on sea, give *Opium, Cocculus, Nux vomica, Lachesis, Sulphur.*

When constipation is attended with a putrid taste and bloody gums, give *Staphysag.*

When patients are constipated, and have a longing for acids and something piquant, give *Sepia.*

N. B. It is well enough to provide one's-self, on sea voyages, with Scotch ale and herrings; also, lemons; as those things are mostly desired by sea-sick patients.

Application of Water is beneficial in this disease; a wet bandage around the stomach, drinking of cold water, and in case of constipation, the use of cold injections and the sitting-bath are generally sufficient to accelerate the cure by the proper remedies.

Administration. — The same as in "Nausea and Vomiting." It is beneficial to take as much exercise on deck as possible, whatever the weather may be, although the patient may not incline to do so at first.

Spasms, and Pain in the Stomach.

(*Cardialgia, Gastralgia, Neuralgia of the Stomach.*)

Diagnosis. — Spasmodic pains and contractions in the pit of the stomach, sometimes slight, sometimes of insupportable violence, and spreading to the chest and back, exciting nausea and vomiting; anguish; coldness of the extremities, and even faintness; belching up of wind often relieves the patient for a time, as, also, vomiting of an acid, limpid fluid, if acidity of stomach or a gouty disposition was connected with it.

Causes.—Any derangement of the nerves of the stomach, either sympathetic, from diseases of the liver, spleen, or pancreas, or more directly from long fasting, the habitual use of *ardent spirits, indigestible food* (new bread, nuts, sweetmeats, chestnuts, cherries, figs, cheese, etc.), *coffee* or *tea*, may cause this disease; especially if, in addition to this, the person exposes himself to cold, damp weather, or if he is of a gouty disposition, which then developes itself on the stomach in this form (*rheumatism* and *gout* of the stomach). Females are particularly liable to this disease, which, in them, appears mostly with derangement of the menses, especially after their cessation (*neuralgia* of the stomach), when it is sometimes associated with fits of fainting, and may end in vomiting of blood. In such cases, the periodical appearance of the disease is frequently observed.

Treatment.—Persons liable to spasms of the stomach must avoid everything which could cause them directly, as mentioned above. Beside this, they should keep their feet warm, and wear a woolen shirt or bandage, or in obstinate chronic cases, a Burgundy pitch plaster on the stomach. Above all, however, we recommend to apply to a homœopathic physician, who, in most cases, is able to eradicate the complaint. For recent cases, or in the attack itself, the following remedies will be found beneficial.

If a person is liable to attacks of this kind, he must be particularly careful in the diet; he must strictly avoid all crude, uncooked vegetable substances, such as salads; also, new made bread, sweetmeats, cherries, nuts, olives and chestnuts; cheese must be avoided, also all kinds of stimulants, tea, coffee, wine, brandies, beer; the use of cold water externally and internally is recommended.

We give, first, a tabular view, to facilitate the choice of the proper remedy.

Spasm in the stomach (*gastralgia*), from

Abuse of *Chamomile tea: Nux vom., Ignatia, Pulsat.*

Abuse of *coffee: Nux vom., Ignatia, Cocculus, Chamomile.*

Abuse of *ardent spirits: Nux vom., Lachesis, Arsenic, Sulph.*

Indigestion: Pulsat., Antimon. crud., Bryon., China, Carbo veg., Nux vom.

Want of exercise, torpid bowels: Nux vom., Sulph.

Excess of mental emotions, as *anger, indignation*, etc.; *Chamomile, Colocynth, Nux vom., Staphysag.*

Loss of animal fluids, causing excessive debility, such as blood-letting, nursing, perspirations, excessive diarrheas: *China, Carbo veg., Phosphoric acid, Cocculus, Nux vom.*

Rheumatism and *exposure to cold and damp weather: Chamomile, Bryon., Rhus tox., Carbo veg.*

A gouty disposition, or where *rheumatism or gout* has fallen upon the stomach; *Ipecac., Bryon., Rhus, Nux vom., Sulph., Bellad., Calcarea.*

Derangement of the menses, if they are too *slight: Pulsat., Cocculus.* If too *profuse: China, Bellad., Platina, Calc. carb.*

SYMPTOMATIC DETAIL.—*Nux vomica.* This is one of the most important remedies in this disease, and it is efficacious almost in every spasm of the stomach, in the beginning; at least there is no risk in giving directly one dose (two, three, or four glob.), as it will procure time for cooler observation and a more correct choice, according to the symptoms. If *Nux vomica* does not give any relief, *Chamomile* or *Cocculus* alternated, every half hour, if necessary, will be of great benefit. The pains requiring *Nux vomica* especially, are: *contracting, pressing,* and *spasmodic,* with sensation of *retraction or clawing* in the stomach, with oppression of the chest, as if it were compressed by a band, with pain extending into the back and loins; nauseous accumulation of water in the mouth, or vomiting of sour liquid or food during the pain, *worse* after a *meal, from using coffee* and *ardent spirits;* from *over-study,* creating thereby constipation, piles, hypochondria, with *irascible* humor, hasty and passionate character. Such persons generally are subject to nervous, pressing headache on one side, with unfitness for exertion, palpitation of the heart with anxiety.

ADMINISTRATION, see at the end of this article.

Cocculus. Often very beneficial, when *Nux vom.*, or *Chamomile* has given but temporary relief, or when there are spasms in the stomach, mitigated by belching up of wind; otherwise, similar to *Nux vom.*

Chamomile. Distension of the stomach, with *pressure* as from a *stone,* or as if the *heart were being crushed* with oppression and shortness of breath; pains are worse at *night* with *great anguish* and *tossing; momentary mitigation* by *drinking coffee.* The patient is *peevish* and *irritable;* pains drive him out of bed. This remedy suits well to be given alternately with *Coffea,* and if then no improvement takes place, try *Belladonna.*

Belladonna. Especially where *Chamomile* was of no avail, although well indicated, mostly in women of a delicate, sensitive constitution, at the time of too *profuse menstruation,* and then alternately with *Platina,* until better. *Bellad.*[cc], alternately with *Coffea*[cc], will be very beneficial in this disease, if the patient is decidedly better, but cannot sleep nor lie quiet. *Belladonna* also suits in such violent pains as to *take away consciousness,* and cause *falling down;* also great thirst, but the pain gets worse after drinking.

Pulsat. Is the principal remedy in mild, sad, tearful dispositions, or where the menses are tardy, producing those spasms. The pains are *shooting;* worse by walking and making a false step; spasmodic pains in the stomach, caused by *fasting,* or *overloading* the stomach; with nausea, *vomiting of food;* not much thirst; pains are *worse in the evening,* with feeling of *chilliness;* frequently loose bowels.

Ignatia. Frequently after *Pulsatilla,* and when there are *pressing pains,* as *from a stone,* especially after a meal or at night; weakness, burning, emptiness in the pit of the stomach, sensitive to touch; aversion to food and drink; cannot bear tobacco; also, pains from mental causes, indignation, etc.; or suits well for persons who have the pains from having fasted too long.

China. Spasms from indigestion, with swelling of, and painful pressure in, the stomach, with rumbling of wind and flatulency; spasms after loss of strength by blood-letting, nursing, diarrheas, etc.

Carbo veg. Follows well after *China,* if the spasms were caused after eating *flatulent* or *spoiled* food; also, spasms occurring in damp and wet weather; particularly if there is a *painful, burning pressure,* with *anxiety,* worse on touch or at night; or contracting, spasmodic pain, forcing the patient to bend double, with shaking; worse when lying down; heart-burn; nausea; the very thought of food sickens him.

Lachesis. *Pressing pains,* ameliorated soon after a meal, but renewed afterward, with *constipation,* dyspepsia, and flatulency.

Lycopodium. Compressive pains, ameliorated in bed during the night; worse in the morning, after a meal, and especially in the *open air.*

Arsenic. *Violent pains* and *anxiety* in the cardia and the stomach; *burning* and spasmodic pains in cardia and stomach; *vomiting after drinking the smallest quantity of liquid;* suitable for spasms in old people, where cancer of the stomach may be supposed to exist, and in drunkards.

Sulphur. *Pressing pains as if from a stone,* mostly after a meal, with nausea, water-brash, or vomiting; *acidity; throwing up of food;* disposition to piles, or accumulation of mucus in the intestines; hypochondriacal, whining mood.

Antimon. crud. See "Indigestion."

Bryonia. *Pressure as from a stone* in the cardia, when eating, or after a meal, with a sensation of *swelling in the pit of the stomach;* pains *worse by any motion;* constipation; rheumatic pains in the head and limbs. In alternation with

Rhus tox. When the *pressure in the stomach and cardia obstructs the breathing,* particularly after taking cold in damp, cold weather. (See "Bilious Rheumatic Fever.")

Staphysag. Spasms in the stomach after anger or indignation.

Calcarea carb. Suitable for plethoric persons, with full red faces or for females who have their menses very profusely; or after *Belladonna* has given partial relief; especially when there is a sensation of *clawing* and retraction in the stomach, worse after a meal, *frequently with vomiting of food;* disposition to piles, constipation, and palpitation of the heart.

Administration.—Dissolve of the remedy selected twelve globules in half a teacupful of water, and give, every thirty or forty minutes, a teaspoonful, until three or four are taken; then wait thirty minutes, and, if not better, select another remedy, and give it in the same manner, until better. This is the mode of administration in the most urgent cases.

When the pains are not so severe, give the medicine at longer intervals; say, from one to two, three, or six hours, until amelioration takes place. In real chronic cases of this disease, give the chosen remedy only evening and morning a dose (four glob.), for two days, and then wait the same length of time, before another remedy is given; if better during that time, no more medicine is necessary.

Application of Water in the form of wet bandages around the stomach, and the use of the sitting-bath, will accelerate the cure; if the feet are habitually cold, apply the cold foot-bath every evening.

Diet and Regimen.—The same as in "Biliousness," and "Gastric Derangement."

If no cold water is applied externally, a mustard plaster, or other heating substances, such as scorched flour, heated bran in small sacks, may be laid on the stomach. The patient is advised to remain as quiet as possible during the paroxysms.

Griping Colic. (*Colica; enteralgia.*) (*Stomach-ache.*)

Diagnosis.—Pains in the intestines, more or less violent; griping, pinching, tearing, or burning, mostly in the region of the navel, yet often spread all over the bowels; severe cases of colic are accompanied by anxiety and cold sweat; stools either loose or confined; when the colic pain is seated in *one* place of the abdomen for a length of time without moving, danger of inflammation of the intestines ensues, which is indicated by the pain, hitherto griping and pinching, becoming *burning*, and fever appearing (see "Inflammation of the Intestines"); vomiting of sour, bilious phlegm, or distension of the abdomen, painful to the touch, often attend the severest cases of colic.

Causes.—These are constitutional or acquired by circumstances; the latter are very many, such as colds, indigestion, worms, constipation, mental emotions; and occupations which require persons to work in deleterious metals, such as lead, etc. According to these exciting causes, the three principal varieties of colic are:

1. *Bilious colic,* with bilious vomiting, severe griping, or shooting or twisting pain in the abdomen; at first relieved by pressure, afterward tender to the touch, with painful distension, cold extremities, restlessness, yellowish cast of the skin and eyes, the face expressing great anguish.

2. *Flatulent* or *wind-colic,* with frequent belching up of wind, with or without relief; swelling of the abdomen, which is distended and painful in different places, as the wind accumulates and moves in different parts of the intestines; the pains come in paroxysms, and are sometimes very severe.

3. *Painter's* or *lead colic,* which commences sometimes before an attack with general lassitude, wandering pains in the bowels and extremities, heaviness in the lower limbs, chilliness, and depression of spirits; the attack itself exhibits the same symptoms as bilious colic, except there is not often vomiting of bile, but great pain and restlessness, during which the patient bends forward, pressing firmly against the abdomen, his extremities feeling cold, and his pulse being small and suppressed.

TREATMENT.—The first thing to be done in any colic, if it is at all severe, is the application of a general warm bath, during which the patient, sitting in a tub, the warm water reaching up to the pit of the stomach, is covered with blankets to confine the hot steam closely around him; after ten minutes, he ascends from the bath and lays down with the blankets, without being dried off, and is covered with sufficient clothes; the warmth then may be kept up by putting heated bricks or hot water flasks around the patient, on the spots where he complains the most; a profuse perspiration will ensue, which relieves the cramp and makes the patient feel easier at once; it must be kept up until every vestige of pain has left for some time. The medicines to be prescribed below may be given, however, from the commencement of the pain, and continued until relief is obtained. We will now give in a tabular view the principal kinds of colic, with their remedies, the symptomatic details of which may be consulted below.

a. Bilious colic: Nux vomica, Colocynth, Chamomile, Bryonia.

b. Flatulent or *windy colic: Pulsatilla, China, Carbo veg., Cocculus, Nux vom., Colocynth, Lycopod., Sulphur.*

c. Painter's or *lead colic: Opium, Bellad., Platina.*

d. Colic with *obstinate constipation* (see "Miserere"): *Opium, Nux vom.*

e. Colic caused by *piles* or *hemorrhoids: Nux vom., Lachesis, Pulsat., Colocynth, Carbo veg., Sulphur.*

f. Colic from an *inflammatory* state of the intestines (inflammatory colic): *Aconite, Belladonna, Hyoscyamus, Mercury, Lachesis, Nux vomica, Arsenic, Sulphur.* (See "Enteritis.")

g. Colic from *worms: Mercury, Cina, Sulphur.* (See "Worms.")

h. Colic from *indigestion* (gastric colic): *Pulsat., China, Nux vom., Bellad., Bryon., Carbo veg.*

i. Colic from *indignation* or *rage: Cham., Coloc., Staphys., Sulphur.*

k. Colic from a *chill: Aconite, Cham., Coloc., Merc., Nux vomica.*

l. Colic from *exposure to cold, damp weather: Pulsat., Bryonia, Rhus tox.*

m. From *bathing: Nux vom.*

n. From *external injuries,* such as *strains* or *blows: Arnica, Bryon., Rhus tox., Carbo veg., Lachesis.*

o. Colic in *children* principally: *Chamomile, Rheum, Coffea, Aconite, Bellad., Cina, Sulphur.* (See "Diseases of Children.")

p. Colic in *pregnant* or *lying-in women: Chamomile, Nux vomica, Arnica, Bryonia, Pulsatilla, Sepia.* (See "Diseases of Women.")

q. In *hysterical women* (nervous colic of women): *Ignatia, Nux vom., Cocculus.* (See the same.)

r. Colic at the time of the *menses* (menstrual colic): *Pulsatilla, Coffea, Veratrum, Cocculus.* (See the same.)

s. Colic in persons with *low spirits: China, Nux vom., Sulphur, Calcarea carb., Stannum.*

Select first, according to the character of the disease, one of the above remedies, and then read its symptoms in the following symptomatic detail. It will be seen above that *Nux vom.* and *Colocynth* are the principal remedies in almost all kinds of colic, and consequently mostly to be used; we recommend, therefore, the careful study of their distinguishing symptoms. Beside these two medicines, *Pulsat.* and *Belladonna* will be found of frequent application.

Administration of these remedies, see at the end of this article.

Symptomatic Detail.—*Nux vomica.* Constipation, *hard* or *difficult stool,* with *pressure in the abdomen as from a stone;* the colic pain is *contractive* or *compressive,* sometimes pinching and drawing; *pressure at the pit of the stomach,* with distension and tenderness of the abdomen when touched; feeling as if the clothes around the waist were too tight; flatulency and severe *griping,* deeply seated in the abdomen, with cold hands and feet, and sometimes sharp and severe *pressure* on the *bladder* and *rectum,* as if wind were about to escape violently, forcing the patient to bend double; beneficial in almost all kinds of colic, where *constipation* predominates, or the patient likes to be quiet, to sit doubly bent, or to lie down on account of violent pains in the loins and head.

Colocynth. This is the principal medicine for colic; *violent,* even the *most violent cutting, pinching, clawing* pains and *stitches* as if from *knives,* with *excessive restlessness, agitation* and *tossing,* sometimes *cramp* in the *limbs, shivering,* either no inclination to stools and *violent diarrhea* and *vomiting of bile* or food, immediately after eating; abdomen either swollen with wind, *flatulency*, or feels *very empty;* however, very tender, as from a bruise. After it are suitable, *Chamomile, Mercury, Belladonna.*

Belladonna. The colic pains are: swelling and *protrusion,* like a pod of the colon between the pit of the stomach and the navel, relieved by pressing upon it or by bending double; pain at the same place, as if the intestines were *grasped by the finger nails;* or *spasmodic constriction* in the abdomen in females, with a feeling of *bearing downward* as if something would fall out, similar to the falling of the womb, or pains connected with this disorder; general characteristic for *Belladonna:* congested, hot head, red face, severe pain in the head, aggravated by movement, cannot bear the light, feels dry in the throat, etc. (See "Materia Medica.") After it *Mercury, Lachesis,* or *Hyoscyamus,* is suitable.

Pulsatilla. Shooting, beating pains in the pit of the stomach; farther down in the abdomen a feeling of heaviness and fullness, with *disagreeable tension* and *distension,* tenderness and pain as if from a bruise when touched; suffering from flatulency (see this article), and consequent colic after indigestion; worse when *sitting, lying,* or in the *evening,* with *shivering;* patient feels better *out doors,* than within; is inclined to, or has diarrhea; *pale face,* with livid circle around the eyes; *pressure,* tension, and aching in the head. After it are suitable, *China, Lycopodium, Mercury, Sulphur.*

China. Excessive distension of the abdomen, as in *tympanitis,* with *fullness* and *pressure,* as if from hard bodies; or spasmodic constriction; pain, with *stoppage of wind* and *bearing down toward the hypochondriacal region;* worse at night, after errors in diet, and in persons weakened by severe loss of animal fluids, such as bleeding, too heavy perspiration, nursing, diarrhea, etc. (See "Pulsatilla.")

Cocculus. One of the principal medicines, particularly in

spasmodic and windy colic, and in those colics of women before or at the time of their menses (see "Female Diseases"); or when there are *constrictive, spasmodic* pains in the hypogastrium, nausea, difficulty of breathing, flatulency, and full, distended stomach; or a feeling of emptiness in the abdomen, with squeezing and tearing in the stomach; nausea; *constipation;* nervous excitability.

Coffea. *Excess in pain, which drives to despair;* great agitation, tossing, grinding of the teeth; coldness of the limbs; moaning, and fits of suffocation.

Ignatia. Colic in the night, waking out of a sleep, with shooting into the sides and chest; difficult, but relieving discharge of wind; suitable for sensitive and delicate women.

Hyoscyamus. Spasmodic and griping pain, with vomiting; cries; pain in the head; hardness and distension of the abdomen, and tenderness when touched.

Chamomile. *Tearing, drawing pains,* with great restlessness; nausea: *bitter vomiting* or *bilious diarrhea;* incarcerated *wind,* with anguish, *tension, pressure, fullness in the pit of the stomach;* one cheek red, the other pale; the colic appears mostly at *night,* toward sunrise, or after a meal. (*Pulsat.* suits after it.)

Bryonia. Fullness and pressure in the abdomen after eating; cutting and *stitching* pains in the bowels, particularly after drinking warm milk; colic pains with diarrhea after taking cold, or in the heat of summer. Alternately with *Rhus tox.,* in bilious rheumatic attacks. (See this article.)

Rhus tox. *Pressure* in the stomach and pit of the stomach; *pain in the abdomen at night;* restlessness and diarrhea of watery and slimy substances. (See *Bryon.*)

Sulphur. Against *hemorrhoidal colic,* when *Carbo veg.,* or *Mercury* has been given without effect; against *bilious colic,* when *Chamomile* or *Colocynth* was insufficient; against *flatulent colic,* after *Chamomile, Calcarea carb., Mercury,* or *Carbo veg.*, was administered; or against *worm colic*, after *Mercury* or *Cina* had been given.

Carbo veg. *Distension* and fullness of the abdomen; difficult belching up of wind; colic after riding in a carriage; flatulent colic, with rumbling in the bowels; discharge of wind of a putrid smell; either constipation, or diarrhea of a putrid smell.

Arsenic. *Excessive pain, with great anguish in the abdomen; intolerable burning*, or sensation of cold in the abdomen; pains are worse at *night*, after *eating* or *drinking; watery or bilious vomiting;* diarrhea, with thirst, shivering, and *excessive debility.*

Veratrum. *Cutting as from knives in the abdomen*, which is very tender to touch; *burning* in the *whole* abdomen; *flatulent colic*, with noisy rumbling of wind, which is discharged with difficulty. (Alternately with *Arsenic*, in severe cases, or with *Coffea* at the time of menstruation.)

Opium. Abdomen hard and distended; tympanitis, with heaviness in the abdomen, as from a weight (*lead* or *painter's colic*); *obstinate constipation*, with vomiting even of fæces and urine; or involuntary stools, of a dark color and fetid.

Lachesis. In *spasmodic* and *inflammatory* colic, when *Colocynth, Belladonna, Cham., Nux vom.*, have been administered without effect; in *hemorrhoidal* colic, and after *mechanical* injuries; after *Carbo veg.*, when there is great weakness, sinking feeling, small, quick pulse; or alternately with *Lycopod.*, if there is great constipation left. (See this article.)

Lycopodium. In *flatulent colic, swelling, fullness*, and *distension* of the pit of the stomach, with colic pain, incarceration of wind, which is not discharged. (Is suitable after *Pulsat.*, or *Lachesis;* see these.)

Platina. In consequence of *fear* or *anger*, or *poisoning by lead*, after *Opium* and *Belladonna;* suitable principally for females, or when the bodily sufferings disappear as soon as the mental distresses begin, or *vice versa;* is afraid of dying; cannot refrain from weeping; *contracting pain in the abdomen;*

pressure in the stomach after eating; also a contracting pain, as if laced too tight; with a sensation of constant bearing down.

Aconite. Extreme tenderness of the abdomen; much anguish, restlessness and tossing, particularly when the pains are located in the region of the bladder; when the bowels seem to retract, with frequent but unsuccessful want to urinate.

Arnica. Contusive pain in the sides of the abdomen in pregnant females; pain from lifting in the abdomen; *fullness in the stomach,* as if one had eaten too much; *stitches in the pit of the stomach,* with *pressure back to the spine,* and *an oppression on the chest,* worse after eating, drinking, and touch; stitches in the left *hypochondrium, taking away the breath; distension and hardness of the abdomen,* with soreness in the sides; better after discharge of urine; diarrhea, watery, or from indigestion.

Mercury. Shooting or violent contracting pains in the abdomen, especially around the navel, with nausea; frequent desire to evacuate, or *slimy diarrhea;* profuse quantity of saliva in the mouth; shivering, with heat, especially in the face; abdomen tender to touch; colic pains, worse in the night; great lassitude.

Cina. Colic pains from worms, especially around the navel, which is tender to the touch. *Cina*$^{cc.}$ in such cases, every half hour repeated (the dose from two to four glob.), is more effectual than the other preparation of *Cina* (see "Worms").

Rheum. Particularly in infants, when the colic is accompanied by diarrhea of a *sour smell* and pressing down before and after the stool; or when there are in adults *cutting pains* in the abdomen, forcing one *to bend over* frequently soon after eating; worse when standing.

Sepia. Colic pains in *pregnant or lying-in women,* or even *spasms,* as if the intestines were turning over; *cutting pains after motion; burning* and *stitches* in the abdomen, which is *hard and distended; pressure and sensation* of *heaviness* in the abdomen, with *bearing down; rumbling of the bowels* after eating; constipation, or greenish diarrhea, especially in children.

Calcarea carb. Contractive, gnawing spasms, or cutting pains in the abdomen; difficulty of discharging the wind, with noisy rumbling of the bowels; cannot bear the clothes tight around the hypochondria; *acidity of the stomach,* with vomiting of food, especially in children when teething; lightish diarrhea.

Stannum. Spasms in the region of the *diaphragm,* as in *hysterical* or *hypochondriacal persons,* with difficulty of ejecting the wind; constipation, or slimy diarrhea, and great weakness. (Compare *China.*)

Administration.—Dissolve twelve glob. of the selected remedy in half a teacupful of water, and give every fifteen or thirty minutes a teaspoonful, for two or three times; then wait the same length of time before giving another remedy, if not better; but if the patient is better, do not repeat the medicine as often. This is particularly the case with *Colocynth,* which is the most frequently-needed remedy. In the most agonizing pains, the alternate use of *Coffea* and *Camphor* in solution, given as above stated, affords temporary relief, until other remedies may complete the cure. In cases where the pains are not so excessive, the medicines must not be repeated as frequently; say, only from two, three, to six hours a dose (four glob.) until better, or until another remedy is needed.

Diet and Regimen.—Persons subject to this complaint must avoid all substances which produce it, such as kale (kohl) and other green vegetables, acidulated drinks, veal, etc. In an attack of colic, give only the mildest nourishment; gruels, toast-water, toasted bread, etc.; no milk, except in worm colic, when *sweet, cold* milk will pacify the worms. Keep the feet dry and warm, also in wet, cold weather, a wet bandage around the stomach and abdomen. In colic from indigestion, a cup of black coffee *immediately* taken is strongly recommended.

Congestion and Stagnation of Blood in the Abdomen.

That process, by which disease is generated and grows, depends upon certain laws, which in no case appear in more constant regularity, than in producing the different kinds of congestions. The three great divisions of the body—head, breast, and abdomen—are, at certain periods of man's life, successively, the places for congestions and stagnation. Thus the head inclines to be congested in childhood, the breast in youth, up to thirty or thirty five years (hence, in this period most all lung-diseases occur), and, finally, the abdomen in middle age, from thirty five to old age (hence in this period so many bowel-diseases, such as hypochondria, piles, dyspepsia, etc., take place). One of the most natural causes for these diseases is *the determination of blood to the abdomen.* We must not increase, by our mode of living, this natural tendency to congestion ; as, if neglected or mistreated, its cure will be very difficult.

Diagnosis.—Persons troubled with this disease have a sensation of heat and burning in the stomach, together with the feeling of heaviness, hardness, and tension in the lower part of the abdomen.

Treatment.—*Nux vomica* and *Sulphur*, are the principal remedies.

Nux vomica. Especially for persons who lead a sedentary life, are *constipated,* have pains in the loins, hips, and back, as if broken and very weak ; hardness and tension of the abdomen ; cannot bear the pressure of the clothing around the waist.

Sulphur. After *Nux vomica* has relieved partially, in all cases, even the most obstinate, where constipation, hypochondriacal and hemorrhoidal symptoms are present ; *Nux vom.*, alternately with *Sulphur*, every second or third day a dose (four to six glob.), until four doses of each are taken, will generally be sufficient to relieve; if not, repeat it after an interval of from eight to fourteen days, during which time no medicine must be taken.

Arsenic and *Carbo veg.* Administered in the same manner, if there is great weakness, with tendency to diarrhea and flatulency.

Capsicum. If the evacuations are soft, trifling, slimy, watery, give twice or three times a dose (four glob.), until better.

Other remedies, to be used successively, but slowly, are: *Pulsatilla, Sepia, Belladonna, Mercury, Lachesis, Lycopodium.*

Application of Water.—The sitting-bath, cold foot-bath, and the wet bandage around the abdomen are beneficial auxiliaries in the treatment of this disease; beside the drinking of cold water.

Diet and Regimen.—Exercise on foot and horseback, regularity of all habits and cheerfulness of mind are necessary.

Diet.—See "Piles."

Inflammation of the Diaphragm. (*Diaphragmitis.*)

This disease resembles pleurisy very much; sharp, shooting pains under the short-ribs; worse on pressing between or below the ribs, on sneezing, or coughing, inhaling, or striking the body; relieved by bending the body forward; frequently there is hiccough present.

Causes.—The same as in pleurisy. We have only to add, that external injuries, such as blows, falls on the ribs directly, or a jarring of the diaphragm by a jump on the heels and feet, or (as in little children it is often the case) a twisting or unnatural turning of the body, are the most frequent causes of this disease.

Treatment.—The same as in "Pleurisy."

The principal remedies are: *Bryonia, Aconite, Nux vomica*

Chamomile. This latter, particularly in infants and children, when they are swollen around the short-ribs, where the slightest touch cannot be borne without screaming or stoppage of breath (see, in "Diseases of Children," "Livergrown"). *Nux vom.*, when *Chamomile* seems to be insufficient, and there is extreme constipation.

If caused by external injuries, *Arnica,* externally, in solution, and internally, in alternation with *Aconite,* every hour or two hours a dose (six glob.) must be used until better.

APPLICATION OF WATER.—Wet bandages around the breast and stomach, beside frquent cold injections, are recommended.

ADMINISTRATION, DIET, AND REGIMEN, the same as in "Pleurisy."

ABDOMINAL INFLAMMATION.

We will now proceed to the inflammations of those organs which lie between the peritoneum, or that serous membrane which envelops all the abdominal viscera. The inflammations of these organs have this one peculiar feature in regard to the pulse, that the higher the inflammation runs, the smaller and more suppressed the pulse appears; sometimes it is only discoverable by hard pressure.

1. *Inflammation of the Stomach.* (*Gastritis.*)

DIAGNOSIS.—This is a dangerous disease, and ought not to be treated by laymen; but, on account of its rapid course, we feel the necessity of introducing it here, in order to enable every one to diminish, or take away entirely its danger, by applying those remedies which have a specific bearing upon it.

Gastritis is characterized by a constant, violent, burning, and stitching pain in the gastric regions, increased by pressure, respiration, or taking any kind of food; beside this, there are heat, swelling, and tension, with pulsation in the region of the stomach; nothing will stay on the stomach, not even pure water; although there is great thirst, yet water is frequently rejected, because sometimes, beside other violent nervous fits and convulsions, hydrophobic symptoms occur, with tetanic spasms, great and sudden prostration; fainting; the pulse gets smaller, more wiry; extremities cooler, and the restless anxiety greater, the higher the inflammation is. Death takes place, either by gangrene (which is announced by sudden cessation of all pain, small, remitting pulse, scarcely perceptible, hands and feet icy cold), or by nervous paralysis, with spasms and fainting fits, together with symptoms of the utmost debility. Signs of improvement are, when the pulse becomes larger and broader, the pains less severe, without ceasing entirely, and the hands and feet warmer.

This disease may, after an improper treatment, pass into chronic inflammation, induration, or ulceration of the stomach.

Causes.—Bilious diarrheas, if suddenly checked; acrid poisons taken into the stomach; abuse of emetics and ardent spirits; transfer of gout; suppressed secretions; external injuries; or drinking of water when heated.

Treatment.—*Aconite* is the first remedy to be given, if the pains are severe, and the heat great in the stomach, or when a chill preceded the affection, or when it was caused by taking cold drinks when overheated.

Administration.—Dissolve twelve glob. in half a teacupful of water; give every twenty or thirty minutes a teaspoonful until ten spoonfuls are taken; if then not better, select another remedy, which must be prepared and given in the same manner, until better, or another remedy is necessary.

Bryonia. Generally after *Aconite* or *Ipecac.*

Ipecac. After *Aconite,* if vomiting predominates, and the disease was caused by indigestion, but the tongue is clear.

Antimon. Under similar symptoms as *Ipecac.;* but the tongue has a thick coating of white or yellowish mucus.

Pulsatilla. After *Ipecac.* or *Bryonia,* or when the disease was caused by indigestion, or a chill in the stomach from having taken ice.

Arsenic. For a similar condition, but there is *rapid failure of strength*, pale, sunken countenance, cold extremities; alternately with *Veratrum*.

Veratrum. For similar symptoms (see "Asiatic Cholera")

Belladonna and *Hyoscyamus*, alternately, if nervous, spasmodic, hydrophobic symptoms appear; drowsiness, delirium, loss of consciousness.

Arnica. In case external injuries were the cause of the disease.

Nux vomica and *Lachesis*, in alternation, if abuse of ardent spirits caused the gastritis; after which,

Lachesis and *Arsenic* may be alternated with benefit.

Cantharis. In the most violent cases, particularly when the burning pain is intolerable; alternately with *China*.

Opium and *Camphor*, alternately, if no remedy seems to ameliorate the case; drowsiness and stupor, particularly in drunkards; afterward give other suitable remedies which will have a better effect.

For gastritis from acrid poisons, see "Poison." After the poison is removed, treat as above.

For the chronic form of the disease, see "Dyspepsia, Cardialgia, Spasms of the Stomach."

Application of Water.—A lukewarm sitting-bath, reaching above the navel, is recommended; in the bath the patient's abdomen is constantly rubbed. After the vomiting ceases wet compresses are applied on the stomach and cold injections used to remove constipation. The chronic form requires strict dieting, the constant wearing of wet bandages, frequent sweatings in the wet sheet, foot and sitting-baths; beside the frequent drinking of small quantities of cold water.

Diet and Regimen.—As during the height of the disease nothing will stay on the stomach, it is better to offer the patient nothing but water; afterward the mildest gruel, made of rice or flour, milk and water, buttermilk, gum-arabic water, milk-toast. Continue this diet for some time before it is changed for a stronger one; and then only soups and mild vegetables.

2. *Inflammation of the Bowels.* (*Enteritis.*)

This disease occurs in two varieties; either *idiopathic,* where no other disease preceded it, or *symptomatic,* when it appears in consequence of other diseases, such as "Typhus," etc. The former is very acute, but of rare occurrence, and involves in its sphere the mucous membrane, as well as the submucous tissue and peritoneal coat—a very painful and dangerous disease; while the latter, not so acute in its course, occurs more frequently, attacking the mucous membrane of the intestines, mostly in portions; being, on that account, not so painful and dangerous, but sometimes leading to ulcerations of the bowels.

DIAGNOSIS of the *idiopathic* or *very acute form.*—Violent burning or pungent pain, permanently on one spot of the abdomen, generally in the region of the navel; increased by the slightest touch or movement; with tension, heat, and bloatedness of the abdomen; obstinate constipation; vomiting of slime or bile, finally of fæces (*ileus miserere*); violent thirst, yet cold drinks do not agree; sobbing, anxiety; restlessness; pulse small, contracted, as in gastritis; urine frequently suppressed.

The fatal termination of this disease occurs under similar symptoms as in gastritis by gangrene; the most violent pain suddenly disappearing, pulse sinking, remittent, imperceptible; involuntary, cadaverously fetid stools.

The symptoms of recovery are the same as in gastritis. In regard to the obstinate constipation which is such a constant symptom in this disease, we would remark that this does not constitute or cause the disease, but is its natural consequence, and disappears as soon as the inflammation, by the proper remedies, is reduced. Any violent attempt, by severe medicines, to effect a passage, would only add to the inflammation, and hasten a fatal result. The best expedient for this purpose is, beside the medicines to be mentioned hereafter, injections of tobacco smoke, which relieve the pain, or lukewarm baths, which destroy the spasms, often remaining after the inflammation is subdued.

Treatment.—*Aconite* must be used first, as directed in gastritis. It is the principal remedy as long as the accompanying fever is intense and the skin very hot.

In severe cases, *Arsenic* and *Veratrum* after it, in a similar manner, as directed in gastritis.

In less severe cases, *Lachesis*, *Belladonna*, and *Mercury*, in alternation, will suffice, if the skin has become cooler, from the application of *Aconite*, but there still remain great soreness of the abdomen and intense thirst.

These medicines must be separately dissolved in water (twelve glob. to half a teacupful), and every two hours, alternately, a teaspoonful given, until three or four teaspoonfuls of each are taken, or until better.

But in the severest cases, when vomiting of fæces appears (*ileus miserere*),

Opium must be administered, every hour a dose (four glob.), and if not relieved within six, eight, or twelve hours,

Plumbum, in the same manner. It is in this stage where injections of an infusion of tobacco, or injecting tobacco smoke, is of the greatest benefit; also a lukewarm bath, to relax the whole system, and facilitate a decided reaction.

Diagnosis of the *symptomatic* or *subacute* form.—This is always a concomitant symptom in typhus, or other malignant fevers; also in consumption of the bowels. The pain of the abdomen consists of a soreness, aggravated by hard pressure, and after cold drinks and indigestible food; the tongue is red, smooth, sometimes shining; loss of appetite; thirst variable; constant dryness in the mouth and throat; nausea and vomiting are more or less present, the more so, the nearer the inflamed portions of the intestines are to the stomach. When the lower parts are more inflamed, which is indicated by the pain in that region, diarrhea of a slimy mucus, often mixed with blood, is present, as in dysentery. This is particularly the case in the beginning of Consumption of the bowels, such as nursing females are sometimes subject to, see "Diseases of Females."

TREATMENT.—If this disease occurs in typhus or other malignant fevers, see their respective chapters. In the commencement of a typhus, if the pain in the abdomen is excessive, give a few doses of *Aconite*, every two or three hours one (four glob.); after which give *Bryonia* and *Rhus tox.* (in a half a teacupful of water, twelve glob. dissolved), every two hours, alternately, a teaspoonful. See "Typhus Fever."

If it resembles a bloody dysentery, after the use of *Aconite* as above, give *Belladonna* and *Mercury* in alternation (dissolve of each twelve glob. in half a teacupful of water), every hour a teaspoonful, until better; after which *Nitric acid* generally suits, particularly if the patient has already taken a good deal of calomel; or *Colocynth*, if bilious, *green* matter is vomited or discharged by the dysenteric operation. For the application of these medicines, and of *Sulphur*, which is important in this disease, see "Dysentery."

If worms are suspected to be the cause of the inflammation of the bowels, or are complicated with it, see "Worms."

If the disease resembles or runs into consumption of the bowels, see "Diarrhea" and "Diarrhea of lying-in Women."

The *chronic* form of this disease requires the same remedies, only administered not so often, because the symptoms are less urgent.

In all severe cases of this kind, it would be indispensably necessary to apply to a homœopathic physician. if one can be had.

APPLICATION OF WATER, see preceding article.
DIET AND REGIMEN, the same as in "Gastritis."

INFLAMMATION OF THE LIVER. (*Hepatitis.*)

DIAGNOSIS.—This inflammation differs according to its place in the liver.

a. When the surface and the convex, or upper part of the liver is inflamed, there are in the right hypochondrium sometimes stitches, at other times burning pains, often as violent as in pleurisy, shooting to the breast bone, the right shoulder-blade, increased by deep respiration, frequently accompanied with cough and vomiting; in this form the patient *cannot lie on the right side.*

b. When the concave, or lower part, and the substance of the liver is inflamed, there is not so much pain, but more a feeling of pressing, heaviness, as of a bag lying in that region; the color of the eyes and face become yellowish, as if jaundice were present; bitter taste, and vomiting; in this form the patient cannot lie on the *left side.*

In both forms general inflammatory fever is present more or less, and the region of the liver sensitive to pressure, and apparently bloated and hot. The first form may be mistaken for pleurisy, as the symptoms are very similar; but, as in such a case the treatment would be the same, no danger can result from such a mistake.

If hepatitis is not well treated, it has the tendency to pass into the chronic state, forming ulcerations, which either appear externally or communicate internally with the intestines or the lungs, causing inflammation of these organs; indurations, adhesion, gangrene, are also issues of neglected hepatitis.

CAUSES.—Summer heat and hot climate predispose to this disease; also, the abuse of ardent spirits; beside, it is excited by external lesions, concussion of the brain, suddenly suppressed diarrhea or dysentery, hemorrhoidal congestion, or strong emetics or purgatives, the abuse of mercury, the presence of stones in the gall-bladder, indigestion, violent passion or anger, particularly when immediately followed by drinking ardent spirits.

TREATMENT.—The following are the principal remedies necessary for the *acute* form of this disease: *Aconite, Chamomile, Bryon., China, Bellad., Mercury, Nux vom., Pulsatilla, Sulph., Lachesis.*

For the species *a.* are more suitable: *Aconite, Belladonna, Bryon., Mercury, Lachesis, Sulph.*

For the species *b: Aconite, Chamomile, Mercury, Pulsat., China, Nux vom., Sulphur.*

For *chronic* affections, such as enlargement and induration of the liver (liver complaint): *Nux vom., Sulphur., Aurum.*

(Other serious chronic diseases must be treated by a homœopathic physician.)

SYMPTOMATIC DETAIL. — *Aconite.* At the commencement of the treatment, when there are violent inflammatory fever, *shooting* pain in the region of the liver, tossing about, fear of death, and anguish; pain seems to be insupportable.

Belladonna. Pressing pains extending to the chest and shoulders; fullness in the pit of the stomach and around the short ribs; difficult and anxious respiration; anxious tossing and sleeplessness; thirst, dryness of the mouth and throat; headache, with clouded sight, and vertigo, with fainting. Suitable after *Aconite*, and alternately with *Lachesis* or *Mercury.*

Bryonia. Pressing pains, with fullness in the hypochondria; *violent oppression of the chest;* rapid and anxious breathing; tongue yellowish and thickly coated, followed by fever and thirst; pains worse by movement; constipation. Suitable after *Aconite* or alternately with *Mercury.*

Mercury. Patient cannot lie long on the *right* side; pains are pressing and shooting; bitter taste in the mouth; thirst and shivering; skin and eyes yellowish. After it *Lachesis* and *Sulphur* are suitable.

Lachesis. If *Belladonna* or *Mercury* is insufficient, or when the patient is in the habit of drinking ardent spirits.

Sulphur. In every case of hepatitis, either at the end of the cure, or when the preceding remedies have produced no perceptible amelioration within a few days.

Chamomile. In hepatitis after taking cold; when caused by violent anger, or when there are dull pressing pains, *not aggravated* by *movement, respiration*, or *external pressure; yellow color* of the skin; *pressure in the stomach;* gastric bilious state of the stomach; tongue coated; bitter taste in the mouth; *fits of anguish*.

Pulsatilla. In hepatitis, from indigestion, alternately with *China;* nausea, bitter taste in the mouth, tongue coated; oppression of the chest; tension around the short ribs; *fits* of anguish in the night, with *loose, greenish*, and *slimy* evacuations.

China. After indigestion, or when there is shooting and pressing: swelling and hardness of the hepatic region; pressing headache; bitter taste in the mouth and yellowish coat on the tongue.

Nux vomica. After a fit of passion, or when there is shooting and beating under the short-ribs of the right side, excessively tender when touched; nausea, with sour and bitter taste; *fits of anguish;* shortness of breath, thirst, vertigo, and headache; suitable for drunkards, and in chronic liver affections, previous to *Sulphur*.

ADMINISTRATION.—Dissolve of the remedy selected, twelve globules in half a teacupful of water, and give every two hours a teaspoonful, until three or four spoonfuls are taken, or until another remedy is indicated by the change of symptoms; as the patient gets better, lengthen the intervals; as soon as greatly relieved, discontinue all medicine for forty-eight hours, when one dose (four glob.) of *Sulphur* may be administered to complete the cure.

In *chronic* hepatitis, give of the necessary remedy only once in twenty-four hours a dose (four glob.), for two or three days; then discontinue six or eight days before the next remedy is given.

APPLICATION OF WATER. — The wet bandage is beneficial; constipation is relieved by cold injections.

The treatment of the chronic form is assisted by the constant wearing of a wet bandage around the abdomen.

DIET AND REGIMEN.—*No meat or meat soups of any kind*, but farinaceous substances; rice and oatmeal gruel, sweetened and made palatable by lemon-juice, lemonade, cold or warm, prunes sweetened or boiled in gruels, baked apples, toasted bread, toast-water, cold water alone. Keep the patient quiet and comfortable as regards temperature.

JAUNDICE. (*Icterus.*)

DIAGNOSIS.—This disease, well known by the yellow color it imparts to all the white parts of the body, is not to be considered dangerous of itself, but becomes only so by neglect, when other serious disorders, hectic fever, dropsy, etc., may follow. In most cases it is the result of neglected liver diseases, or is caused by taking cold which affected the liver; also, by worms or gall-stones, obstructing the gall-duct, or is induced by excessive mental emotions. In jaundice the bowels become constipated, and if fæces pass, they are hard and whitish; the urine is orange-colored, and the skin dry, or, if moist, it is from weakness, and the perspiration imparts a yellow color to the patient's linen. Sometimes a slight fever accompanies these symptoms, which increases toward night, remitting or even intermitting in the morning; this is the case in the milder form. In the severer forms of this disease, accompanied with high fever, the brain becomes affected, which, if not relieved soon, may cause the death of the patient (see for the treatment of such a state, "Inflammation of the Brain").

TREATMENT.—The principal object must be to increase, by degrees, the healthy action of the skin; the patient, therefore, ought to keep warmly covered in bed in a warm room, and take, for the first three or four days, *Mercury*, morning, noon, and night a dose (four glob.); if not better at the expiration of four days, give *Hepar*, in the same manner; but if signs of amelioration appear, give it at longer intervals; this course generally removes the disease in eight or ten days, during which time the patient must keep in an equal, warm temperature and perspiration. In very obstinate cases, *Lachesis*, *Nitric acid*, *Sulphur*, may be given afterward in the same manner.

Jaundice, caused by a fit of passion, requires *Chamomile*, followed by *Nux vom.*

If it is caused by the abuse of *Mercury*, or *Calomel*, give *China*, *Hepar sulph.*, *Lachesis*, or *Sulphur*.

If a child becomes yellow from having taken rhubarb too often or too much, give *Chamomile* or *Mercury*.

If persons are liable to jaundice upon every trifling occasion, give *Lachesis* and *Sulphur*, every week one dose (four glob.), alternately, to eradicate the disposition.

If jaundice is complicated with fever, see "Inflammation of the Liver."

APPLICATION OF WATER. — Lukewarm sitting-baths, wet bandages around the chest and stomach, and the sweating in the wet sheet are powerful auxiliaries in the treatment of this disease; constipation is relieved by cold injections.

DIET AND REGIMEN, as in "Hepatitis."

INFLAMMATION OF THE SPLEEN. (*Splenitis.*)

DIAGNOSIS.—Sharp, pressing, or shooting pains in the left side, below the short-ribs; the spleen on pressure is painful, and when pressed upward excites cough, and nausea in the stomach, sometimes vomiting of blood; if fever is present it is very high, with all the concomitant symptoms of inflammation of internal organs. The region of the spleen is enlarged and congested.

CAUSES.—Similar to those of inflammation of the liver, beside the abuse of *quinine* or *Peruvian bark;* also, living in a marshy region causes congestion of the spleen, and consequently inflammation, under otherwise trifling circumstances.

TREATMENT.—We have an acute and chronic form. For the *acute, Aconite, Bryonia,* and *China* are the principal remedies, to be administered as directed in hepatitis.

If vomiting of blood is present, or sometimes even the blood is discharged by the stools, *Arnica, Rhus tox.,* and *Arsenic,* followed by *China,* are necessary, one remedy after the other, in the same manner as above.

For the *chronic* form, *enlargement, induration* of the spleen (fever cake), *Sulphur, Calcarea carb., Ferrum, Lycopodium, Carbo veg.* are the principal remedies; administration as directed in the chronic form of hepatitis; but it is strongly recommended to procure the aid of a skillful homœopathic physician for its treatment.

APPLICATION OF WATER, DIET AND REGIMEN, as in "Hepatitis."

WORMS.

Every part of the system can, under favorable circumstances, create and sustain worms, or other imperfectly organized animals; thus, the skin, liver, lungs, kidneys, even the brain and eyes, in some animals, are favorable places for their generation, the species of animals varying according to the organ attacked. *Worms* are most frequently found in the intestinal canal; there are three kinds of worms met with, the *Ascaris,* or pinworms (ascaris vermicularis), *Maw-worms* (ascaris lumbricoides), and the *Tapeworm* (tænia), of which latter there are two varieties:

a. The *broad one* (tænia lata), varying from three to twelve feet in length, seldom comes away entire, but in joints; and

b. The *solitary tapeworm* (tænia solium), with long and slender joints, sometimes reaching the length of thirty feet.

DIAGNOSIS.—It is frequently not an easy matter to decide

positively on the presence of worms in the system, as most all those symptoms which could lead to such a conclusion are also met with in other diseases, save the one symptom, surest of all, that is, the passage of some worms, or undoubted pieces of them. This uncertainty in the diagnosis of the worm disease is no less annoying and embarrassing for an allopathic practitioner; as his prescriptions are dangerous, and in most cases, without good or decided result for the little patient, as with the worms their cause is not always expelled. Homœopathy, on account of its guiding principle, avoids either of the two dangerous issues, and, prescribing for the ostensible symptoms as they reflect the inward disease, cures and eradicates this surely, safely, and mildly. Merely expelling the worms, by remedies which have no *specific* bearing upon the worm disease, is of no essential use, and requires often enormous quantities of poisonous and dangerous stuff before one of the worms is sickened, killed, or expelled. Yes, I have seen the foundation of painful chronic diseases laid by the over-medication in the presumed or real presence of worms; there are even cases where children have died under the operation of those drugs, which allopathists consider necessary to apply in such dangerous doses. The most irrational, nay, a real lottery business, is the use of those manifold nostrums, in the shape of lozenges, syrups, etc., which generally contain one or more specific anti-worm remedies; for instance, worm-seed, or pink-root, which given in small and not offensive doses would produce salutary effects, but in the combination of dangerous purgatives expose the little patients to death or misery; at least, the smallest number escape unhurt, most of them receiving injuries of the abdomen, the bad consequences of which impede not a little the future development of the child.

Worms, as such, are not dangerous. They have no teeth, and consequently cannot eat children up alive. It is true, they can and will disturb the quiet and rest of a child, and make it pick at the nose, or cough, or cry out suddenly, or even have fits, etc.; yet all this is only produced by the worms having been made restless, by the presence of sickness in the system, which causes them to touch the walls of the intestines, usually avoided by them—living in and of the mass of mucus and other nutritive substances, with which the system had been indiscriminately, and in too large quantities burdened. As soon as the system recovers from its own disease, either from cold or irregularity of diet, the worms return to their usual, unobtrusive quiet again, giving no signs of their existence, nor causing alarm. Every person, more or less, has worms without the least injury to the system. Neither is it absolutely the quantity of them which is the most dangerous quality of this disease; a few worms can cause as many fits, or other spasmodic symptoms, as whole clusters of them. It depends altogether on the accompanying disease; and this it is which we will have to treat, before we can expect the worms to leave the system (which I have seen frequently, after a dose of homœopathic preparation of *Sulphur*), or to be absorbed (digested and reduced to mucus, from which they originated). This latter is the most common result of homœopathic medicines in this disease. In such cases, the children show signs of improvement, as soon as their abdomen becomes reduced in size and hardness; their complexion improves, they become more agile, grow better in height, and sleep quiet.

And this result is always attained by the judicious use of homœopathic medicines in this disease, in whatever form it may appear; for instance, as fits, diarrhea, scrofula, etc. Fits, occasioned by worms, are not in the least dangerous, and only become so by unwisely dealing with them.

The principal symptoms, by which the presence of worms in the system is indicated, are the following: the complexion of the patient is pale and changeable; livid circles around the eyes; accumulation of saliva in the mouth in the morning, and when not having taken nourishment for some time; irregular appetite; nausea; fetid breath; great hunger; picking and boring at the nose, with sneezing; abdomen enlarged, but not hard; frequent distressing pain in the stomach, in the region of the navel, which forces the patient to draw up the limbs against the abdomen, or lie on the stomach when going to sleep; pupils of the *eye dilated;* bleeding at the nose; starting, as if from fright, during sleep, also grinding of the teeth; disposition to spasms, and unusual emaciation. The surest sign, however, is the discharge of worms, or parts of worms.

Signs of *tapeworm*, in particular, are: a sensation, as of something suddenly rising from the left side into the throat and falling back, or as if a lump in one or the other side was making an undulatory motion; dizziness, particularly in the morning, before eating.

Signs of *ascarides*, or *pin-worms*, especially, are: itching in the anus, more in the evening or at night; difficulty of making urine; tenesmus; apparent hemorrhoidal complaints; discharge of mucus from the rectum, bladder, or vagina (fluor albus).

Signs of *maw-worm*, or *lumbricus*, particularly, are: all the above general symptoms of worms, but frequently stomach-ache, which is relieved after drinking sweet, cold milk.

Diseases caused by the Presence of Worms.

Infancy is the age, when, on account of the general predominancy of nutrition, laxity and weakness by accumulation of mucus in the intestines preponderate; and consequently, those remote causes for the generation of worms, which may be favored even by circumstantial ones, such as flabby constitution of the child, damp habitation, and other epidemical and endemical influences.

This variety of the remote causes of worms gives rise to an equal variety of diseases, flowing from the same source (the worms), yet different, according to their exciting causes.

Thus, these diseases vary, from the most trifling illness, to the most severe colics, and dangerous fevers. The worms create, operating on the *nervous system* by sympathy, convulsions, all kinds of spasms, epilepsy, St. Vitus's dance (*chorea*), somnambulism, periodical paralysis, insanity, fury.

On the *vascular* or *blood system:* fevers, congestions to bowels, hemorrhages, eruptions on the skin, appearing in irregular blotches of a scarlet color.

On the *reproductive system* (the intestines themselves): pains, spasms, increased secretion and accumulation of mucus, diarrhea, dysentery, worm colic.

TREATMENT.—The principal remedies for the diseases produced by worms on the *nervous system*, as above stated, are: *Ignatia*, *Cina*cc., *Nux vom.*, *Hyoscyamus*, *Belladonna*, *Spigelia*, *Sulphur*.

On the *vascular* or *blood system : Aconite*, *Belladonna*, *Hyoscyamus*, *Cina*, *Ferrum*, *Mercury*, *Sulphur*, *Silicea*.

On the *reproductive system*, or the *intestines : Aconite*, *Belladonna*, *Cina* and *Cina*cc., *Mercury*, *Sulphur*, *Spigelia*. (For the detail of these medicines, see below.)

Especially against *tapeworms*, the most suitable remedies are: *Mercury*, and *Sulphur*, to be given every four or six days, alternately, a dose (six glob.) after which *Calcarea carb.*, *Graphites*, *Stannum*, may be given in the same way, if necessary. *Cupr. oxyd. nigr.* is strongly recommended. See Boston Quart. Homœop. Jour., Vol. I., p. 138.

Against *ascarides* (*pin-worms*): *Aconite*, and *Ignatia*, or *China* and *Mercury*, or *Calcarea carb.*, and *Ferrum*, or *Cina* and *Sulphur*, alternately, every second or third evening a dose, until better. An injection every evening of an ounce of pure sweet oil (olive oil), without any other admixture, is an excellent adjunct against these troublesome worms. The ascarides lodge never higher up in the abdomen than the rectum; therefore, can be expelled easily, or killed.

Against *maw-worms*, or worms in the intestinal canal, are

generally appropriate: *Aconite, Belladonna, Hyoscyamus, Mercury, Cina* and *Cina*^cc., *Sulphur, Silicea, Spigelia, Ferrum, Ignatia, Nux vom.;* but in particular diseases caused by maw-worms, as follows:

a. For *colic,* with *fever:* *Cina*^cc., *Aconite, Belladonna, Hyoscyamus, Mercury.*

b. For *colic* with *convulsions:* *Cina*^cc., *Belladonna, Hyoscyamus.*

c. For *colic* with *diarrhea* and voracious appetite: *Spigelia, Nux moschata.*

d. For *fever:* *Aconite, Spigelia, Silicea.*

For *diarrhea,* frequent but small stools, mostly at night, pale face, and listlessness, require: *Nux moschata.*

For *slow fever, in scrofulous* children: *Silicea.*

Symptomatic Detail.—*Aconite.* In the commencement of all cases, where considerable fever exists; restlessness at night; irritability of temper; also, in cases without fever, when there is, from the presence of ascarides, continual itching and burning at the anus; and then alternately with *Ignatia.*

Administration.—In fever, every two or three hours a dose (infant children above one year of age three glob.), repeated two or three times, until the fever abates, when another remedy will be necessary. In cases of ascarides, alternately with *Ignatia,* every evening a dose (two or three glob.).

Ignatia. In pin-worms, or ascarides (see *Aconite*). In *maw-worms,* when there are spasmodic twitchings in the muscles of the arms, as if the St. Vitus's dance was commencing. In this latter case, alternately with *Sulphur,* every evening a dose (two or three glob.).

Sulphur. At the end of every case of worm affection, after other remedies have either subdued the fever, or mitigated the nervous symptoms. Give every evening one dose (two or three glob.), for three evenings, and then wait from six to eight days, before another remedy is applied, or the same repeated, if necessary.

Cina. This is one of the most important remedies, particularly when there is boring at the nose, fever (after the application of *Aconite*); irritability; restlessness at night; desire for things which are rejected when offered; pale, bloated face, with livid circles around the eyes; craving for food, even after a meal; the child wants bread, potatoes, and other gross victuals; colic; griping; distension and hardness of the abdomen; discharge of *pin* and *large* worms; diarrhea; weakness of the limbs; the child cannot stand any more on its feet; spasmodic movements in the limbs.

ADMINISTRATION, see *Aconite*.

Cina^{cc}. When the children are very nervous, cry out in their sleep, or have *severe* colic pains, give every one or two hours a dose (two or three glob.), until better, or another remedy is necessary. Where children cry out in the night, groan, and are restless, give every evening only one dose (two or three glob.), until better.

Spigelia. In severe cases of worm colic, fever, and diarrhea, with craving appetite and chilliness, or where the symptoms appear regularly at the same time of the day.

Administration in acute cases, the same as *Aconite* in fever. In chronic cases, every evening a dose (two or three glob.)

Hyoscyamus. In worm fevers, when the patients are very nervous, restless, cry out, want to run off, and stool or urine passes off involuntarily.

Administration as in *Aconite*.

Belladonna. Worm colic after the administration of *Aconite*, when great pains remain in the stomach, which are relieved by lying on the bowels, starting in the sleep, sensibility to light, headache; on awaking, the child does not know where it is, etc. Particularly useful in scrofulous children, with distended abdomen and red cheeks, or where red blotches, like erysipelas, appear on different parts of the body. In such cases, in alternation with *Silicea.*

Administration in *acute* and *chronic* cases, the same as *Aconite.*

Mercury. In *worm diarrhea,* swelling and hardness of the abdomen, and when there is unusual flow of saliva from the mouth.

Administration as in *Spigelia,* after which it is suitable.

Nux vomica. Worm symptoms with constipation (the child has frequent, but insufficient calls to stool), and irritability.

Administration as in *Mercury.*

China. In worm diarrhea, when it has already lasted some time; distension of the abdomen; debility; great appetite; pains in the stomach after every meal. Suits well in alternation with *Veratrum,* particularly when the stools are light-colored.

Administration as in *Mercury.*

Ferrum. When there is vomiting and accumulation of watery fluid in the mouth.

Silicea. If a worm fever assumes the slow, chronic form, with or without diarrhea, particularly in scrofulous children.

Administration as in *Sulphur.*

Diet and Regimen.—In worm fever, adhere to the diet recommended for common fever. In severe worm colic, give as a palliative, cold, sweet milk, from time to time. In diarrhea, avoid acids, fruits, and all indigestible articles; give, rather, soups of mutton or lamb, with rice. Avoid, in chronic worm diseases, heavy, gross nourishment, such as too much bread and butter, potatoes, heavy puddings, pies, raw or boiled vegetables; but meat-soups of any kind, meat, roasted or broiled, plenty of cold water and milk, are beneficial. Beside, bathing in cold water, and exercise in the open air. In worm fever the wet bandage and sitting-bath are recommended.

CONSTIPATION. COSTIVENESS.

This term must not always be taken in the absolute sense as a diseased state of the bowels; as there are persons who naturally have only every two or three days an evacuation—a habit which frequently promotes rather than disturbs general health, if the latter is not interfered with by an unwise use of medicines, such as taking pills or aperients of a drastic or saline nature. As a general rule, we can consider it the normal state of the bowels, to have one evacuation every day. This ought to become a fixed rule and habit, as it frequently corrects costiveness of the bowels, without the use of any medicine.

Some occupations of life predispose to costiveness, particularly those which allow but little exercise. Persons, under such circumstances, must abandon these occupations, if possible, for a length of time, take a great deal of exercise in the open air, change the diet (see below), and make use of cold water, externally and internally, in large quantities (see "Application of Water"). Nothing is more injurious than the continued use of medicinal aperients. They render the bowels, in time, more costive and torpid. The best expedient for facilitating an immediate action on the bowels, if wanted, is an *injection*, either *of cold water*, if the person otherwise is in health or the patient prefers it, or lukewarm water, sweet oil, or lard, and a small piece of castile-soap dissolved in it, if the constipation has been very obstinate, or a quick evacuation is wanted, as in children, when they have fits, etc.

In most cases of acute diseases, constipation is only one of the many symptoms constituting the disease; because it disappears as soon as the whole complex of symptoms has been taken away.*

* One of the most striking cases of this kind, showing in a high degree the truth of the above statement, presented itself to me a few years ago, in a lady who had been persuaded to take castor oil, three days

If, however, constipation is the only or principal symptom in a disease, as in *miserere, lead colic*, etc., we have remedies which combat it more safely and successfully than all the aperients commonly used. Cases of this kind, however, must be treated by experienced homœopathic physicians.

TREATMENT.—We will now give first a tabular view of the causes and complications of constipations, with their principal remedies, the detailed symptoms of which follow below.—These must be consulted before a selection is made.

Constipation in general, or a *disposition* for it: *Bryon., Nux vom., Lachesis, Lycopodium, Sulphur, Sepia.*

In persons who lead a *sedentary life: Bryon., Nux vom., Sulphur, Opium, Platina, Lycopodium.*

In *drunkards: Lachesis, Nux vom., Opium, Sulphur.*

In *old persons*, or those of weakly constitutions, where constipation often *alternates with diarrhea: Antimon. crud., Conium, Opium, Phosphorus.*

In *pregnant women: Nux vom., Opium, Sepia.*

In *nursing infants: Bryon., Nux vom., Opium, Sulphur.*

In *lying-in women: Bryon., Nux vom.*

In *consumptives: Stannum, Silicea Sulphur.*

By *traveling* in a carriage: *Platina, Opium.*

---

after her confinement, although in former cases of this kind she always had suffered very much after its use, from irritation of the intestines. After the administration of the castor oil, a violent and painful diarrhea appeared, threatening fearful consequences for the life of the patient. This was, however, soon removed, by the exhibition of *China, Mercury*, and *Pulsatilla*, and her health decidedly improved, from day to day, her appetite and strength returned, and she moved about as if she was well; yet there was no disposition for evacuating, until on the *twenty-second day* after the last evacuation, when it appeared, without any artificial means, in a perfectly healthy condition. During the eight days previous to it, the patient had been allowed a good nourishing diet, and enough of it, too.

I have frequently had cases where patients had no evacuations for eight, ten, or twelve days; but I never have experienced their suspension for twenty-two days, except in the above case.

During *sea-voyages: Cocculus, Nux vom., Silicea.*

From poisoning by *lead:* See "Painter's Colic."

From abuse of *purging medicines: Opium, Nux vomica, Lachesis.*

From abuse of *quinine: Pulsat., Carbo veg., Veratrum.*

Symptomatic Detail.—*Bryonia.* In all recent cases of constipation during *fevers* or *bilious attacks,* where headache, chilliness and rheumatic pains predominate; particularly, also, in *warm weather;* the patient is of a nervous, irritable temperament. After it, or in alternation with it, *Nux vom.*

Nux vomica. Is of the most frequent application in *hypochondriacal persons,* or those suffering from *piles;* also, after derangement of the stomach, when there is *frequent* but *ineffectual effort* to evacuate, or a feeling as if the *anus were closed* or *contracted;* ill-humor, fullness of the head, cannot bear the clothes tight around the waist. After it, or in alternation with it, *Sulphur.*

Sulphur. In all cases of *habitual costiveness,* or where *Nux vom.* was insufficient.

Opium. In all cases where there is *great torpidity* of the bowels, and a feeling as if the *anus were closed,* but *without* the frequent and ineffectual efforts to evacuate, as is the case in *Nux vomica;* the patient only feels full in his bowels, has congestion to the head, with dark redness of the face, slow and full pulse; this remedy is of frequent application in children, old persons, pregnant women, drunkards, and hypochondriacal persons.

Sepia. In cases where there are, beside constipation, *flashes of heat, sick-headache,* a pressing down, particularly in pregnant women, or where *Nux vomica, Opium,* and *Sulphur* have been insufficient.

Platina. In nervous females, and weakly hypochondriacal persons, where the stool only appears in small pieces, followed by tenesmus and tingling in the anus; shuddering, and a sensation of weakness in the abdomen; sometimes, also, a constrictive pain in the abdomen, and ineffectual desire to evacuate. Compare *Nux vomica.*

Lachesis. A very useful remedy in obstinate constipations during fevers, particularly where abscesses of internal organs are existing or presumed to exist, as in the liver, mesenteric glands, etc., or in alternation with

Lycopodium. Where an obstinate disposition to constipation is present, from constitutional causes, such as scrofula, which had fallen on the bowels after it disappeared from the skin, etc.; if, in such cases, these two remedies remove the costiveness, but the disease attacks the lungs and produces cough, which is worse when a part of the body gets cool by exposure, give *Hepar sulph.* See "Dyspepsia."

Antimon. crud. In cases where *constipation* and *diarrhea* alternate, if one ceases the other sets in; the stools are never regular.

Phosphorus. If *Antimon.* is insufficient, or when the patient is of a consumptive habit, or has the consumption.

Stannum. If *Phosphorus* does not suffice, or when there is frequent but ineffectual desire to evacuate, particularly in consumptives.

Silicea. Same as *Stannum,* when this is insufficient, or in children whose stomachs are distended and hard, indicating worms or swollen glands; also, in dyspeptic persons, with heart-burn, sour taste in the mouth, etc.

Cocculus. See "Sea-sickness" and "Colic."

Conium. For *old* and *weakly* persons, who are troubled with frequent but ineffectual efforts to evacuate (after *Nux vom.*); also, in scrofulous children, where the mesenteric glands are swollen (after *Silicea*), particularly accompanied with soreness of the abdomen.

Pulsatilla. In similar cases, where *Nux vomica* would suit, but the temperament is mild and phlegmatic; or after derangement of the stomach by fat food, the patient appearing morose and silent; also, after abuse of *quinine,* either with or without the return of the fever and ague, and then in alternation with

Carbo veg. This remedy, particularly, when persons have become very *much debilitated,* complain of *rheumatism, piles,* or have the *consumption.*

Veratrum. After *Opium,* when there is great torpor in the bowels, deficiency of expulsive power; or where the abdomen becomes *very tender to the touch* (and then in alternation with *Arsenic*); see "Bilious gastric Fevers;" also, after abuse of *quinine,* when there is great congestion to the head and hypochondriacal feeling.

Administration.—In cases where constipation exists as the only troublesome symptom, give the medicine selected in quick succession and large doses; for instance, *Nux vomica,* every three or four hours a dose (six to eight glob.) for one or two days, until relief is obtained, or another remedy is chosen; or *Lachesis* and *Lycopodium,* in alternation, three times a day a dose (six glob.); but where constipation is habitual or constitutional, the remedies must be administered at longer intervals; for instance, *Nux vomica,* every evening a dose (four glob.), for three or four days; then discontinue an equal length of time without taking medicine, after which either repeat it or select another remedy, if necessary, which in most cases will be *Sulphur.*

Application of Water, internally and externally, is an important auxiliary for the cure of constipation. When the latter is not of very long standing or not very obstinate, the injections can be made of cold water, of which two or three every day may be taken; the sitting-bath in such a case may be of cold water also; but if the constipation is very obstinate, take for the above-named applications milkwarm water, and let the sitting-bath reach above the navel, and lengthen the time of application; let the patient use it for half-an-hour or upward. In inflammatory diseases, fevers, etc., the injections must be made of cold or cool water.

Diet and Regimen.—These are important agents in the cure of constipation ; first of all is the habit of attending to the calls of nature carefully and regularly, at a certain time, say after breakfast, though there should be no actual result from it; secondly, the careful avoidance of all nourishment which is confining in its character, such as salted meats, cheese, rice, wheaten flour, except these things are mixed in a sufficient quantity with their opposites, such as have a loosening quality, fresh meat, and soups made of it, green vegetables, and fruits, except almonds or nuts. But the chief promoter of a healthy action on the bowels is the frequent and liberal use of cold water, internally and externally, with bodily exercise in the open air. The cold and ice water can be drank freely during and after a meal, without the least inconvenience, and ought to be preferred to the use of wines, brandies, tea or coffee.

Diarrhea. Looseness of the Bowels.

This complaint varies so much in regard to time of duration, form and cause, that we are obliged to give here a general view of its varieties. It is either recent, lasting only for a few hours or days, or is chronic, lasting for months or years. The discharge itself may vary as regards consistency or character, either watery, fluid, fecal, slimy, mattery, bilious, or bloody (see "Dysentery"). Sometimes a diarrhea is dangerous ; at other times salutary, as in biliousness or after indigestion (see these articles). In general, however, the popular idea of the harmless or beneficial nature of diarrheas, which the common practice of the old school of medicine has freely propagated, must be restricted, in so far as any diarrhea is of itself an indication of a diseased state of the intestines, and no disease ought to be created or wished for where we can do without it. It has been, and is yet, to a great extent, a common expression that a good cleansing of the bowels is necessary, etc. ; now, these ideas, when carried out in practice, lead sometimes to awful consequences, while the good which they may occasionally produce might have been obtained by mild and rational means. See "Constipation" and "Biliousness." On the other hand, it is just as dangerous to stop a diarrhea suddenly by violent means, such as brandy, paregoric, or astringents generally, as thereby the disease is not cured, but merely its natural outlet stopped; as if an ulcer could be cured by covering it over to confine and hide the matter, which it has to discharge. It is always fortunate if such a diarrhea reappears.

Treatment.—We will now give first a general view of the varieties of diarrhea, as regards causes, form, and appearances, with their principal remedies, whose detailed symptoms may be found below, and must be consulted before a choice is made.

Diarrhea without pain: *China, Phosphoric acid, Ferrum, Secale.*

With *griping* or *colic* pain: *Mercury, Colocynth, Chamomile, Rheum, Pulsatilla, Bryonia, Rhus tox., Arsenic, Sulphur,* (See "Bilious colic.")

With *tenesmus*, during or after the discharge, in the anus: *Aloes, Ipecac., Mercury, Belladonna, Nux vomica, Sulphur.* (See "Dysentery.")

With *vomiting:* *Ipecac., Veratrum, Arsenic, Rhus tox.* (See "Cholera.")

With *debility:* *China, Arsenic, Ipecac., Veratrum, Secale, Phosphorus.* (See "Cholera Morbus," and "Asiatic Cholera.")

Of *mucus* and *blood:* See "Dysentery."

Of *bile:* See "Bilious Gastric Derangement;" beside, *Aloes, Bryonia, Rhus tox., Arsenic, Mercury, Pulsatilla.*

Of watery (rice-water) liquid: see "Cholera Asiatica."

After *eruptive fevers*, such as small-pox, scarlet, measles, etc.: *Pulsatilla, China, Phosphoric acid, Arsenic, Sulphur.*

After *sudden mental emotions:* after *joy: Coffea, Aconite, Pulsatilla;* after *fright: Chamomile, Veratrum; fear* of cholera and other dangers: *Chamomile;* after *grief: Phosphoric acid, Ignatia;* after *anger: Colocynth, Chamomile, Nux vomica.* (See "Mental Diseases.")

After *indigestion:* from partaking of *milk: Bryonia, Sulphur;* of *acids* or *fruits: Lachesis, Pulsatilla, Arsenic;* of other indigestible substances, fat meats, etc., *China, Pulsatilla,* coffee without milk. (See "Indigestion.")

After the abuse of drugs: of *Mercury* or *calomel: Hepar, Pulsatilla, China, Carbo veg., Nitric acid;* of *magnesia: Pulsatilla, Rheum;* of *rhubarb: Pulsatilla, Mercury, Colocynth;* of *tobacco: Pulsat., Chamomile, Hepar, Veratrum;* of *quinine: Pulsatilla, Carbo veg.*

After *cold* or *iced drinks: Pulsatilla, Carbo veg., Arsenic.*

After *taking cold, cold on the bowels: Dulcamara, Chamomile.*

In *summer: Bryonia, Mercury, Arsenic.*

In *autumn* and *spring,* during the changeable weather: *Bryonia, Rhus tox., Dulcamara, Carbo veg.*

In *weak* and *exhausted* persons: see "With Debility."

In *consumptive* persons: *China, Phosphorus, Calcarea, Ferrum.* (See "Consumption.")

In *chronic* diarrhea, of a scrofulous character: *Iodine, Phosphorus.*

In *aged persons: Secale, Antimon. crud., Bryonia, Phosphorus.*

In *pregnant* and *lying-in females: Phosphorus, Antimon. crud., Dulcamara, Pulsatilla, Sepia, Rheum.* (See "Female Diseases.")

In *children*—by *worms, teething,* and *scrofula:* see these articles.

Symptomatic Detail.—*Antimon. crud.* Watery diarrhea, from disordered stomach, with foul tongue and nausea.

Aloes. Bilious papescent stools, the whole body becoming

hot during the evacuation, with a feeling of sickness in the region of the liver; evacuations of fecal matter, bilious, not watery, not very profuse, having a peculiar putrid smell.

Dulcamara. In *most all diarrheas from taking cold,* or when there are greenish, or yellowish, slimy, or watery evacuations, particularly at *night,* with colic and griping pains in the region of the navel; great thirst, *nausea,* debility, and restlessness.

Colocynth. *Bilious* or *watery* diarrhea, with *severe cramp-like pains* (see "Bilious Colic" and "Dysentery"); or after *Chamomile,* when caused by anger or vexation.

Chamomile. *Bilious, watery,* or *slimy* diarrhea, of a *green* (*grass-green*) or *yellowish white,* curdled appearance, like *scrambled eggs,* with or without *vomiting of bile* (see "Biliousness"); griping, tearing colic; distension and hardness of the abdomen; fullness in the pit of the stomach, and under the short-ribs; bitter taste in the mouth; this medicine is particularly useful in diarrheas from cold, fear, anger, vexation, and in those of infants (see "Diseases of Children"), when they draw up the legs, cry, toss about, want to be carried, etc.

Rheum. *Sour smelling* evacuations, with ineffectual effort *before* and *after,* at the same time *contractive colic* in the abdomen, and *shuddering* when evacuating; grayish brown evacuations, *mixed with mucus;* very useful in diarrheas of *infants,* particularly when they cry, toss about (see *Chamomile*), and in diarrheas of *lying-in-women.*

Ipecac. Diarrhea of *fomented* evacuations, greenish, yellowish, putrid, *bloody or slimy;* dysenteric, when there are discharges of white flakes, and great tenesmus (see this article), or diarrhea with vomiting (see "Cholera Infantum," "Cholera Morbus," and "Asiatic Cholera").

Veratrum. In all diarrheas resembling the different varieties of *cholera* (see these articles); or where there is great *debility* or *griping pains,* as if *knives were cutting the intestines,* which happens often in fevers.

Secale. In *cholera,* or when *painless* evacuations are attended by *great weakness;* in *old people,* particularly *females,* where drowsiness ensues, in alternation with *Belladonna.* (See "Cholera Asiatica.")

Carbo veg. In *cholera* (see this article), or where there are *thin, light-colored* evacuations, of a *putrid* or *fetid smell,* particularly in *children;* or after taking cold in wet weather; also, after abuse of *quinine,* in alternation with *Pulsatilla.*

Arsenic. *Burning evacuations,* with *severe colic pains,* alternately with *Veratrum;* or *fetid, putrid, indigested* diarrhea, alternately with *Carbo veg.;* or *watery, slimy, burning* evacuations, principally after *midnight,* when *Dulcamara* or *China* have afforded no relief; or in *cholera* (see this article).

Bryonia. Diarrhea from the heat of summer (summer complaint of children), or where *bilious rheumatic* (see this article) symptoms accompany the bowel complaint, alternately with *Rhus tox.*

Rhus tox. In *cholera infantum* (see this article); or in bilious rheumatic disorders. See *Bryonia.*

Pulsatilla. In all diarrheas from indigestion or disordered stomach, where, after some griping pain, *watery, green,* or *bilious slimy* stools appear, particularly at *night;* sometimes the color changes, frequently from yellow to white, or the discharge is mixed with blood; bitter taste in the mouth, and foul tongue; in diarrhea from abuse of *quinine* and *calomel.*

Mercury. In critical diarrhea after fevers or bilious states of the stomach, when it threatens to become too debilitating and irritating; this critical diarrhea generally commences with griping pain and rumbling of the bowels, after which a copious, bilious, slimy, and frothy evacuation of a very fetid smell follows, with signal relief; yet this may recur in a short time after, and finally, if not relieved by *Mercury,* run into a dysentery. *Mercury* suits for almost any diarrhea when accompanied with griping in the bowels before, and tenesmus or burning in the anus after the discharge.

Nitric acid. Diarrhea after taking too much calomel or mercury, particularly when the stools are *bloody*, with tenesmus at the anus, sometimes of a fetid smell.

Nux vomica. *Frequent but scanty evacuations* of watery and greenish, lightish substance, with colic and tenesmus, and then in alternation with *Mercury.*

Ignatia. Diarrhea of a bloody slime, with rumbling in the bowels, or after continued grief.

Belladonna. Frequent, small evacuations of mucus, sometimes with fever heat in the head, pressing down (see "Dysentery"); or in those congestions to the head which follow severe diarrheas, or accompany them in old persons, and then in alternation with *Secale.* (See this remedy.)

Hepar sulph. In diarrheas of children, when they smell sour, are lightish, greenish, yellowish, bloody, slimy, and like dysentery; also, in those of nursing women. (See "Diseases of Females.")

China. Diarrhea after *eating* (*lienteria*), or in the *night;* also, when it is very debilitating, with rumbling in the abdomen. (See "Cholerina.")

Phosphoric acid. Diarrhea *without* pain, after *grief* and *distress* of mind; or when it passes involuntarily. (See "Cholerina.")

Ferrum. *Painless* evacuations after *eating* and *drinking,* or discharges in the night, with griping, flatulency, thirst, pain in the stomach, back, and anus. (See "Ascarides.")

Hyoscyamus. *Watery* diarrhea; *involuntary discharges,* particularly in the *night.*

Sulphur. In most cases where other remedies seem to have failed, particularly when there are *frequent* stools at *night,* with *griping,* of a slimy, watery, frothy substance, and of a sour and fetid smell, or bloody; also, if a diarrhea returns easily on taking the least cold.

Phosphorus. In chronic diarrhea without pain, particularly in the diarrhea of consumptives.

Iodine. In chronic diarrhea of a whitish color, in scrofulous persons, and which will not yield to any other remedy.

ADMINISTRATION.—In *recent* cases dissolve twelve glob. of the selected medicine in half a teacupful of water and take after every evacuation a teaspoonful until better, or another remedy is necessary; children half the quantity. In *chronic* cases take every evening and morning a teaspoonful of such a mixture, or if taken in the dry state three or four glob. at a dose.

APPLICATION OF WATER in some forms of this diseased state of the body is beneficial, particularly where by a reaction on the skin we can support the effect of the proper remedies. And this can be done in chronic, debilitating, and painful diarrheas by the application of the wet bandage, at the same time being well covered for the purpose to excite perspiration; sometimes sitting-baths are also necessary.

DIET AND REGIMEN.—Acids or acidulated drinks, fresh vegetables, and fresh meats and meat soups are forbidden; allowed are, rice, toasted bread, boiled milk, and gruels; no coffee and spiritous liquors. Cold water can be drank, if it is otherwise not injurious. Keep quiet as much as possible, even to lying down.

DYSENTERY. BLOODY FLUX.

DIAGNOSIS.— This complaint is, properly speaking, not a diarrhea; as no fæces are discharged, but only mucus and blood, accompanied by constant urging to go to stool, violent tenesmus in the anus and rectum, or severe pains in the abdomen, if the disease is located higher up in the intestines. As long as this irritation or inflammation of the mucous membrane of the intestines lasts, no fæces are discharged; but when these make their appearance, even mixed with bloody mucus, the dysentery may be said to be at an end, or at least ameliorated.

Its causes and course vary; sometimes it appears suddenly,

sometimes is preceded by diarrhea and other gastric rheumatic symptoms.

We distinguish a *white* dysentery, where only *light-colored* mucus (scrapings of the intestines) are discharged; this is soon followed by the *bloody* dysentery, when the blood comes from the highly-inflamed mucous membrane. In such cases more or less fever is always present. If the patient is relieved, the fever subsides, and gradually with it the pains, and frequent urgency of the calls, the skin becomes moist, and sleep and rest ensue. Death may come from gangrene and exhaustion, but happens very seldom, under a judicious homœopathic treatment. Very severe cases of dysentery ought to be treated by a skillful homœopathic physician. The causes of this disease may be local, by irritating the intestines directly in eating and drinking, or general, by suppression of perspiration (hot days and cool nights promote this cause), or by an epidemic influence, which affects in a similar manner the mucous membrane of the intestines, as the influenza-miasm attacks the nose and bronchia; also, low, marshy regions, where intermittents prevail, incline to the propagation of dysentery, which is sometimes very fatal at such places.

Treatment. Principal remedies are *Aconite, Aloes, Belladonna, Mercury, Colocynth, Ipecac., Nux vom., Bryonia, Rhus, Sulphur, Nitric acid, Carbo veg., Arsenic.*

Aconite. In all cases at the commencement, when there is fever, pain in the head, neck and shoulders, heat and thirst alternate with shivering. This is particularly the case when we have cold nights and hot days.

Aloes. Discharge of mucus by the rectum, looking like membranes; *bloody stool, with violent colic;* diarrhea with *tenesmus;* violent *burning* in the rectum; congestion of blood to the abdomen.

Belladonna. After *Aconite,* or in the beginning, when there is dryness in the mouth and throat, tenderness of the abdomen, and blood passing with the mucus; constant feeling of bearing down.

Mercury. This is by far the most important medicine in this disease, and beneficial in all stages, but particularly when there is *violent tenesmus* before and after the evacuations, as if the *intestines would force themselves out*, and yet nothing but *pure blood*, sometimes streaked with *white mucus* or *greenish matter* appears; at other times the evacuation resembles scrambled eggs. Concomitant symptoms are: violent colic, *nausea*, *shivering* and shuddering, cold perspiration on the face, great exhaustion and trembling of the limbs. (It alternates well with *Aconite* or *Belladonna*, if there is fever, and with *Colocynth*, if the discharges are mixed with green, bilious matter.)

Colocynth. After *Mercury*, the principal medicine, when the colic pain appears periodically, and is excessive; the discharges are mixed with green matter or lumps. In such cases, alternate with *Mercury*, if this remedy had not been given already.

Ipecac. Is also of great benefit in this disease, when it occurs in the fall, or when the mucus or slime appears first, afterward only mixed with blood. After, or in alternation with it, give *Colocynth*, if necessary.

Nux vomica. *Small*, *frequent evacuations* of *bloody slime*, with heat and thirst, mostly in summer; alternately with *Mercury*, when there is great *downward forcing*.

Bryonia and *Rhus*. In alternation, under the same conditions as stated in the article on "Diarrhea."

Sulphur. In the most critical cases, where no other remedy seems to afford relief; after *Mercury*. It must be allowed to have its effect at least thirty-six hours, before another remedy is given.

China. Dysentery in *marshy* countries, or when the discharges are *very offensive*.

Nitric acid. One of the best remedies, after *Belladonna*

and *Mercury* have been given without effect, particularly when the discharge is either mucus without blood or blood without mucus; in either case, however, the tenesmus which follows, is violent.

Carbo veg. and *Arsenic.* In alternation, if the discharges become putrid in smell and involuntary; stupor ensues; red or bluish spots appear on the skin; the patient is very weak, and his breath begins to be cold; the pains in the bowels are *burning.* *China* may follow these two remedies, if the putrid smell of the discharges will not change.

Administration.—Dissolve twelve glob. of the selected medicine in half a teacupful of water, and give every hour or half hour a teaspoonful, or, if the discharges are not so frequent, after every discharge a teaspoonful, until six, eight, or ten teaspoonfuls are given, when the medicine must be omitted for a couple of hours, to await its effect. If then necessary, either repeat the same or select another remedy, if the symptoms have increased. But as soon as an amelioration takes place, discontinue all medicine, even if there is yet frequency of stool and violent pain at times. If very restless at night, give *Belladonna*$^{cc.}$ and *Coffea*$^{cc.}$, every hour a dose (four glob.), for four hours.

If the disease becomes more *chronic*, give the medicine at longer intervals, say three times a day, finally only once a day. Cold water injections are of the greatest benefit, if the patient can bear them, and the dysentery is in its inflammatory stage.

Application of Water.—The effect of the proper remedies may be greatly supported by using water externally and internally. In recent cases perspiring in the wet sheet, the wet compress at the same time over the abdomen, afterward an ablution and sitting-bath in milkwarm water is generally sufficient, particularly when the dysentery was caused by getting cold. But if the pains are very severe and obstinate, these must first be subdued by the wet compress, very frequently changed; as soon as the pains have decreased, the above process for perspiring may be commenced.

The patient should drink a great deal of cold water and receive frequent injections of cold water, as long as the tenesmus is great.

DIET AND REGIMEN.—The patient ought to lie in or on the bed constantly, even during convalescence, if possible, well covered, but not too much heated. For food, if wanted, toasted bread, softened in water or black tea; for drink, toast-water, or small quantities of warm lemonade, in the inflammatory period, and when not taking *Acon.* at the time.

Gruels of oatmeal, rice-flour, or farina, are allowed.—Meats or soups of meat, eggs, and all animal food, are strictly forbidden, even during convalescence. Wine and spirits are real poison, in this disease, and long after it.

After diseases.—If *dropsy, paralysis, or rheumatism* follow the dysentery, when it has either been treated badly, or was suppressed by allopathic remedies, see these articles, or send for a homœopathic physician in time.

CHOLERA MORBUS.

This disease, well known under the above name, occurs mostly during the summer, in all parts of the country, north and south, resembling in its appearance the much dreaded Asiatic cholera, from which, however, it entirely differs, in character and result. (See "Cholera Asiatica.")

DIAGNOSIS.—Cholera morbus generally attacks suddenly, without any precursory symptoms, with vomiting and purging, accompanied with pains in the stomach and bowels, anxiety and tenesmus; sometimes the vomiting and urgency to go to stool are very violent and incessant, at other times less so. In very violent cases, exhaustion soon follows, pulse becomes small, scarcely perceptible, extremities cold; finally spasms and convulsions appear.

At first, the discharged substances consist of the contents

of the stomach and of bile; afterward of a watery, lymphatic liquid; and finally nothing is thrown up; when violent retching and gagging, with urgency to go to stool, remain. The discharges from the bowels consist first of fæces; afterward of a watery, bilious liquid; each stool preceded and accompanied with violent, burning, cutting colic, especially in the region of the navel.

CAUSES.—Intense heat in the summer; irritable temperament; teething in children (see "Cholera Infantum"); sudden suppression of habitual discharges, such as menstruation or diarrheas, or of cutaneous eruptions and gout; errors in diet, such as eating unripe, watery fruit, or drinking acrid, sour liquids, beer, etc.

TREATMENT.—The principal remedies in this disease are: *Chamomile*, *Ipecac.*, *Arsenic*, *Colocynth*, *Dulcamara*, *China*, *Veratrum*.

In the beginning, give *Ipecac.* (administration as below); if not better within half an hour, give *Veratrum* and *Arsenic*, in alternation, in the same manner; but if this treatment does not succeed within one and a half or two hours, select from among the remedies described below one which is more homœopathically suitable, and give it as stated under "Administration."

SYMPTOMATIC DETAIL.—*Chamomile.* In the beginning of the disease, or when the tongue is coated yellowish; colic in the region of the navel; pressing pains from the stomach up to the heart; great anguish; cramps in the calves of the legs; watery diarrhea and sour vomiting; particularly after fits of passion, and with an irritable temperament.

Ipecac. When *vomiting predominates*, alternately with painful diarrhea. It is generally *always* given in the beginning of the disease, in alternation with *Veratrum*.

Arsenic. *Violent vomiting*, and *diarrhea* of watery, bilious or slimy, greenish, brownish, or blackish substances, with severe pains n the abdomen, great *restlessness, sudden pros-*

tration, cold extremities, and clammy sweat. In alternation with *Verat.*

Veratrum. For the same symptoms as those mentioned under *Arsenic*, only that the pains in the bowels, especially around the navel, are *violent, cutting*, as from *knives;* also, pains or cramp in the calves of the legs; *prostration* is *very great.* See "*Ipecac.*" and "*Arsenic.*"

Colocynth. Green vomiting, with *violent colic;* the stools at first greenish and bilious, afterward become more colorless and watery.

Dulcamara. In cholera morbus caused by iced drinks or exposure to sudden changes of the temperature; frequent greenish stools, with bilious vomitings; great debility and severe pains in the abdomen.

China. Cholera morbus from indigestion; vomiting and diarrhea after eating ever so little (*lienteria*); painful eructation, with oppression on the chest; rumbling in the bowels; flatulency.

Administration.—Dissolve of the selected remedy twelve globules in half a teacupful of water, and give every ten or fifteen minutes a teaspoonful, until four teaspoonfuls are taken, or another remedy is necessary, which must be prepared and given in the same manner.

Application of Water.—The patient should drink as much cold water as possible, even if it should excite more vomiting. He then should be put in a sitting-bath, during which time the extremities are constantly rubbed; if he has cramps in his bowels, give an injection of cold water. After the vomiting ceases he is rubbed dry and covered in woolen blankets with a wet compress on his abdomen; in this position he remains until perspiration sets in, after which he takes an ablution in milkwarm water.

Diet and Regimen.—For a drink, thin oatmeal gruel or cold water; if wanted. After the diarrhea has ceased and reaction has taken place, and if the patient is feverish, give gruels with lemon-juice. In general, treat as stated in "Bilious Fever."

Beside, consult the article on "Asiatic Cholera."

ASIATIC CHOLERA. (*Cholera Asiatica.*)

This disease appeared hitherto among us as an epidemic. Before it, the star of Allopathy grew pale, and is ever since on its downward course; with it Homœopathy battled most successfully, and ever since her banner floats unfurled in every clime.

DIAGNOSIS. — Sudden prostration of strength; diarrhea of watery substances (rice-water discharges, without smell or color; similar, profuse vomitings, which follow each other quickly. Although these evacuations may give the patient a little relief, it is only momentary; his prostration increases constantly until cramps appear in the feet, hands, limbs, and arms, sometimes in the bowels and breast; insatiable thirst, with a burning sensation under the sternum (in the region of the heart). Agonizing restlessness precedes the last stage— that of collapse, in which, to the above symptoms are added, cessation of circulation of the blood in the extremities, which assume an icy coldness, while the heart palpitates violently, no pulse is perceptible; tongue and breath grow cold, agonizing oppression in breathing; hollow, hoarse, and shrill voice; blue lips and nails; livid countenance; sunken eyes; shriveled skin on hands and feet. During all this time, the secretion of urine is stopped. Finally, the skin of the patient is covered with a cold, clammy perspiration. Up to this time, the patient was perfectly conscious, although feeble; but now he sinks into stupor, with bloodshot, upturned eyes, and expires.

Although Asiatic cholera presents itself in the form of a diarrhea, yet it is not such; because no fecal matter is found in the discharges; its nature consists in a decomposition of the blood, produced by an unknown agent (miasm or animalcula), and aided by mental and physical debilities, such as fear, care, overpowering sympathy, weakness of body and mind by night-watching, exposure, etc. This decomposition of the blood in its solid and liquid parts (coagulum and serum) may be the work of days, hours, or minutes. Generally, however, it commences in the early morning hours, at which time most of the cholera attacks begin. The watery part of the blood (serum) escaping from the blood-vessels, passes into the stomach and bowels, whence it is ejected in violent gushes, or runs from the bowels in streams. Thus we see that the first appearances of *cholera asiatica* are those of a hemorrhage of the white part of the blood; a view with which the consequent symptoms in the following stages of the disease can easily be harmonized. The cramps in the muscles of the extremities and bowels are caused by the cessation of the action of arterial blood on the muscles, and cease immediately, as soon as the arterial irritation reaches them again. It would carry us too far, to explain all the following symptoms of the disease; nor would it be of any practical use.— This, however, we must state yet, that in that form of Cholera Asiatica, called the *sicca* or dry cholera, where no discharge from the stomach and bowels takes place, the disagreement with the above theory is only apparent; because, by the suddenness of the attack, the decomposition of the blood is rendered so general and great at once, that the cramps follow immediately, before the serum has time to escape.

Prevention. — During a cholera epidemic, a person must not give way to fear and despair, which debilitate the system too much, allowing, thereby an easier entrance to the enemy. The best remedy against the weakening thoughts is a constant and vigorous activity of body and mind, which draws our attention away from disease and death to our duties and objects of life. Necessary, above all, is regularity in all our actions, in sleeping and waking; moderation, but sufficiency in eating and drinking. The most substantial nourishment is the best, such as beef, mutton, potatoes and bread; the best drink is cold water or ice-water, which, with dry bread in sufficient quantity, is the best calculated to appease tha craving and gnawing appetite, and the rumbling of the bowels, which, in time of cholera, almost every one feels daily. A flannel bandage, even in summer, covering stomach and bowels, is strongly recommended. To be avoided, are; over-exertions of body or mind, grief, anger, fear, as well as great muscular labor, running, walking to exhaustion, and sexual excesses. Beside these precautionary measures, every one ought to have a firm reliance in the will of God, who has placed within our reach a safe and sure remedy against this disease.

The best medicine for prevention is *Sulphur*, which, in the thirtieth dilution, may be taken every week twice, six globules each time in the evening. This remedy, more than any other, destroys within the system the liability of attack, by diminishing the psoric diathesis, more or less inherent in every one.

Cure of an Attack of Asiatic Cholera.—Not every diarrhea, in time of cholera, is real Asiatic cholera, yet it predisposes to it; and we must, therefore, *immediately* and energetically attend to it. The first and most imperious duty in such a diarrhea is to lie down; as the horizontal position is indispensable to a speedy cure. With the rice-water discharges or vomiting, commences the first stage of the disease, in which *Camphor* is the specific remedy, having actually the power of killing or destroying the animalcula or malignant agent which has infested the system. The application of the *Camphor* must be *effectual* and *immediate*, in the following manner:

Cover the patient, up to the chin, well and abundantly, particularly his feet, do not allow his arms out of bed; then give him quietly, without showing anxiety by unnecessary hurry, of the tincture of *Camphor,** every two, three, or five minutes, one drop, on a little piece of sugar; also, after fifteen or twenty minutes, some brandy and water, if he can retain anything on the stomach. As soon as the patient begins to get warm, and to perspire, give the doses less frequently, and discontinue them altogether when he perspires freely. A few doses of brandy and water will then do him good and strengthen him. In this perspiration the patient must remain without change for eight or ten hours, when he will generally have a good appetite for a lunch of cold beef or mutton, with salt, dry bread and cold water. If, however, the slightest indisposition yet remains, he must not leave the bed, as a relapse might take place. During the reaction, following the use of the camphor, frequently a headache ensues from congestion to the head, which in children and middle-aged persons disappears after the exhibition of one or two doses of *Belladonna* (for children three glob.; for adults six glob.); in aged persons, when stupor is combined with it, *Secale corn.* (thirtieth dilution) is yet necessary, three hours after *Belladonna* is given.

If costiveness follows the use of camphor, a cup of coffee without milk, and twenty-four hours afterward a dose of *Sulphur* (six glob.) is indicated. If the diarrhea is not entirely checked, but changed into a dysenteric one, with straining and bloody tinge, *Mercury* will suffice, followed by *Sulphur*, twenty-four or thirty-six hours afterward. If by the *Mercury*, however, the dysenteric stool is changed into the choleroic, the use of *Camphor* is necessary again, followed by one or two doses of *Veratrum alb.* (twelfth dilution).

If, however, the cholera proceeds into the *second stage*, where cramps appear in different parts of the body, *Veratrum* and *Cuprum* are necessary; the former, when the cramps

* The tincture of *Camphor* ought to be made out of one part of the gum to five parts of alcohol.

are more in the extremities and bowels; the latter, when in the breast, or when great oppression in breathing is present. It is frequently best to give these two remedies alternately, in the following manner: Dissolve of each remedy twelve or sixteen globules, in four tablespoonfuls of water, and give every fifteen minutes a teaspoonful (each remedy having its separate teaspoon), giving less frequently as the symptoms decrease in violence. In this stage, it is not so much the diminution of diarrhea or vomiting, which indicates an amelioration, but the greater regularity and less rapidity of the pulse, which always will be followed by a discontinuance of the cramps, although these may yet threaten to break out again.

If these remedies are not successful within four or six hours, or if the cramps are more in the calves of the legs, where the slightest motion will excite them, or when stupor threatens, which is particularly the case in old persons, or when the diarrhea still continues, *Secale corn.* must be given, in the intervals of half an hour a teaspoonful dissolved in water like *Veratrum* and *Cuprum.* If a few doses are given, wait an hour or two, if the case does not grow worse; if, however, there is a great deal of nausea or retching, increased by motion of head or body, *Tabacum* (six glob.) must be given, at any time during the attack.

If in this stage congestions to the lungs and heart appear, indicated by violent stitches in the side, almost preventing respiration, and producing restlessness and great anguish, give *Cuprum* and *Hydrocyanic acid* (*Prussic acid*), in alternation, every ten or fifteen minutes a dose (dissolved in water, a teaspoonful as a dose. N. B. *Prussic acid* must be given in the second dilution).

The covering of the patient during the second stage ought still to be warm, but already more according to the feeling of the patient; his drink, cold or warm water, left to his choice. Ice pills may be given to him freely, or injections of ice water if the bowels are cramped; rub slightly the cramped parts with the hands; warming bottles, and all the other heating apparatus heretofore applied, are not of much use, although a homœopathist may allow them as not interfering with his medicine.

If the disease should go into the *third stage* (*collapse*) the scene and treatment change entirely. No pulse, livid countenance, hoarse voice, and sunken eyes characterize this period. Yet our hope is not gone; particularly in cases which, up to this stage were treated strictly homœopathically, or where the disease ran quickly through the first stages. This period generally lasts much longer than any of the former, and medicines must be given at longer intervals. The disease frequently stays in this stage for two or three days, almost unaltered; a slight improvement in the pulse is sometimes perceptible only within two days. In such cases, the medicine must not be changed or repeated often. The principal remedy is *Carbo veg.*, in the thirtieth dilution, prepared as *Veratrum* above, of which for the first six hours, every hour a teaspoonful should be given. If a great deal of burning remains in the stomach, with drinking frequently, but little at a time, *Arsenic*, thirtieth dilution, prepared similarly, may be alternated with *Carbo veg.* But if thus four or six teaspoonfuls of each remedy have been given, their use should be discontinued for ten or twelve hours—particularly if the pulse has shown evidence of returning during that time. The improvement of the pulse is, in this stage, the most important amelioration; the coldness of the surface is not of so much importance, as it often remains for a longer time without injury. If, after twelve hours, the patient's condition is not much improved, the same remedies may be repeated, and in this manner continued for a couple of days, when, in most cases a healthful reaction takes place.

The covering, in this stage, must be altogether left to the feelings of the patient, and only so much put over him as decency requires, as the patient generally refuses all covering, and is, restless. To try to warm patients in this stage by external means, is not only useless, but cruel; as they actually complain of burning up internally; such means only hasten dissolution. We rather recommend to wrap the patient in a sheet, wrung in cold water, which may, after a few hours, be repeated, if he desires it. But, in such a case, the patient ought to be covered beside with a blanket or two, to follow up the beginning reaction. Cold drinks, particularly ice water, are preferable in this stage.

In the period of convalescence, which is usually very short, great care ought of course to be taken in diet and exercise—rice and other gruels, afterward small quantities of broth, meat, and vegetables.

If a typhoid fever appears, it must be treated accordingly.

In that torpor or stupor which sometimes succeeds a severe attack of cholera, when the patient cannot easily be aroused, is very weak, pulse slow, yet the expression of his countenance is natural, *Spiritus nitri dulcis* is of the greatest benefit, as *laurocerasus* is in those cases of stupor or lethargy, which border on paralysis of the brain, or on exhaustion of the nervous system, where the expression of the countenance is indicative of great suffering, the patient very weak, pulse slow, eyes half-closed, in continual lethargy, only broken by deep sighs and moaning.

We must mention here yet a disease, called *cholerina*, which often precedes and follows cholera. It is a diarrhea of fecal matter, accompanied with rumbling of the bowels, generally caused by the constitutionality of a cholera season, under debilitating influences of mind and body, such as *fear* and *grief*. If caused by the latter, *Phosphoric acid* and *China*, in alternation, after every evacuation a dose (six glob.) will suffice; if excited by fear, *Chamomile* (six glob.), a few doses; if, however, attended with bilious rheumatic symptoms, tending toward a typhoid state, such as headache, pains in the limbs, arms, and back, with occasional chilliness, *Bryonia* and *Rhus*.

in alternation, two doses of each, every two hours one (six glob. a dose), and then waiting twenty-four hours, will change the symptoms, so that then either *Sulphur* will suit, or, if the diarrhea still continues, *China* and *Phosphoric acid*, in alternation, as above stated.

Sulphur frequently takes away that disposition to diarrhea, so common in times of cholera. It ought to be taken only twice, on two succeeding evenings, or one evening and the next morning a dose (six glob.); after which no medicine of any kind should be taken for twenty-four or forty-eight hours.

We would recommend to every one, to have with him, in cholera times, a small bottle of *Camphor*, *Veratrum*, and *Cuprum*, in case of need; if not necessary, it certainly increases the feeling of safety.*

* In the cholera epidemic of 1849, which raged in Cincinnati worse, perhaps, than in any other city of the same size, every homœopathic family was provided with a small case of four vials, containing ***Camphor***, ***Veratrum***, ***Cuprum***, and ***Sulphur***, as the principal remedies for the prevention and cure of cholera. Printed directions accompanying these remedies enabled persons to make immediate use of them, when necessary; thus preventing entirely the application of allopathic medicines before the homœopathic physician could arrive. These simple but effective means kept the homœopathic practice free from many obstacles and difficulties, and made its results so glorious, and, even in the history of homœopathy, unrivaled. The average loss which was sustained by the homœopathic practice, in 1849, amounted to only three and a half per cent., viz: of 2410 patients treated homœopathically, 85 were lost. In 1850 the attack of cholera in Cincinnati was not so severe; the cases generated not so much by epidemic influence as by indigestion, and other weakening causes. Such cases, however, were more difficult to manage, as the exciting cause could not be so easily removed, being of a material nature; yet the same homœopathic medicines proved entirely successful; even more so, in the aggregate, than the previous year. The loss, of patients treated by us during that time, was not more than three per cent.; the ratio of other practitioners, as nearly as could be ascertained, was about the same.

The above description and treatment of Asiatic cholera is carefully made after our own experiences during these two epidemics, in which nearly two thousand cholera patients were attended by us.

PILES. HEMORRHOIDS.

DIAGNOSIS.—The piles form on the anus tumors or lumps, which protrude externally (*external piles*), or remain inside the rectum (*internal piles*). These lumps either bleed (*open piles*) or do not bleed (*blind piles*). The cause of the piles is a constitutional taint, which breaks out at certain times in this local affection of the rectum, and is then called the piles. It becomes an important disease, when a bad, or mere external treatment suppresses the outward piles, without curing the internal disposition. This latter, consequently, not unfrequently attacks more important organs, such as the lungs, brain, etc., where it generates incurable diseases. Just as detrimental to general health is the painful and abominable practice of the surgeons, of cutting off these lumps or tumors. It is a blessing, however, that in most cases such operations are of no avail.

CAUSES.—The use of strong and heating drinks, coffee, liquors, highly-seasoned food, sedentary habits, costiveness, suppression of long-continued discharges, etc., are among the exciting causes of this disease, and ought, consequently, to be strictly avoided in its treatment.

TREATMENT.—In all cases of piles, begin the treatment with

Nux vomica, as the principal remedy, which suits for all varieties of this complaint. After it, particularly in chronic cases, alternately with it, give

Sulphur. These two remedies are mostly sufficient to effect a cure; given alternately, every evening a dose (four glob.) until better. If they do not suffice, give of the following remedies, *Ignatia*, *Sepia*, *Belladonna*, *Hepar*, *Colocynth*, one after the other, in intervals of twenty-four or forty-eight hours.

The cure of chronic piles must be directed by a skillful homœopathic physician; as there are too many and too various constitutional considerations to be observed, which could not be given in a work like this.

Application of Water in this disease is of the greatest benefit. It is generally sufficient during a homœopathic treatment to direct the patient to make use of the sitting-bath, the cold bandage around the abdomen, and injections of cold water to remove constipation; beside, advise him to drink freely of cold water.

Diet and Regimen.—The same as stated in the article "Constipation."

Itching of the Anus.

If it occurs in children, it is caused by the so-called pin-worms (see "Ascarides"). In such a case give *Aconite, Nux vom., Cina, Cina*^{cc}, *Ferrum, Sulphur, Silicea, Calcarea*, every other evening a dose (three glob.) of one remedy for one week, until better or another remedy is necessary. If this course is insufficient, give the child every morning, for several days, a drop of the tincture of *Urtica urens*, in a little water. If caused by piles, *Nux vomica* and *Ignatia* are the principal remedies, given as stated under the heading "Piles." Beside these medicines, the washing or sponging in cold water, or even cold water injections are of the greatest benefit. Sometimes sweet oil, used in the same manner as the water, will be of use.

Falling of the Body. Prolapsus Ani.

By this term is meant the protrusion of a portion of the lower intestine or rectum. It occurs more frequently in children than adults, caused by severe strainings when at stool. The rectum can easily be brought back again by a gentle pressure of the thumb and fore-finger, greased or oiled for that occasion, the patient bending forward during the operation, and reclining on his back after it. We have remedies which diminish the tendency to this troublesome disease.

Treatment.—*Ignatia* is the principal remedy, and must be given once in twenty-four hours (four glob.) for six or eight days; then discontinue eight days, and if not better, give

Mercury, in the same manner. After that, *Nux vomica*, and *Sulphur*, in the same manner, until better. *Sepia*, *Lycopodium*, *Colocynth*, are also suitable to be given, if necessary, in the same manner.

Externally, wash with cold water, and make frequent use of the sitting-bath, as stated in "Piles."

DIET AND REGIMEN.—As in "Diarrhea." If this treatment is of no avail, consult a homœopathic physician.

RUPTURE. HERNIA.

A protrusion or swelling in the inguinal region or groin, generally indicates a rupture, by which the intestines descend, thus forming the outward swelling. As a disease of such consequence and importance is beyond the sphere of an exhausting discussion in a domestic work, we must limit our remarks about a few dangerous points, to which the disease may run at times, leaving the treatment of the rupture itself to the combined efforts of the surgeon and homœopathic physician, who must be consulted.

Sometimes an *incarceration* of the rupture takes place, when the tumor becomes very painful, inflammation in the surrounding parts ensues, with vomiting, quick and hard pulse, and fever. If the rupture cannot be brought back, or the inflammation reduced by other means, mortification and consequent death are unavoidable.

First try the reduction in the following manner: place the patient on his back on the bed, grasping the swelling with one hand gently, and rub and press it with the fingers of the other hand, pressing upward toward the body constantly, sometimes even in a rotary manner. Continue these efforts for half an hour; if the swelling is repressed, keep it in its place with the palm of the hand for some time, giving, beside, the following medicines:

Aconite. If the fever is *very high*.

Nux vomica, followed in two hours by

Opium. If the *strangulation* of the rupture continues, and afterward in alternation with *Nux vomica* until better.

Also, *Lachesis, Belladonna, Rhus, Arsenic, Veratrum,* can be given in extreme cases, if necessary; one after the other, every two hours one remedy, until better.

Application of Water.—Cold injections are frequently of the greatest benefit in incarcerated rupture, as also the application of cold water or ice, even in the most desperate cases.

Administration.—Dissolve of the necessary remedy twelve globules in half a teacupful of water; give every fifteen or thirty minutes a teaspoonful, for two hours, or until better.

Diet and Regimen.—As in fevers. Complete rest in a horizontal position is indispensable, and a truss must not be worn until all soreness has subsided.

Dropsy of the Abdomen. (*Ascites.*)

As this is one of those diseases which require a most skillful medical attendance, in order to secure a successful termination, we cannot pretend to give more than what is necessary to a knowledge of its rise and progress. This will enable persons to be aware of the danger in time to seek for help, when it is yet possible to render it successfully.

Diagnosis.—A swelling and tension of the abdomen, which follows the position of the patient; a fluctuation inside the abdomen is distinctly felt by the palm of one hand while clapping gently against one side, when the other hand presses the opposite side of the abdomen, in the lowest part of which the fluctuation is felt the strongest, while the patient is standing erect. Urine is scanty, brown like beer (peculiar to ascites); stools are scanty and dry; also, the skin, tongue, and mouth dry; when the water is collected in a sack (*hydrops saccatus*), the swelling is unequal in the beginning; the urine less scarce and brown. As the disease progresses, the feet and other parts swell successively; fever and dry cough appear, which consume the strength more and more, until death ends the misery.

Causes.—As such, we find previous acute fevers, scarlet or other eruptions, diseases of important abdominal organs, especially the liver, badly treated, intermittents of too long standing, which debilitate the absorbing vessels, gout, abuse of spiritous liquors, mechanical lesions, such as blows on the abdomen, falls, etc.

This disease sometimes lasts very long, according to the causes, and the constitution of the patient.

A pregnancy, not closely watched in its progress, may be mistaken for a dropsy of the abdomen; but, in such a case, a skillful physician must decide.

Treatment.—As this disease can be cured, if early attended to in the right manner, we recommend every one to apply immediately to a good physician. Until one can be procured, give,

Arsenic and *Sulphur*, in alternation, every four days one dose (six glob.), followed by *Apis mellif.* in the same manner

The tapping may be allowed in cases where the accumulation of water is very rapid; but no one must trust in it as a curative means; the necessary internal treatment must therefore be continued, until cured entirely.

Diet and Regimen.—As in all chronic diseases, the usual homœopathic diet.

External Injuries of the Abdomen.

On receiving large wounds in the abdomen, do not despair immediately, as a great many are cured who received the severest cuts and shots in the abdomen, if only properly treated. Clean the wound with lukewarm water, and replace the intestines as soon as possible, handling them not with the hands, but with clean linen cloths. If the patient is faint, from loss of blood, give *China;* if frightened, *Coffea,* and afterward *Arnica.* Sew up the wound carefully with a silken thread waxed, leaving an opening on the lowest corner, which must be covered with scraped linen, dipped in a mixture of *Arnica* (twelve drops to a teacupful of water). If diarrhea ensues, give *Colocynth* alternately with *China.*

If a child has swallowed a button, or any other metal substance, do not give it aperient medicine, in the hope of purging it out of the system more quickly; this is impossible; on the contrary, the substance will come out less quickly, as the liquid state of the fæces prevents them from carrying it along. In the meantime, observe carefully each stool to be sure that the substance has passed. If a needle is swallowed, it may work itself through a different part of the body; in such a case, give *Silicea,* every six days a dose (four glob.).

If live animals are swallowed, such as frogs, insects, etc., let the patient drink plenty of sweet oil.

CHAPTER XV.

AFFECTIONS OF THE URINARY AND GENITAL ORGANS.

We invite the special attention of our readers to the study of the anatomical position and structure, as well as the physiological bearing, of the organs named in the above heading, as it will be important for the true diagnosis of their diseases, which are various and severe.

Inflammation of the Kidneys. (*Nephritis.*)

Diagnosis. — In the region of the kidneys (on both sides of the spine, above the hip, and below the short ribs), appears a pungent, pressing pain, shooting downward to the bladder; difficulty of urination; stranguria, or ischuria (the latter only when both kidneys are inflamed, which rarely ever occurs); the urine scanty, red, and hot, sometimes bloody; the testicle drawn near to the abdomen on the affected side, painful and swollen; the foot on the same side sometimes spasmodically affected and benumbed; in severer cases, high fever, thirst, full hard pulse, constipation, vomiting; colic pains; the pains in the kidney are worse when lying on the affected part and the back; also when standing and walking.

If this inflammation is not cured entirely, the kidney hardens and indurates, or suppuration takes place, which leads to the formation of abscesses and their opening, either outside through the skin, or inside in the intestinal canal. This chronic affection of the kidneys requires medical skill for its successful termination.

The principal causes are: stones or gravel in the kidney; violent blows and concussions, or any other external injury bearing on this part; excess in the use of wines and liquors; lying on the back for a long time; lifting heavy loads; suppression of piles, and their congestion transferred to the kidney; the use of acrid diuretics and the abuse of Spanish fly, sometimes even when only applied as a blister, externally.

TREATMENT.—*Camphor*, when the disease is caused by the application or use of Spanish fly (*cantharis*), or when no urine passes or only in a slender stream very slowly, with burning in the urethra and bladder. Give in such a case one or two drops of Camphor spirits, on a lump of sugar, every hour or two hours, until better.

Aconite. If the fever is high, give several doses (four glob. each) of this remedy, every hour one, before the following remedies are resorted to.

Cantharis is the principal medicine, when there are shooting, tearing, and incisive pains, *painful emission of a few drops of urine only*, or *complete ischuria;* sometimes urine mixed with blood.

Belladonna. In most cases, where the pains are worse periodically, shooting from the kidney down into the bladder, with great anguish and colic; in fleshy women, at the time of change of life (critical age), when the menses stop. (*Hepar sulph.* will suit after *Belladonna*).

Nux vomica. When this disease is caused by suppressed piles, or when there is any other abdominal congestion, with tension, distension, and pressure in the kidney.

Pulsatilla. In delicate females, whose menses have stopped or are very scanty; also, when the urine appears turbid, leaving a purulent sediment.

Arnica, externally and internally, if caused by external injuries; after it the above remedies may be resorted to.

N. B. If nephritis is caused by the pressure of stones in the kidneys, the fever which usually accompanies this disease does not appear so quickly, but, instead of it, the foot and thigh of the affected side become numb, and the testicle retracts; sure signs of stones in the kidneys or the ureter. In such a case apply on the most painful spot, where the stone is lodged, narcotic, warm fomentations of hops mixed with tobacco leaves; as soon as the stone or gravel reaches, in its descent, the bladder, the pains and inflammation caused by them cease at once. Beside this external treatment, give the patient the above medicines, as indicated.

If the kidney indurates, which is known by the patient complaining of a sensation of weight in the loins or sometimes by a feeling of numbness in the foot of the side affected, give *Mercury*, every evening a dose (four glob.).

If suppuration takes place, which is known by a sensation of heaviness, accompanied by throbbing in the region of the kidney (the latter symptom ceases when the matter, mixed with blood, is discharged with the urine), give *Lachesis* and *Hepar* alternately, every evening a dose (four glob.), for eight days, or until better; apply to a homœopathic physician.

ADMINISTRATION. — Dissolve, of the necessary medicine, twelve globules in half a teacupful of water, and give every half-hour, hour, or two hours, a teaspoonful until better, or until another remedy is needed.

APPLICATION OF WATER. — Tepid sitting-baths, frequently repeated, will accelerate the cure and support the effect of the proper homœopathic remedies.

DIET AND REGIMEN, as in fevers generally; but particularly wines, liquors, and beer are prohibited in convalescence.

INFLAMMATION OF THE BLADDER. (*Cystitis.*)

DIAGNOSIS.—Burning pains in the region of the bladder, with external swelling; tension; heat and pain on touch; urine red and hot; difficulty or inability of making water;

constipation, with tenesmus; fever, with a hard pulse; in some cases, vomiting and hiccough.

The issue of this inflammation is either resolution, indicated by a thick urine, or suppuration discharged with the urine, or abscesses and fistulae from the bladder outside, or induration, which leads to a thickening of the bladder, impeding, thereby, its action, and leading to various chronic disorders; or, if fatal, gangrene takes place.

Its causes can be external injuries; suppressed piles and retarded menstruation; rheumatic, gouty, or syphilitic transfers; stones in the bladder; pressure on the bladder in pregnancy, or during the birth of the child; the use of irritating drugs, as *Cantharides*, etc.

TREATMENT. — Beside the remedies recommended in "Inflammation of the Kidneys," give

Hyoscyamus, when spasms of the neck of the bladder set in, impeding the flow of urine.

Carbo vegetabilis and *Arsenicum*, when the patient complains very much of *burning* during urination, which *Cantharides* failed to cure.

Dulcamara, when this disease returns on the slightest exposure to cold.

Sulphur and *Calcarea*, when the disease becomes chronic.

ADMINISTRATION, APPLICATION OF WATER, DIET AND REGIMEN, the same as in "Nephritis."

STRANGURY, DYSURY, ISCHURY, AND ANURY.

These four terms signify only different degrees of the same affection.

In *strangury*, the discharge of urine is *painful* and *difficult*.

In *dysury*, *difficult* and *incomplete*.

In *ischury* and *anury*, it is totally *suppressed*.

Strangury and dysury are troublesome, but not dangerous complaints, while the true ischury, or total retention of urine, ranks among the most dangerous diseases, and kills, either by gangrene or rupture of the bladder, effusing the urine into the abdomen ; in its chronic form, however, the urine can be absorbed and carried into the circulation, producing, thereby, eruptions on the skin, and making the perspiration, saliva, etc., smell urinous.

The causes of these affections are various. Mechanical injuries or impediments, such as gravel, stones, callosities and strictures, spasmodical, or caused by syphilitic disorders; tumors in these parts ; falling of the womb, or its dislocation ; congestion of every kind ; paralysis of the bladder ; the use of ardent spirits, Spanish fly, violent diuretics, etc.

Treatment. — For *strangury*, and *dysury*, if caused by the abuse of *ardent spirits*, *Nux vom.*, *Pulsatilla*, and *Sulphur;* if by the use of Spanish fly, *Camph.*, *Puls.*, *Apis mel.*, *Acon.*; if by *suppressed piles*, *Nux vom.*, *Pulsatilla*, *Sulphur;* if by *taking cold*, wet feet, etc., *Dulcamara*, *Nux vom.*, *Mercury*, *Puls.*, *Bellad.*, *Apis mel.;* if after a *fright*, *Acon.;* if after a *fall*, *blow*, etc., *Arnica;* if in *pregnant females*, *Cocculus*, *Pulsatilla*, *Nux vomica;* if in *children*, *Pulsatilla*, *Aconite*, *Belladonna*, *Mercury*.

For *ischury* and *anury*, if it is *spasmodic*, *Nux vom.*, *Pulsatilla*, *Opium*, *Hyoscyamus;* *inflammatory*, *Aconite*, *Cantharides*, *Belladonna*, *Nux vom.*, *Pulsatilla* (see "Cystitis"); *paralytic*, *Hyoscyamus*, *Dulcamara*, *Arsenic*, *Lachesis*.

Administration the same as in "Inflammation of the Kidneys" (*Nephritis*).

Application of Water ; beside the frequent use of sitting-baths of a cool temperature, it will be beneficial to cover the parts affected with wet bandages during the time between the sitting-baths.

Diet and Regimen the same as in nephritis ; beside this, in *strangury* the drinking of large quantities of cold water, or the moderate use of gum-arabic, dissolved in water, is strongly recommended. In cases of disease of the bladder, consult, as soon as possible, a homœopathic physician.

INCONTINENCE OF URINE. (*Enuresis, incontinentia urinæ.*)

This troublesome disease exists in three varieties:

1. It is a *complete* or *paralytic* incontinence of urine (*enuresis completa s. paralytica*), when the patient is constantly troubled with an involuntary dribbling of urine, owing to a variety of causes, all having the tendency to paralyze, more or less, the contractive power of the muscles around the neck of the bladder. Instances of this kind are; apoplexy; consumption, and paralysis of the spine; too great distension of the bladder by long retention of the urine; surgical operations on the bladder; paralysis, or weakness of the bladder, particularly in old age; difficult and hard parturitions. This form of incontinence of urine requires the most careful attention of a homœopathic physician. We only mention some of the principal remedies for this form of *enuresis*, with which a treatment may be commenced: *Hyoscyamus, Belladonna, Causticum, Conium, Arsenic, Lachesis.*

2. Or it is an *incomplete* or *spasmodic* incontinence of urine (*enuresis incompleta s. spastica*), where the urgency to pass urine is so sudden and great, that the patient is immediately forced to yield. This form occurs very frequently, caused by continual irritation in the bladder, or some contiguous part, either by stones, gravel, worms, (ascarides), (see "Worms"); menstrual or hemorrhoidal congestion; gastric derangement, with rheumatic or gouty complication; scirrhous tumors in the bladder, rectum, prostate glands; ulcers, fistulas; also, from mechanical pressure of the pregnant or dislocated uterus (see "Diseases of Females"); or, lastly, by the bad habit of urinating too frequently, diminishing, thereby, the size of the bladder.

The principal remedies for this complaint are: *Belladonna, Causticum, Cina, Hyoscyamus, Ignatia, Pulsatilla, Rhus, Lachesis, Mercury.* (Compare each remedy in "Materia Medica.")

ADMINISTRATION of these medicines as in nephritis.

3. The urine escapes *involuntarily* only *in the night* (*wetting the bed*), (*enuresis nocturna*). This occurs mostly in children, and depends on bad habits, uncorrected in early years, or on local irritations, such as worms (see this article), or other derangements, enumerated under the form No. 2 (see their treatment). If it is a bad habit, try to correct it, by diminishing the quantity of drink allowed in the evening, by laying the child on its side while asleep, by awakening it several times during the night in order to pass urine, or even by chastisement in the morning, the effects of which will be remembered, even in the sleep. Beside, use the following remedies: *Silicea*, every third evening a dose (three glob.), for two weeks; if not better,

Sepia in the same manner; if not better.

Sulphur, *Arsenic*, *Carbo veg.* in the same manner, one after the other.

Application of Water; the cold sitting-bath in the morning, and in the evening a cold sponge-bath are beneficial auxiliaries in the treatment of the above diseases.

Diabetes.

Diagnosis.—Any secretion of urine, the excessive increase of which has a weakening, morbific effect on the whole system, may be called a diabetes; although the quality of the urine be not altered, its appearance shows that it contains more water, it being colorless (*nervous urine*); cases of this kind either correct themselves, or are in connection with hysteric or hypochondriacal diseases, the cure of which will, also, take away this form of diabetes. But where the urine is not, or not much, increased in quantity, however changed in quality, having a *sweetish* taste, and containing *saccharine* (sugar) matter (*diabetes melitus*), as high as an ounce in a pound, it is necessary to institute an early and earnest treatment for this disease, which, in its commencement, can be cured easily, and only becomes fatal by neglect. But, as such a complaint is too important in its progress and issue to be treated domestically, we here only indicate the remedies, with which a rational treatment may be commenced.

TREATMENT.—*Phosphoric acid, Carbo veg., Conium, Mercury, Sulphur.* The first of these medicines is almost a specific, as also the two last ones, which may be given in alternation; give, every evening, a dose (four glob.), for one week, and then wait a week for its effects.

APPLICATION OF WATER; the sitting-baths used in this disease must be made of water with the chill taken off; beside these, the wet bandage around the abdomen, changed at least twice a day, is recommended; the patient is advised to drink large quantities of cold water.

DIET.—Only bread, roasted meats, and soups of meat, are allowed; *no* vegetables whatever; the patient must keep in an even temperature.

PILES OF THE BLADDER. (*Hemorrhoides Vesicæ.*)

As the pile disease consists in a congestion, which can tend to any part of the system, and produce piles, where the nature of the attacked organ admits of it, it is not strange to speak of piles of the bladder, because this organ allows the same disorganization, in this respect, as the rectum. They are also either *blind*, or *open, running* piles.

DIAGNOSIS.—If they are *blind*, or not *running*, they create great difficulty in making water, strangury, ischury, sometimes spasms, and inflammations of the bladder (see these articles), with consequent induration and suppuration.

If they are *open, running* piles, the blood coagulates in the bladder, obstructs the passage of urine, and may contribute to the formation of stones.

TREATMENT.—Consult a homœopathic physician, if possible. If not, use the following remedies: *Nux vomica, Pulsatilla, Sulphur,* beside all those recommended in the articles on *strangury* and *ischury*, in the same manner as there stated.

APPLICATION OF WATER; the frequent use of the sitting-bath and the drinking of cold water will be beneficial.

POLYPUS OF THE BLADDER.

The neck of the bladder is the place most favorable to the generation of this kind of fleshy excrescences, where they occasion frequent obstructions in urinating, producing similar symptoms to those exhibited in piles, and stones of the bladder. Their existence, however, is rendered beyond doubt, as soon as fleshy particles of a round form, with a stringy substance attached to them, pass from the bladder; females are subject to them more than males.

TREATMENT.—If possible, consult a homœopathic physician for this disease, as the cure depends too much on constitution to make a prescription of remedies, for a domestic work of this kind, possible. To commence the treatment, however, give *Calcarea carb.*, every third or fourth evening a dose (four glob.), for four or six weeks.

N. B. I once cured polypus of the bladder with *Chamomile;* the case was a complicated one, where the concomitant symptoms strongly advised its use. No other remedies had been used before; after the exhibition of *Chamomile,* the polypus passed off altogether.

Staphysag. is recommended after *Calcarea carb.*, in the same manner.

APPLICATION OF WATER; the frequent use of the sitting-bath will support the effect of the proper homœopathic remedies.

GRAVEL AND STONE IN THE BLADDER. (*Calculus.*)

DIAGNOSIS.—It is sometimes very difficult to be certain of the existence of a stone in the bladder, as it produces all the symptoms recorded under *strangury, ischury,* and *piles of the bladder.* (See these diseases.)

The only sure guide in establishing a true diagnosis, is the examination by a competent physician or surgeon. In gravel, the diagnosis is easier, as some of it will pass, from time to time, clearly showing the nature of the disease.

TREATMENT.—The treatment for a *stone in the bladder* can not be given here, as such a disease must not be left to domestic practice.

The best remedy for *gravel* is *Sarsaparilla,* either in a homœopathic preparation (four glob.), or, if not at hand, of the tincture of Sarsaparilla, every evening one drop on sugar, until better. Beside this remedy, those stated under "Strangury" are recommended.

HEMORRHAGE WITH THE URINE.

(*Hœmaturia. Mictus cruentus.*)

DIAGNOSIS.—The blood comes with the urine, either mixed with it, like dark beer (then it proceeds from the kidneys, *hœmaturia renalis*), or it is separated from the urine, coagulated (then it comes from the bladder (*hœmaturia vesicalis*), or the blood comes alone, without urinating (then it proceeds from the urethra, *stymatosis*). In the first case, pains are felt in the region of the kidneys; in the second, the region of the bladder is painful; and in the third case, the pains are in the urethra.

CAUSES.—This disease occurs always in consequence of other diseases, already located there, to which we refer the reader. These are: inflammation of the kidneys and bladder, and their causes, mechanical and external, stones and gravel, strangury, etc.

TREATMENT.—The principal remedies are: *China, Ipecac., Arnica, Pulsatilla, Lycopodium,* to be given as stated under "Strangury."

AFFECTIONS OF THE PENIS.

If the front of the penis—the glans and the prepuce—is inflamed, red, and swollen, give, when caused by friction, *Aconite* and *Arnica,* in alternation, every two or three hours a dose (four glob., infants half a dose), until better; keep quiet on the bed or a couch; abstain from all meat diet, and bathe, if necessary, with cold water alone, or water and milk; if caused by want of cleanliness, give *Aconite* (four glob.), alone, and bathe. If it was caused by the touch of poisonous plants, give, in the same manner, *Belladonna* and *Rhus*, after *Aconite* has been given. If a burning discharge appears from the urethra, give *Mercury*, and if not better in twenty-four or thirty-six hours, give *Capsicum*, and in a few days after, *Hepar;* if the parts become hardened, callous, and bluish, give *Lachesis* and *Arsenic*, in alternation.

Diet and Regimen.—Nothing but milk and water, dry toast, and gruels.

N. B. For syphilitic disorders, chancres, and gonorrhea, see these articles.

Affections of the Testicles.

Inflammation, with painful swelling of the testicles, from

External injuries: Aconite and *Arnica*, as above, under the "Affections of the Penis;" *Arnica*, also, externally.

Gonorrhea suppressed: Pulsatilla, externally and internally, as above; *Mercury, Nitric acid.*

Metastasis of the mumps: see this disease; *Pulsatilla* is the principal remedy; also, *Mercury* and *Nux vom.*

Abuse of Calomel: Pulsatilla and *Carbo veg.*, in alternation, as above.

If necessary give *Sulphur* after the above remedies have ameliorated, but not altogether cured.

Diet and Regimen as in "Affections of the Penis."

Hydrocele, or dropsy of the scrotum: if in infants shortly after the birth, wash with a mixture of six drops of *Arnica* tincture, in a teacupful of water, three or four times a day; if in older children, the same, externally, and *Pulsatilla*, every evening a dose (three glob.) internally; if in adults, *Pulsatilla, Silicea, Sulphur*, each remedy for eight or twelve days, every fourth day a dose (four glob.) during that period, until better, and if not, apply to a homœopathic physician.

Diet and regimen as usual in chronic diseases, when treated homœopathically.

Seminal Weakness.

(Pollution. Impotence. Onania.)

These diseases are very weakening, and frequently fatal to happiness, health, and even life. As their introduction here would carry us beyond the sphere of a domestic treatise, we advise our readers not to neglect, for a single day, the above complaints, which explain their nature in their names, but to have the advice of a skillful homœopathic physician at once.

Eruptions on the Genital Organs.

Eruptions on the glans; *Bryonia, Rhus;* on the hairy part, *Lachesis;* on the penis, *Graphites, Phosphoric acid;* on the prepuce, *Sepia, Silicea;* between the thighs, *Petroleum.*

Prurigo on the scrotum (tetter) requires, mostly, *Sulphur, Dulcamara, Nitric acid, Petroleum, Thuja.*

Administration.—Every evening a dose (four glob.), and thus every medicine used for four days, before another one is commenced; if it is not better, wash with a solution (twelve glob. in half a teacupful of water) of the same remedy during its internal use.

Diet and Regimen as in chronic diseases.

Erysipelas of the scrotum requires *Belladonna, Rhus,* and *Arsenic,* in the same manner as stated under "Erysipelas." (See "Diseases of the Skin.")

Diet and regimen as in "Erysipelas."

Syphilis.—Gonorrhea.

We can only mention here the commencement of the treatment for these complaints, as inveterate or chronic disorders of this kind are so complicated and difficult of treatment, as to require the utmost attention of a skillful homœopathic physician

a. Syphilis. Chancre.

If infection has taken place, and a slight soreness manifests itself on the glans, with a pimple which soon becomes a small ulcer, marked by its hard surface and elevated edges, take, internally, *Mercury*, three times a day (six glob), and wash, externally, with a solution of *Mercury* (twelve glob. in half a teacupful of water), until the advice of a physician can be obtained.

b. Gonorrhea. Clap. Gleet.

If, after infection, a soreness of the whole urethra ensues, with inflammation of the glans in particular, take *Aconite*, every two or three hours a dose (four glob.), for six or eight times, and after it, if a running appears, *Mercury*, every three hours a dose (four glob.), until medical aid can be procured. Outwardly, use cold water bathing; to subdue pain and inflammation, keep *perfectly quiet*, and abstain from all meat diet.

Diet and Regimen are alike for both complaints: no meat whatever; but milk, water, and bread; the most perfect rest.

Application of Water.—In the above diseases the frequent use of tepid sitting-baths, the application of wet compresses and the drinking of cold water are particularly recommended as beneficial auxiliaries of the proper homœopathic remedies.

CHAPTER XVI.

DISEASES OF FEMALES.

THERE are diseases peculiar to the female sex, whose distinctive character is founded in the different physical organization of the female from the male. It shall be our endeavor to be as minute in treating of them as the object of this work will allow, although a great many of them must, and will, always demand the especial attendance of a physician, on account of their importance to life and difficulty of treatment; yet a right knowledge of their nature will diminish fear, and create confidence and trust—a great lever in surmounting medical difficulties.

1. MENSTRUATION.

With the appearance of the menses (*courses*) the age of puberty commences with the female, and various changes take place in the mental and physical development; such as change of voice, expansion of the chest, enlargement of the breast, a marked reserve in manners, and an increased attention to outward decorum and appearance. This time generally comes, in northern climates, between the thirteenth and fifteenth year; in southern, between the eleventh and thirteenth. The same difference of time is observed in the disappearance of the menstrual discharge, which takes place, in the northern climates, generally between the forty-third and forty-fifth year; in the southern, between the forty-first and forty-third year. The menses appear quite regularly in a healthy female, every twenty-eight days (a slight deviation of from two to three days earlier or later does not constitute of itself disease), and last, at an average, five days, although this is no absolute rule.

We cannot recommend too strongly a strict adherence to the general principles of Hygiene, as the departure from these lays, in most cases, the foundation to those derangements in the menstrual functions which prove so fatal to the life and happiness of a female. And here we may remark that, in the course of a long practice, we have found the wearing of thin-soled shoes to be the most fruitful source of the decay of female beauty, and the decline of female health. The damage of tight lacing (although considerable) is nothing in comparison with the fatal habit of appearing, in all kinds of weather, in thin-soled shoes; the consequences of the latter are beyond description, fearful, and destructive. Almost all diseases which follow a stoppage of the menses, consumption, fluor albus, etc., can be traced to this source. Let reform set in!

Obstructions of the First Menses.

When the menses do not appear, although the time of puberty has come, the young girl will show signs of deranged health which demand our immediate attention. She has, perhaps, frequent bleeding at the nose, congestions to the head, flushed face, constriction of the chest, palpitation of the heart, etc. If these symptoms manifest themselves, give first,

Pulsatilla. If, beside other symptoms, she looks rather pale, is slender and feeble, melancholy and sad; feels better in the open air.

Bryonia. If she looks flushed in the face, her nose bleeds frequently, inclined to constipation.

Veratrum. If she is chilly, and inclined to diarrhea.

Sulphur. If either of the above remedies have not brought on the menses.

Administration. — Of the selected medicine, give every evening a dose (four glob.) for four nights, then discontinue four days, and give *Sulphur* in the same manner. If not better in four or six weeks consult a physician.

Diet and Regimen.—Let the diet be simple, but nutritious; exercise as much as possible; apply warm foot-baths before going to bed.

Chlorosis. Green Sickness.

Diagnosis.—Pale, white color of the skin, cheeks, and lips; chilliness, lassitude, yet easily excited on the least exertion; weak, slow pulse, difficulty of breathing, and palpitation of the heart when exercising; swelling of the feet; no appetite, but sometimes an immoderate desire for unusual things, earthy substances, as chalk, etc. The blood is thin, watery; if not cured, general dropsy and consumption, or nervous diseases can set in. It is mostly a disease appearing in young girls, when the first menses do not appear, or after several hemorrhages, or other diseases, carrying with them great loss of life-sustaining fluid.

Treatment. — If it occurs in young girls, the treatment mentioned for obstruction of the first menses, in the preceding article, will suit; yet, after *Sulphur*, we would recommend *Calcarea carb.;* if it occurs, however, after severe sickness, or hemorrhages, give *China* and *Carbo veg.;* every other evening a dose (six glob.), alternately, for at least five or six weeks. In both cases, if the above medicines do not relieve, apply to a skillful physician without delay.

Application of Water.—The frequent use of the sitting-bath in the morning, and the sponge-bath in the evening are very beneficial; during the night the patient can apply the wet bandage around the abdomen; but during menstruation all application of water must be omitted.

Diet and Regimen.—Let the diet be very nutritious, exercise plentiful, particularly in open air; if mineral springs are chosen for a summer resort, give the preference to the chalybeate, containing iron.

Suppression of the Menses. Amenorrhea.

Or their *temporary cessation*, when once well established. This occurs either suddenly, by taking cold (from wet feet mostly), overheating, violent mental emotions, faults of diet, etc., and often produces violent congestions to the chest, head, or stomach, with cramps, convulsions, inflammations, etc.; there is no disease which could not appear in consequence of it; or the menses have gradually disappeared, without creating any immediate symptoms in the female economy, giving rise to suspicion of pregnancy.

TREATMENT. — Beside the remedies recommended in "Obstructions of the First Menses," which will be of the greatest benefit here, and of which *Pulsatilla* is the principal, we recommend

Aconite. In alternation with *Bryonia*, every hour or two hours a dose (four glob.), in a sudden check of the menses, producing congestions to the head and chest, or *Cocculus*, in alternation with *Veratrum*, in the same manner, if severe cramps in the abdomen are present.

Opium. If all the blood seems to have rushed to the head, producing *heaviness there*, with a dark redness of the face, and drowsiness, alternately with *Apis. mel.*

Cuprum. In spasms of the chest, and in alternation with *Veratrum*, if, also, the *abdomen* suffers; or with *Opium*, if the *head* is congested, and with *Apis. mel.*, if faint at the *stomach*.

If the menses have been checked by mental agitation or depression, take those remedies recommended for fright, fear, etc., in "Affections of the Mind." See this article.

ADMINISTRATION the same as in *Aconite*, above.

APPLICATION OF WATER.—See "Chlorosis."

Painful Menstruation. Menstrual colic. (Dysmenorrhea.)

The causes of these tormenting distresses of females are generally laid in the early part of womanhood, and owing chiefly to improper treatment of other diseases, suppression of eruptions or habitual discharges, rheumatic disorders, colds, etc. The pains either appear before or during the flow of the menses, sometimes resembling real labor pains, with bearing down and forcing; at other times as a constant aching in the loins, hips, and limbs. They generally diminish in violence as soon as the regular flow has commenced, but not always.

TREATMENT. — If possible, lie down, cover well, and take *Coffea, Pulsatilla,* and *Veratrum,* in alternation, every half hour a dose (four glob.) *until better.* If this does not suffice take *Nux vom.*, if the *forcing* pains predominate; *Cocculus,* if *colic pains* in the abdomen appear, with shortness of breath; *Chamomile,* if with discharge of dark-colored blood, there are pains, like labor-pains, together with colic pains and tenderness of the abdomen, in alternation with *Apis mel.*

If a profuse perspiration sets in while in bed, do not leave it soon after the pains cease, nor cool off too quickly, else the pains return. Avoid the use of heating substances, either externally, or internally, save a warm brick on the feet or stomach.

ADMINISTRATION.—As above under *Coffea,* etc.

DIET.—No coffee for the first two days.

Menstruation too Early.

If the menses appear too early, say every two or three weeks, the disorders causing it are too complicated frequently to be prescribed for in a domestic treatise; apply to a physician; yet the cure may be commenced with the following remedies:

Ipecac. Almost a specific in all passive hemorrhages where feebleness, dullness, nausea, and coagulated discharges prevail.

Ignatia. Where the menses return every two weeks, spirits are depressed; in alternation with *Ipecac.*, if its symptoms are also present.

Belladonna. Heat and pains in the head, with cold feet and dryness of the throat; bearing down in the abdomen.

Calcarea carb. is almost a specific in this disease, where with the menses a diarrhea or frequent discharges from the bowels appear, with pains in the bowels; suitable after *Belladonna.*

Sulphur. If the menstruation is *too early* and *too profuse.*

Natrum muriaticum. If *Calcarea carb.* is insufficient.

ADMINISTRATION.—Just before, or in the beginning of the menses, one or two doses of the selected medicine every three hours one dose (six glob.); after the menses are over, take one more dose and then wait until the next appearance of the menses, and observe whether they are more regular, as regards time.

Menstruation too Late and too Scanty.

Pulsatilla is the principal remedy, when the above difficulty exists, and also when the menses appear irregular, sometimes too late and too profuse (as this is the case particularly at the critical period—change of life), sometimes too early and too scanty. In the former, *Lachesis* alternates well with *Pulsatilla.* In most all cases,

Sulphur is necessary, to complete the cure.

Compare, also, "Suppression of the Menses," "Obstruction of the First Menses."

ADMINISTRATION, DIET, AND REGIMEN, the same as stated there.

Menstruation too Copious. Flooding. (Menorrhagia.)

In cases of this kind, causes mental and physical may operate, to enumerate all of which here, would be impossible

We content ourselves in directing the reader to the various sources, where he can find their remedies.

If *mental* causes, such as fright, fear, etc., exist, give the remedies stated under "Affections of the Mind," for the several exciting causes.

If *external injuries*, see this chapter. In cases of this kind *Arnica* is the first remedy, after which others may be selected.

In general, however, *Ipecac.* is the principal remedy (see Menstruation too Early"), followed by *China*, if there is great weakness, buzzing in the ears, faintness when raising the head off the pillow; *Belladonna*, if there is downward pressure; *Pulsatilla* and *Lachesis*, if it occurs during *change of life;* also, in such a case, or in aged women, *Ipecac.* and *Secale.*

Chamomile. If dark, clotted blood is discharged, accompanied by colic-like labor-pains, violent thirst, coldness of the extremities, headache with clouded sight, and humming in the ears.

Coffea and *Camphor*, in alternation, when there is, beside the above symptoms, *exceedingly painful colic.*

Platina. After *Belladonna* or *Chamomile*, when the discharge is too profuse, or of too long duration, of *black* and *thick blood*, with great nervousness, sleeplessness, and constipation.

Secale. Particularly with *great weakness* and *coldness of extremities.*

If real *flooding* ensues, resisting the above medicines, the application of *cold water*, or *pounded ice*, over the lower part of the abdomen, externally, is necessary to coagulate the blood in the vagina and uterus, which stops the hemorrhage. There can be no fear of getting cold in doing this, if it is done well; always keep the patient lightly, but well covered. In such a case, the patient must lie with the hips higher, at least not lower than the shoulder. This treatment will be effectual in the severest cases of flooding.

Administration.—Dissolve six globules of a remedy in six teaspoonfuls of water, and give every fifteen, twenty, or forty minutes a teaspoonful, sometimes in alternation with another, and lengthen the intervals as the patient gets better, when no medicine is needed any more.

Diet and Regimen.—The drink must be cold and not stimulating; except when faintness appears, with deadly paleness of the face, no pulse, and cloudiness of sight, give wine and brandy, in frequent, small quantities. *Camphor* and *China*, in such cases, are of the greatest benefit. The patient ought to lie perfectly quiet.

Menstruation of too long Duration.

Compare "Menstruation too Copious," and give of the selected medicine every evening and morning a dose (six glob.) until better. (See, also, next article, on "Change of Life, or Critical Period.")

Diet in such cases must be highly nutritious. It is best to consult a physician early.

Critical Period. Cessation of the Menses. (Change of Life.)

This period, commencing about at the age of forty-five years, forms one of the most important in the life of a female. If not guided through this critical time by the counsel and aid of a skillful physician, she gathers the seeds of endless miseries, or even early death. This period may be a blessing to her, as well as a source of great distress; as after it her health either becomes more confirmed, or disorganizations in internal organs are formed, which soon carry her off. Without enlarging further on the subject, we recommend the early and constant advice of a skillful physician during this time, which generally lasts from one and a half to two years.

First, an irregularity of the courses is experienced; they stop for three months, then reappear with great violence, then stop for four or six months, during which time the woman shows more or less symptoms of congestions; piles appear; the limbs swell; pruritus (violent itching of the private parts) frequently sets in, also cramps and colics in the abdomen; asthma and palpitation of the heart; sick-headache; hysterics; apoplexy, etc. These maladies are so various, and continually changing and complicated, that they require the constant watchful care of a family physician. Do not neglect them.

TREATMENT.—We can here only give general rules: eat and drink moderately; sleep in airy, well-ventilated rooms; avoid violent emotions or exercise, but contrive to be busy mentally and bodily; shun exposure to inclement weather, wet feet, etc. (See "Hygiene.")

Pulsatilla and *Lachesis* are, in this period, the principal remedial agents, of which take every six days one dose (six glob.) alternately, unless other remedies are necessary. If diseases otherwise occur, see their respective chapters.

PROLAPSUS UTERI. (*Falling of the Womb.*)

A great deal of abuse has taken place, of late, with this disease, which has almost become as fashionable, as neuralgia, etc., through the neglect and ignorance of practitioners, who call every feeling of pressure which they cannot cure a "falling or dislocation of the womb," supported by the feelings of the patients, who really believe they have such a complaint, while in the majority of cases, they have only the peculiar sensation of forcing or bearing down, which results often from congestion to the womb, caused by other inherent chronic ailments. These ought to be ascertained and cured, and the poor sufferer not tormented with endless and senseless supporters and bandages, explorations by speculums, attempts to replace the womb, etc., by the practitioners who frequently afterward assert that they have replaced the womb, what really they could not have done, because it was not dislocated. If after all the patient is not cured, and the same feeling returns, it is said, "A relapse has taken place; we must replace it again;" and so the poor sufferer, confiding in her medical attendant, never receives relief. There are, undoubtedly, cases of falling of the womb, which require manual replacement; but these occur mostly after mechanical injuries, falls, blows, missteps, etc., or after severe labor in childbirth, and an examination gives unequivocal signs of dislocation. To such cases, the above remarks have no reference. I have seen frequent cases of the former kind, however, which were pronounced and treated by eminent physicians as prolapsus uteri, where no dislocation whatever existed; in women, too, who never had children, and who had not suffered external injuries. These patients were cured without external helps of pessaries and supporters, and became entirely healthy by a rational internal treatment, after their several chronic maladies, congestions to the womb, neuralgias, and indurations of the womb, etc., had been removed. Yet they frequently would, during the early part of the treatment, insist upon it, that they had a falling or dislocation of the womb; judging from their own feelings, and having been indulged or strengthened in them by their former physicians.

Treatment.—If a falling of the womb, or its dislocation is certain, from the preceding external injuries above stated, and the consequent constant feeling of downward pressure, less when lying, worse when moving or walking, compelling her to lean forward; the patient ought to lie down, and remain quiet, in a horizontal position, sometimes for weeks. During that time, let her take,

Belladonna and *Sepia*, alternately, every other morning a dose (six glob.) until better, or until one week has elapsed, when the patient discontinues the medicine for one week, yet remains lying; after which, she may repeat the same, or take,

Nux vom. Afterward, *Calcarea carb.* in the same manner.

Sometimes a dose of *Platina, Cocculus,* and *Ignat.* may be given, if the patient exhibits great nervousness, with constipation.

Application of Water; the wet bandage, often renewed, as also frequent sitting-baths of short duration, will be of great benefit.

Diet.—The usual homœopathic diet in chronic diseases.

Leucorrhea. Fluor Albus. (*Whites.*)

This troublesome and weakening complaint consists of a discharge of mucus, variously colored, and of different consistency, from the private parts. It occurs, generally, between the age of puberty and the critical period, and is seldom seen later than this, except when discharges of this kind are excited in consequence of the disorganization of the womb. If it manifests itself in children, or even in infants, it is either on account of want of cleanliness of these parts, or local irritations, such as are produced by pin-worms (ascarides), etc.

Weakly females, of a nervous, relaxed, or excited temperament, are more prone to it; and the more our present state of society becomes over-civilized, with its legion of pleasures, inactivity of body, idle and late hours, bad literature, and immoderate use of tea, coffee, and spices of all kinds (we mention here, only as an instance, the increased use of vanilla), the more easily will this disease be engendered.

It would carry us too far, to go into the practical detail of a disease which requires the most skillful attention of a medical attendant; and we earnestly recommend an application to him in an early stage of the disease.

Beside this we recommend cold water, in all its various applications, as the best means to restore the tone and strength of the weakened parts of the system.

The principal medicines to be taken domestically, are:

Pulsatilla. Discharge thick, like cream, sometimes creating an itching around the affected parts.

Cocculus. Discharge of a reddish hue before and after menstruation, with colic and flatulency.

Sepia. After *Pulsatilla;* parts become excoriated; discharge yellowish, greenish, fetid.

Calcarea carb. *Whitish, corrosive discharge* in *children;* in adults it is milky before menstruation or after lifting; particularly in fat, corpulent females.

Sulphur. If none of the above remedies should prove sufficient.

Administration.—Four doses of a remedy selected, every evening one dose (six glob.); then abstain from taking medicine for four days, and if not better at the end of that time, select another remedy, and take it in the same manner.

Application of Water; frequent tepid sitting-baths of short duration (from six to ten minutes), are very beneficial in the treatment of this disease; toward the end of the cure the wet bandage may be applied, to strengthen the parts affected. At that time injections of cold water in the vagina are also recommended.

Diet and Regimen.—Diet must be nourishing, but not flatulent (see "Dietetic Rules"). Avoid the causes which excite this complaint; particularly colds and excitements of any kind.

Pregnancy.

As this state of the female is an entirely physiological one, it must not be considered abnormal of itself. It only becomes so, by deviating from the rules of health. As regards diet, a pregnant female may live as she has found it for herself most beneficial heretofore. She must abstain, however, from excesses in diet, which previously would not have injured her, for the sake of the welfare of a being bound to her by the most endearing ties; the moral and physical health of this expected offspring depends upon its mother's actions.

Be careful in all things; careful in not making a misstep, in not dressing too tight, in not sitting up too late at night; in walking too great a distance, and in eating and drinking, be careful and moderate. But enjoy life, as far as is possible within these conditions; and the reward will be the happiness of others.

Exercise in the open air is good and necessary, but it must not be too violent; for instance, on horseback, etc.; walking in the open air is the best. Do not walk out immediately after dinner; but early in the morning or at night. Do not take purgative medicines. Daily sponge-baths of cold or tepid water are very beneficial, as also the drinking freely of cold water, particularly when inclined to constipation; the latter, if become annoying, must be relieved by sitting-baths and cold injections.

We will now consider the most common ailments during pregnancy.

Diseases during Pregnancy.

Pregnant females, even if ever so healthy otherwise, are liable to diseases to which pregnancy, as such, predisposes. These we will treat of in particular; while, for other ailments, we refer the reader to their respective headings, giving here only the most suitable medicines:

For *moral affections* (see "Affections of the Mind"): *Aconite, Pulsatilla, Belladonna, Platina, Lachesis, Stramonium, Veratrum.*

Headache: Belladonna, Bryonia, Nux vomica, Platina, Veratrum, Cocculus.

Toothache: Chamomile, Belladonna, Pulsatilla, Mercury, Sulphur, Sepia.

Convulsions and spasms: Belladonna, Hyoscyamus, Ignatia, Chamomile, Platina.

Dyspepsia: Nux vomica, Pulsatilla, Sepia, Phosphorus.

Constipation: *Bryon.*, *Nux vom.*, *Opium*, *Lycopod.*, *Sepia.*

Dysury and *strangury* (*scanty and painful urination*): *Nux vomica*, *Pulsatilla*, *Cocculus*, *Sulphur.*

Diarrhea: *Antimon. crud.*, *Phosphorus*, *Pulsatilla*, *Mercury*, *Sepia.*

Piles (*hemorrhoids*): *Nux vom.*, *Ignatia*, *Aconite*, *Sulphur.*

Incontinence of urine: *Pulsatilla*, *Belladonna*, *Stramonium*, *China*, *Silicea.*

Sleeplessness: *Coffea*, *Belladonna*, *Nux vomica*, *Hyoscyamus*, *Opium.*

Fainting (*hysterics*): *Ignatia*, *Pulsat.*, *Aconite*, *Bellad.*

Melancholy (*low spirits*): *Aconite*, *Pulsatilla*, *Ignatia*, *Belladonna.*

Piles or *hemorrhoids:* *Nux vom.*, *Sulphur*, *Ignatia*, *Sepia.*

Cramps in the *abdomen:* *Bellad.*, *Nux vom.*, *Pulsat.*

Cramps in the *back:* *Ignatià*, *Rhus tox.*, *Kali carbonic.*, *Bryonia*, *Belladonna.*

Cramps in the *hips:* *Colocynth*, *Rhus.*

Cramps in the *legs* (*calves*): *Veratrum*, *Secale.*

Cramps in the *feet:* *Calcarea carb.*

Pain in *right side* (see article "Liver"): *Chamomile*, *Aconite*, *Pulsatilla.*

Heart-burn (*sour stomach*), *Water-brash:* *Nux vom.*, *Phosphoric acid*, *Pulsatilla*, *Sulphur.*

In all the above diseases, compare their respective chapters.

Nausea and Vomiting during Pregnancy.

This distressing complaint is present during pregnancy in some females; in others it is wanting. It begins usually about six weeks after conception, and lasts up to the fourth, fifth, even seventh month, more or less violently. It is of a constitutional origin, and cannot be taken away easily, as the exciting cause still exists. The same may be said about the spitting of frothy saliva, with which some women are troubled.

Exercise in the open air, cheerful society, strengthening food, and refreshing drinks, such as ale, lemonade, or salt fish, sardines, smoked herring, are frequently means to alleviate the sufferings. The following medicines, also, often have a good effect:

Ipecac. If bile is thrown up, coated tongue, loss of appetite.

Nux vomica. If with sickness at the stomach there is headache, constipation, pressure in the stomach.

Arsenic. Vomiting after eating and drinking; great weakness.

Pulsatilla. Sour vomiting; white, coated tongue.

Petroleum. (See "Sea-sickness.")

Natrum muriaticum. Nausea and vomiting with loss of appetite and taste: water-brash, acid stomach and painfulness of the pit of the stomach.

Application of Water.—See "Sea-sickness" page 307.

Administration.—Give of the selected remedy three or four doses (four glob. each) a day, for two or three days in succession before the application of another remedy.

Pruritus. (Itching.)

This distressing disease of the private parts often takes away rest and comfort from the pregnant female, and must be removed as soon as possible. Try first, frequent washings and compresses of cold or warm water, and if not better, wash with a solution of borax and water, three or four times a day.

Treatment.—*Bryonia, Carbo veg., Graphites, Mercury, Pulsatilla, Sepia, Silicea, Sulphur, Rhus, Sarsaparilla,* are the principal remedies.

See their application recommended under "*Pruritus,*" in "Diseases of the Skin."

Varicose Veins.

A complaint which consists in an extension of the veins on the lower extremities, owing to the pressure of the pregnant uterus on the large veins of the abdomen, impeding the speedy return of the venous blood upward, creating, thereby, stagnation. If they are not painful and large, frequent washing in cold water is sufficient, as they speedily disappear after the birth of the child. But when they are very large and painful, the patient should lie down for a few days, and apply beside, if necessary, a bandage or laced stocking, to compress the extended veins. This bandage should be applied in the morning, when the least swelling is present.

The following remedies can be taken with benefit, every three days one dose (six glob.), changing the medicines every week, until better: *Arnica, Nux vomica, Pulsatilla, Arsenicum, Lycopodium, Carbo veg., Lachesis.*

Spots on the Face during Pregnancy.

Yellowish or brownish spots on the face, which often appear in pregnant females, require the use of *Sepia,* every eight days one dose (six glob.), for five or six weeks or until better; if not, *Sulphur* in the same manner.

Miscarriage. (*Abortion.*)

Miscarriage can take place at any time between the first and seventh month. If it occurs after the seventh, it is no longer so called, but *premature birth;* as at this period the child can be saved, and the object of pregnancy be gained, to give birth to a living child. But if the child is born before the seventh month, it cannot live; thence the name "*miscarriage.*" The more advanced the pregnancy is, the less is the danger which might result from a miscarriage. The oftener a woman has miscarried, the more her constitution inclines to new misfortunes of the same kind. Miscarriages are more liable to occur again at the same time of pregnancy, at which the former or last one happened; if once past that period, the danger to miscarry diminishes. Miscarriage can become a habit; it sometimes appears epidemically, in so far, at least, as in certain seasons the uterine congestion generally increases (menses appear more frequently and profusely, hemorrhages take place spontaneously, etc.), and in the same ratio, the possibility and occurrence of abortion multiplies.*

If a woman approaches the time where formerly she had miscarried, she must be careful not to provoke a return by walking great distances, lifting, running down stairs, riding over a rough road, etc. These practices might excite at any time a miscarriage in females who never were predisposed to it; certainly much more in those already predisposed. A weakening, luxurious mode of living, late hours, great mental excitement, are causes of miscarriage, and must be strictly avoided.

The premonitory symptoms of a miscarriage are: chilliness, followed by fever and pressing down sensation, which afterward increases to labor-pains; cutting, drawing, mostly in the loins and abdomen. A discharge of bright-red blood either immediately issues from the vagina, or coagulated, dark blood appears afterward in spells; frequent repetitions

* I observed this phenomenon, on the approach of the Asiatic cholera in Cincinnati in December, 1848, when there was a sensible increase of miscarriages and hemorrhages of every kind, increasing during the spring of 1849, and being at its height in July and August, when the cholera was raging the most fearfully. Women miscarried at this time who never before had had any predisposition to it, although mothers of many children; premature births occurred without any apparent cause, bodily or mentally. After that time, the tide of the disease turned, and with it the abortions decreased in number; also, other kinds of hemorrhages. Undoubtedly, the small quantity of positive electricity in the atmosphere caused a general debility in the nervous system, and consequent muscular and vascular laxity, which even involved, in its general effects, the uterus in all its functions. Hence the epidemical appearance of abortions. Such facts must only be known and recognized as such, and it becomes an easy task to prevent misfortune.

of these efforts of nature are usually necessary to expel the fœtus; varying in duration from two hours to two days.

TREATMENT.—As soon as the above symptoms appear, even if in a slighter degree, the patient must lie down and keep perfectly quiet, without moving; if the attack is brought on by mechanical injury, a fall, blow, misstep, or walking, lifting, etc., take

Arnica. Twelve globules dissolved in half a teacupful of water, every fifteen or twenty minutes a teaspoonful, until better, or until after one hour another remedy becomes necessary.

Secale will be the next remedy to be given, in the same manner as *Arnica*, particularly in females who have miscarried more than once; in older ones, or in those who have a weak and exhausted constitution, when the discharge consists of dark, liquid blood, and the pains are but slight.

China, in alternation with *Secale*, becomes necessary, when the loss of blood is considerable, and weakness and exhaustion evidently increase; buzzing in the ears; cloudiness of sight; loss of consciousness; fainting when raising from the pillow.

Hyoscyamus, if the patient falls into spasms or convulsions of the whole body, with loss of consciousness, discharge of light, red blood, worse at night.

Crocus, if dark clotted blood is discharged, increased by the least exertion, with sensation of fluttering or motion around the navel. If other remedies fail, this sometimes will help.

Ipecac. becomes a necessary remedy, in alternation with *Secale*, if with *flooding* there is nausea, fainting, cramps.

Platina and *Belladonna* in alternation, either at the beginning, or after *Ipecac.* has failed to relieve, and the pains are in the loins and bowels, severe bearing down, as if the intestines would be forced out; sensation in the back, as if it were broken; very pale or flushed face; discharge of dark, thick, clotted blood.

ADMINISTRATION the same as stated in *Arnica*.

DIET AND REGIMEN. — As in "Menstruation too Copious," "Flooding," which article may also be consulted, if the above remedies are insufficient for the *flooding*. After the fœtus has passed away, treat the patient in the same manner as would be necessary after a regular birth. The patient must keep the bed for the same length of time as in regular child-bed. This fact must be well remembered.

Do not neglect to procure a physician, if possible, immediately.

N. B. *Premature birth*, or a birth occurring after the seventh, and during the eighth month, must be treated as a regular birth; but frequently needs medical aid, which ought to be procured.

PARTURITION. REGULAR BIRTH.

This is a physiological and healthy process, setting in at the end of the ninth month of pregnancy, by contractions of the womb, called labor-pain, which, at first slight, increases, by degrees, in violence and strength, until the child is expelled. If labor occurs after the ninth month (sometimes it delays for two weeks), it becomes harder on account of the child becoming larger, and its head more closed, consequently less compressible.

Labor-Pains.

The following medicines will be of benefit to correct the irregularity and painfulness of labor pains:

For *nervous trembling, fear* and *anxiety, before or during labor-pain: Acon., Coffea, Bellad., Ignatia.*

For *ineffectual* or *spasmodic* pains; *Coffea, Chamomile, Nux vom., Secale.*

For the *absence of labor-pains: Pulsatilla, Secale.*

For *excessively painful labor-pains: Coffea, Aconite.*

For *sudden cessation of labor-pain*, with congestion to the head, redness of the face, drowsiness: *Opium.*

Administration. — Every half hour a dose (four glob.) until better, or another remedy chosen.

During the progress of labor, and any time after delivery, cold water may be drank freely by the patient, if she wishes it. Decidedly objectionable, during this time, are all warm drinks and alcoholic liquors, so frequently offered to the patient with a view to assist labor.

Cramps. Convulsions. Spasmodic Pains.

These are nervous symptoms, which frequently appear during labor, retarding the quick and successful delivery. In such cases, give

Chamomile. If acute, cutting pains extend from the loins to the hypogastrium, attended with spasms.

Belladonna. If the pains bear down most violently, so that convulsive motions of the limbs ensue; great agitation, constant tossing; red and bloated face; profuse sweating or dry, heated face.

Hyoscyamus. Severe convulsions, with loss of consciousness, great anguish and cries, with oppression of the chest.

Stramonium. Trembling of the limbs and convulsions, without loss of consciousness.

Ipecacuanha and *Ignatia* in alternation, when the patient complains of a confused feeling in the head; sensation of suffocation; convulsions.

Cocculus. If the whole body is cramped or convulsed, particularly the lower part of the abdomen, with heat and redness of the face; in alternation with *Belladonna.*

Administration.—Every fifteen, twenty, or thirty minutes, one dose (three glob.) until better or another remedy is required; if the medicine is taken in water, dissolve twelve globules in half a teacupful, and give every fifteen or twenty minutes a teaspoonful.

ADHERENCE OF THE AFTER-BIRTH. (*Placenta.*)

When, within half an hour, after delivery, no more pains appear, to expel the after-birth give *Pulsatilla* and *Secale,* alternately, every fifteen or twenty minutes a dose (three glob.), until new contractions ensue, after which, the placenta will soon appear. If the patient's head is congested, full, red, give of *Belladonna* four globules in preference to the above remedies.

TREATMENT AFTER DELIVERY.

Perfect rest and sufficient covering are the first necessities after delivery. No change of clothes or position ought to take place within the first eight or ten hours after delivery; during this time the patient generally enjoys a good sleep, into which she may be allowed to fall one hour after delivery; nothing restores the lost strength better than a good, quiet sleep.

If *flooding* threatens, rub the region over the womb by regular frictions with the hands, until the womb contracts again, and after-pains appear, which diminish the danger of flooding; or else give her *Belladonna,* if there is a great deal of bearing down; *Chamomile,* if there is coldness of the limbs and pains around the abdomen.

China and Ipecac., in alternation, in the worst cases, when the above remedies do not succeed; or,

Pulsatilla, if the discharge of clotted blood appears at intervals, ceases, and reappears; also, *Crocus, Platina,* and *Sabina.* As the last remedy, apply cold water in wet bandages, which must be frequently renewed, or pounded ice on the abdomen, which allays the flooding soon. (See "Mentruation too Profuse, Flooding.")

AFTER-PAINS.

These are necessary evils, as their beneficial effect in contracting the womb more perfectly is too evident. Yet, they sometimes become harassing and almost unbearable; in such cases use the following remedies:

Arnica, as the first medicine, to soothe the irritability of the womb after such heavy exertions; next, or in alternation with it,

Pulsatilla, almost a specific for these pains; or, if not better,

Chamomile and *Nux vom.*, in alternation.

Secale, in weakly persons, or those who have already had many children.

Coffea, if the pains seem to be so severe that the patient almost despairs.

ADMINISTRATION.—Every half hour or hour a dose (four glob.), until better.

DURATION OF CONFINEMENT.

If thus far this process is a perfectly healthy one (and neglect or mismanagement only can make it a source of suffering), its remaining part—that of confinement in bed after delivery—passes off, generally, in the same healthy manner. During this time, usually fourteen days, positively *no visitors* should be admitted *on any consideration*. In the best case, where nothing is wanting in regard to appetite, strength, or milk, and other natural discharges, the patient must not be allowed, before the fifth day, to sit up, and then, during the next five or six days, only as long as is necessary to have the bed made and aired. The reason is, to give the womb ample time to reduce and replace itself in its proper size and location; this can *safely* be done only while lying. Attending to this advice, *literally*, may save years of misery. The diet, during that time, may be more substantial, if wished for, and if the mother and child feel well otherwise.

BREASTS. NIPPLES. SECRETION OF MILK.

It is of the utmost importance for happiness and health,

that the greatest care should be bestowed upon the breasts and their secretions, the milk, the fountain of life for a being so dear to a mother. Months before the birth of the child, the breasts, which sometimes already enlarge at that time, must be prepared for their future duty, by washing them, every day in cold water, particularly the nipples, so as to harden them for the service to come.

Milk-fever generally, if it is not too severe, passes off without injury, and requires no other action on our part than to watch the patient closely, day and night, attending scrupulously and kindly to her wants, because mental excitement, at this period, often becomes fatal.

If, however, chilliness is followed by a very high fever, flushed face, etc., give *Aconite* in alternation with *Coffea,* if great restlessness is present; every hour a teaspoonful of a solution made of twelve globules in half a teacupful of water. *Bryonia, Belladonna,* and *Rhus* are afterward necessary, one after the other, every six or eight hours a dose (four glob.), if the pain and swelling in the breast, still continue. The child may continue to draw the breast, or it may be drawn by the nurse or a breast-pump.

DIET very light; gruel, toast, and tea.

Sore Nipples.

The soreness and tenderness, even bleeding of the nipples, require, at first, applications of

Arnica tincture, six drops of it to half a teacupful of water; wash with it every time *after* the child has nursed. If no better in eight days, and the nipples *inflame, swell,* and threaten to *ulcerate,* give

Chamomile, particularly when the pains seem to be insupportable, like toothache; every four or six hours a dose (four glob.), until better. If the nipples ulcerate or suppurate, dissolve of

Silicea, twelve globules in half a teacupful of water, and wash three or four times a day, or after every nursing; if not better in four or six days, take the following medicines, one after the other, in the same manner as *Silicea*, until one relieves, when all medicines must be discontinued until worse again: *Mercury, Sulphur, Graphites, Lycopodium, Calcarea carb.*

DIET as usual.

Ague in the Breast. Gathered Breast.

Give immediately, *Chamomile* and *Bryonia* in alternation, every hour a dose, four glob., for four hours; after which discontinue for four hours and let the fever pass off by perspiration, without giving any more medicine; if the fever will not disappear, however, or returns, give

Aconite and *Belladonna*, particularly if the breasts are swollen, hard, and very tender; externally apply hot brandy cloths. If lumps remain in the breast, rub with sweet oil, or lay over the breast a plaster of beeswax and sweet oil.

If a *gathering* of the breast cannot be avoided, abstain from applying the warm poultices as long as possible, as it would only implicate a still larger part of the breast within the suppurating sphere; give, during this time,

Phosphorus and *Hepar*, in alternation, morning and evening one dose (four glob.), until better, or until four doses of each are taken, after which discontinue the medicine, awaiting its effects for at least three or four days; if no signs of improvement are visible, give

Mercury and *Lachesis* in the same manner; and then again *Phosphorus* and *Hepar*, until the abscess has opened, or the swelling is diminished.

After the abscess has opened and discharged the matter, give

Silicea, internally, every evening and morning a dose (four glob.); externally, a wash on the breast, three times a day, made of twelve globules of *Silicea* in half a teacupful of water, well shaken. This remedy may be followed, in two weeks, by

Sulphur, internally, same as *Silicea,* and in alternation with it, until the breasts are healed.

DIET, nourishing, but not stimulating.

Deficiency of Milk.

Beside using drinks which have a tendency to increase the milk, such as milk-punch (milk with brandy), beer and milk, tea or coffee with milk, give

Pulsatilla, Causticum, Calcarea carb., each one for a week, every third night a dose (four glob.).

Suppressed Secretion of Milk.

If the secretion of the milk is suppressed suddenly, either by mental or physical causes, great injury is to be feared, if the proper measures are not adopted immediately; one of them is to take

Pulsatilla, twelve globules dissolved in half a teacupful of water, every two or three hours a teaspoonful. If congestion to the head, lungs, or abdomen takes place after the milk has disappeared, give *Belladonna* and *Bryonia,* in alternation, in the same manner as *Pulsatilla.*

If *mental emotions* were the cause, give

Aconite, Coffea, Chamomile. (See in "Diseases of the Mind," for the consequences of fear, fright, etc.)

If *taking cold* was the cause, give *Chamomile, Bryonia,* and *Rhus,* particularly when the head and limbs ache, in the same manner.

If *diarrhea* sets in, give *Pulsat., Bryonia, Rhus, Bellad.*

Milk Bad, too Thin, or repugnant to the Child.

Give the mother *Cina, Mercury, Silicea,* every third day a dose (four glob.), each remedy for ten days; *Silicea,* particularly if the child *vomits* immediately after sucking.

Excessive Secretion and involuntary emission of Milk. Weaning.

Internally, give *Pulsatilla, Bryonia, Belladonna, Calcarea,* in succession, each remedy for thirty-six hours, every twelve hours a dose (six glob.). Externally, wash with spirits of camphor, and wear constantly cotton batting. This is the best external application which can be used to stop the secretion of milk at the time of weaning the child.

State of the Bowels.

On account of the great changes going on at this time in the female organism, whereby a great quantity of liquids is discharged from the womb and breasts, their secretion in the intestines and discharge by the stool is retarded, mostly for five days after delivery; if a stool is forced, artificially, before that time, it must operate injuriously, as that much liquid is taken away from places where nature needed it most. If after the lapse of five days, no motion on the bowels has appeared, give of

Bryonia, four doses, every three hours one (six glob.), and await its effects twenty-four hours, after which, give *Nux vomica* in the same manner, if necessary.

Sulphur after that, if necessary, in the same manner. An injection, either of lukewarm water, and two tablespoonfuls of sweet oil, or the same with a little castile-soap dissolved in it, may be given on the sixth day, if necessary, and as often afterward as needed.

If *diarrhea* sets in the principal medicines are: *Rheum, Phosphoric acid, China, Pulsatilla.* For closer examination of the symptoms and their exciting cause, see article "Diarrhea."

But there is one kind of diarrhea peculiar to nursing women, which is frequently connected with the *nursing sore mouth* (see this below). The discharges from the bowels are whitish, curdled, smelling sour and musty, being copious and frequent, but not very painful. This diarrhea is the beginning of consumption of the bowels, and must be attended to immediately. I have found the following remedies almost specific in such cases:

Nux vomica, and *Hepar*, alternately, every three hours a dose (six glob.), until better, or until six doses of each are taken; at the same time the patient must lie on the bed or couch.

Diet.— Black tea, dry toast, rice, afterward, beef-steak and roasted mutton. (See, beside, "Consumption of the Bowels.")

Sore Mouth of Nursing Women.

In some females this complaint is constitutional; it is caused by the peculiar irritation which nursing has upon their digestive organs; if let alone, it sometimes becomes so bad as to force us to discontinue nursing, or to send the patient to mountainous places (the higher the better), where the digestive organs become stronger and more able to resist this weakening influence, occasioned by the constant loss of fluid (milk). The following remedies, however, will be used with benefit:

Mercury, *China*, in alternation, every evening and morning a dose (four glob.), for a week.

Nitric acid, every other evening a dose (four glob.), until better, or for a week; and, afterward,

Borax, *Nux vom.*, *Sulphur*, in the same manner. (Beside, see article on "Stomacace."

Diet and Regimen.—Diet nutritious, but not flatulent, as frequently a diarrhea accompanies this complaint, which requires particular attention. See foregoing article.

Exercise in the cool, fresh air (but not fatiguing exertion by walking), riding out in a carriage, etc., are beneficial· also, cold bathing, or sponging.

Discharge from the Womb during Confinement.

(Lochia.)

This bloody secretion from the womb is called the "Lochia," and lasts, generally, from nine to fourteen days, becoming gradually paler from the beginning, until finally a lightish, mucous discharge is left, which diminishes in quantity, until it also disappears.

This is the natural process; the deviations from it are ab nomal, and require attention. If the discharge is *suppressed* entirely, and fever, pain, and congestion follow, particularly in the abdomen and head, give *Bryonia, Pulsatilla, Hyoscyamus, Platina, Secale, Veratrum.*

(Another means to make it reappear again is, to apply on the womb warm fomentations of hops in a bag, or compresses dipped in warm water.)

If it is *too profuse*, or of *too long duration, Ipecac., China, Secale, Calcarea carb., Pulsatilla, Bryonia, Platina.* If the white lochia becomes bloody again, *Rhus.*

Administration the same as in "Menstruation too Profuse, Flooding."

Diet and Regimen, also, the same.

Pain. Inflammation in the Abdomen.

Metritis and Puerperal Fever.

If the abdomen becomes very sensitive to the touch or by movement, shooting pains, fever, headache, give immediately *Bryonia* and *Belladonna,* twelve globules of each dissolved separately in teacups half full of water, every two hours a teaspoonful, alternately; send for the physician *immediately;* if the lochia had stopped, apply, externally, a bag filled with hops dipped in hot water and wrung out well. If perspiration ensues, encourage it until the pain has disappeared.

General Complaints during Confinement.

For *sleeplessness*: *Coffea.*

For *colic*: *Chamomile, Bryonia, Pulsatilla, Sepia, Verat.*

For *convulsions* (spasms): *Ignatia, Hyoscyamus, Platina.*

For *retention of urine*: *Nux vom., Bellad., Pulsat.*

For *debility*: *China, Phosphoric acid, Veratrum, Calcarea carb.*

For *falling off of the hair*: *Lycopodium, Calcarea, Natrum mur., Sulphur.*

For *white swelling* (milk leg): *Belladonna, Rhus, Lachesis, Arsenic, Sulphur.*

N. B. For further information and the administration of medicines in the above diseases, see their respective Chapters.

CHAPTER XVII.

TREATMENT OF CHILDREN.

Apparent Death of a New-born Infant.

(Asphyxia.)

When a new-born infant, either from exhaustion or other causes does not breathe, or at least very imperfectly, order a warm bath, and while that is being prepared, rub the spinal processes, from the neck down to between the shoulders, up and down, gently but firmly for some time, and blow the breath gently into its mouth from time to time, if it does not breathe.

In the bath, pursue the same manipulations, and give a few drops of a solution of *Tartar emetic*, one grain in half a teacupful of water. If the child looks blue in the face (strangled), give *Opium*, in the same manner prepared, on the tongue, and by injection.

When the child revives, but looks still pale and exhausted, give *China*, one glob., every two hours, for six hours.

Diet of a New-born Infant.—After washing and dressing, the infant wants sleep, into which it falls as soon as it is warm enough. Put it in the mother's bed; near her, if possible. After having slept for six or eight hours, lay it on the breast, even if no milk were there, and feed it afterward with molasses and water (under no circumstances bread and water), or milk and water, half and half, and sweetened with loaf sugar.

Wash its mouth after feeding every time with cold water; it prevents the *thrush*.

Colic. Crying of Infants.

Examine well whether pins, sticking the little sufferer, are the cause.

If no cause is apparent but the universal one (colic), give *Chamomile* and *Belladonna*, in alternation, every half hour or hour a dose (one glob.) on the tongue.

If the child bends its body double while crying, and retracts its thighs, give

Chamomile when the face is red; or *Belladonna*, when the face is pale. If the child has greenish stools at the same time, give *Chamomile*. If it has loose evacuations, of a *sour* smell, give *Rheum*. If these will not suffice,

Ipecac. and *Jalappa*. All in the same manner. For great restlessness, sleeplessness, and feverish heat, with crying, give *Coffea* cc. and *Belladonna* cc., in the same manner.

Sometimes a tepid bath relieves the infant's sufferings, when nothing else will do it, or the application of the wet sheet, to do which, the infant is simply wrapped in a wet napkin or towel and well covered.

Elongation of the Head.

This deformity of the infant's head is only temporary; wash it with *Arnica tincture* and water (six drops to a teacupful); in a few days it will disappear.

Snuffles. Obstruction of the Nose. (*Coryza.*)

Give *Nux vomica*, one glob. in the evening, and *Sambucus* the next evening, if not better; in that manner alternate, until relieved.

If the nose runs water, give *Chamomile;* and if this does not relieve, *Calcarea*, every other night one or two globules;

Carbo veg., when it is worse, every evening, and

Dulcamara, when worse in the open air;

Tartar emetic, when there is rattling of mucus in the chest, worse at night.

Swelling of the Breasts of Infants.

Do not press or handle rudely these delicate swellings; as they contain nothing, the least of all milk, to be squeezed out. It is an inflammation, and must be treated like any other inflammation of glands. First, we should try to reduce the swelling; which can be accomplished, in most cases, by covering it with a lint, dipped in sweet oil. If this will not succeed, wash it several times with warm brandy and water, and give the child internally, *Chamomile* and *Belladonna*, alternately, every evening and morning a dose (one glob.). If it still grows larger (I have seen them of the height of one inch and more), keep on it a bread-and-milk poultice, and after the gathering opens, treat it like any other abscess; inwardly, give *Mercury* and *Hepar*, every evening one glob., alternately.

Restlessness. Sleeplessness.

If without any apparent cause, the child cannot sleep, give it *Coffea*$^{cc.}$ and *Belladonna*$^{cc.}$, alternately, every hour one glob., which in most cases will have the desired effect. If not, however, give

Chamomile, if the restlessness is attended by flatulency and griping; the child starts and is feverish, with redness of *one* cheek.

Pulsatilla and *Ipecacuanha*, if it arises from overloaded stomach.

Opium, if the face of the child looks red and bloated.

Application of Water, see “Colic of Infants,” page 417.

Inflammation of the Eyes.

This is a frequent complaint among infants. Do not expose the eyes to a light too strong, nor to cold draughts of air. Drop a few drops of the mother's milk into the eyes several times a day. Beside, give *Aconite* and *Belladonna*, in alternation, three times a day one glob., for several days.

If this course does not succeed, give

Chamomile, when the eyelids are swollen and glued together in the morning with yellow matter.

Mercury and *Pulsatilla,* in alternation, if small, yellowish ulcers are perceived on the margins of the eyelids, with discharge of yellowish matter.

If not better, give *Euphrasia* and *Rhus,* in the same manner; and, at last, *Sulphur,* every other evening one glob., for a week, particularly in scrofulous children.

Thrush, or Sore Mouth of Infants. (*Aphthæ.*)

This disease appears commonly in the first month after birth, and consists in the formation of small, white flakes on the tongue and around the gums. At first they are not very numerous, but soon multiply and run together, covering sometimes the whole tongue and mouth and extending down the throat.

Causes.—The principal cause of this disease is a constitutional taint, and not, as is frequently believed, the want of cleanliness only, although the latter may contribute to its development.

If children are nursed by the bottle or spoon, the use of improper food may give rise to it; consequently this disease attacks more frequently such infants than those nursed exclusively by the mother.

Treatment.—Wash immediately the mouth and tongue with *Borax,* dissolved in water and sugar (do not rub with the dry *Borax*); cleanse well all spots with a cloth dipped in the solution, and then wash the mouth well with another clean cloth, dipped in clean, cold water. If *Borax* is used in the dry state, too much of it remains in the mouth, creating there the same disease which had to be cured; because it is the true homœopathic remedy; in the above described manner, however, cases of thrush have been cured, which were previously treated for a length of time with pulverized

Borax, without the least beneficial effect. If Borax had been used too freely, the irritation following its use, will subside by the exhibition of *Chamomile* and *Coffea,* twelve globules of each, dissolved in half a teacupful of water; every three or four hours a teaspoonful, until better. Afterward, if necessary, give the child *Mercury,* and *Sulphur,* every three or four days, alternately, one glob.

Heat. Red Gum. Heat Spots.

This is an eruption of red pimples on the face, neck, and arms, sometimes over the whole body, caused mostly by keeping the child too warm.

In most cases, this eruption disappears quickly, without medicine, if the child is not kept too warm, and bathed regularly.

If the child is restless, give *Chamomile, Aconite, Bellad., Rhus, Arsenic, Sulphur,* every evening one glob., and every day another remedy, until relieved.

Excoriations. Rawness of the Skin.

Belladonna, if it occurs in very fleshy infants, and when there is fiery redness, in alternation with *Rhus tox.*

Chamomile, if the children are very restless. Every evening one glob., for three or four days; then discontinue the medicine for four days.

Mercury, Sulphur, Lycopodium, Carbo veg., and *Silicea,* in the same manner, if not better.

Wash often in cold water, and dry well; after which, use externally fine wheaten starch, or a weak lotion of *Arnica tincture.*

Jaundice.

This disease sometimes occurs in children when they have taken cold or been purged too frequently with castor oil. In such cases give

Chamomile and *Mercury*, in alternation, every evening one glob., until better.

Nux vomica. In the same manner, if the child is restless and costive.

Hepar. If the above remedies do not suffice, every other evening one glob.

Erysipelas.

(See "Erysipelas," under "Diseases of the Skin.")

This disease claims the attention of a homœopathic physician. Yet the following remedies may be given, until one can be procured:

Belladonna and *Aconite*, alternately, every three or four hours one glob.; after the fever has subsided,

Belladonna and *Rhus*, in the same manner.

The parts affected must be kept dry by dressing them with lint.

Convulsions or Spasms.

Order immediately a warm bath, and while that is preparing, select from among the following remedies that which is suitable.

Belladonna. In almost all spasms the first remedy. Give, in preference, the *Belladonna*$^{cc.}$, in the following manner: put directly two glob. of it on the tongue of the child; then dissolve twelve glob. in four teaspoonfuls of water, mix well, and give every fifteen minutes a few drops on the tongue.

After the bath (which may last from five to ten minutes), wrap the child, without drying off, in heated flannel, and lay it with its head higher on a pillow made of quilts, and, if possible, covered with oil-cloth.

If the spasms will not cease, keep the child's feet and legs in warm water, at the same time pouring a stream of cold water on the crown of its head, until consciousness returns. This process must be *repeated frequently*, although the first attempts have proved inefficient; it has been tried with the greatest success.

If by this time the child has not yet recovered from the fit, order an injection to be made of lukewarm water, and a tablespoonful of sweet oil, together with a little soapsuds (castile soap and water) to be given, and select another remedy, which administer in the same manner as *Belladonna*cc..

Chamomile. Convulsive jerkings, moaning, eyes half open, *redness of one cheek.*

*Cina*cc. If worms are to be suspected.

*Coffea*cc. In weakly and nervous children, subject to frequent fits.

Ignatia. When the fits return in regular intervals, followed by fever and perspiration.

Ipecac. When the breathing is short between the fits, nausea, and frequent spasmodic stretchings.

Opium. In fits after *fright,* when the breathing is labored, the face dark, flushed, almost blue.

Hyoscyamus, in convulsions from sudden fright, the muscles of the face twitch, and the mouth foams ; involuntary evacuations of fæces.

Stramonium, when the convulsions were caused by sudden fright, or in fevers from repelled eruptions ; and

Sulphur, when caused by repelled chronic eruptions.

If, after the fit, the child sleeps with its eyes half open, give *Hellebor.*, and *Belladonna,* as directed under "Hydrocephalus," page 425.

TEETHING. (*Dentition.*)

With seven months, the two middle teeth of the lower jaw appear; shortly after, the two corresponding ones in the upper jaw. From this time the little organism is constantly putting forth teeth, until, at the end of two or two and a half years, the first dentition, consisting of twenty teeth, is completed.

The process of teething excites in the little ones a variety of diseases, which, if not well treated, too often prove fatal. The mother can do a great deal, in directing the mode of her living, in eating, drinking, and acting, so as not to make her milk another source of suffering for the sickly sufferer. (See "Hygiene.")

The gums swell and are painful; yet the child wants to bite and press something hard on the teeth, to relieve the intolerable itching and irritation underneath the gums. Give it an ivory ring. If fever appears, with restlessness, retching, etc., give *Coffea*$^{cc.}$ and *Belladonna*$^{cc.}$, alternately, every half hour or hour, half a teaspoonful (twelve glob. having been dissolved in half a teacupful of water).

Chamomile and *Belladonna.* If convulsive jerkings or twitchings occur in the sleep.

Cina. If with teething it has a dry, spasmodic cough, or signs of worms; rubbing at the nose.

Aconite. If the fever is high.

If a diarrhea of a yellowish color occurs, it is not objectionable at first; but if it becomes of a whitish, slimy color, and curdled, give *Coffea, Ipecac., Calcarea carb.;* if of a greenish or grass-green color, give *Chamomile* and *Cuprum.*

If *convulsions* ensue, treat as stated in that article, page 421.

If the teeth are tardy in breaking through, do not lance them (it can only be of use where they are much swollen and *heated*), but give *Calcarea carb.*, every evening two glob., for a week; then discontinue a week, and give *Sulphur,* in the same manner.

Give the child frequently cold water to drink.

If *constipation* occurs during teething, give *Bryonia* and *Nux vomica,* alternately, every evening a dose (two glob.) for six days; beside, an injection of cold water every day.

CONSTIPATION.

It is a bad practice to give children physic, castor oil, etc., which, although it may temporarily relieve the patients, renders them afterward more constipated than ever; when an injection, which would be quite as efficient, is so easily administered. First, however, give the following medicines:

Bryonia, Nux vomica, and *Opium*, in succession, each remedy for one day, and three doses (two glob.), of each in a day. If not better, give *Sulphur*, in the same manner.

Allow as much cold water as they will take, and rub their stomachs every evening well with sweet oil.

If the above treatment does not produce the desired effect, give an injection of simple cold water, which, if ineffectual, may be followed by one, consisting of tepid water and sweet oil, having dissolved in it a small piece of castile soap.

Diarrhea of Infants.

If it has a *sour smell: Rheum.*

If it looks greenish, even grass-green: *Chamomile, Cuprum*

If with *colic* and a red face: *Chamomile.*

If with *colic* and a pale face: *Belladonna.*

If not relieved after these, give *Sulphur.*

If the diarrhea always appears in the heat of summer: *Ipecac., Nux vomica, Bryonia, Carbo veg.*

If from *cool weather: Dulcamara, Antimon. crud.*

If with great emaciation and weakness: *Arsenic, Carbo vegetabilis.*

Administration.—After every operation, one glob. of the selected medicine. For further information, see "Diarrhea."

Fevers of Infants.

Always give *Aconite*, two glob. first; in two or three hours *Chamomile* and *Coffea*, in alternation, every one or two hours two glob. (or in water, as usual); and lastly, *Belladonna*, in the same manner.

By that time, the fever must have shown its character, or the child will be well.

Diet.—Give a thirsty child as much cold water as it wants.

DROPSY OF THE BRAIN. (*Hydrocephalus.*)

Children with large heads, and of a scrofulous taint, are more subject to this disease than others, as their brains are more liable to congestions. The most trivial derangement of the bowels, sudden change in the atmosphere, teething, eruptive and other fevers; in fact, all diseases which may befall children, can, under certain circumstances, take their final and fatal issue through the dropsy of the brain, if timely aid does not prevent such a result.

DIAGNOSIS. — Whenever a child becomes drowsy, its head hot, feet cold, with or without nausea and retching, and *sleeps with eyes half open*, be careful and give it immediately the following remedies:

TREATMENT. — *Bellad.* and *Hellebor.* (of each twelve glob. in half a teacupful of water), every hour or two hours a teaspoonful, until four teaspoonfuls of each are given, or until the child becomes more lively. If the same drowsiness reappears, repeat the same medicine; if the third time, it appears, give *Opium* and *Sulphur*, in the same manner, and afterward *Bryonia* and *Hellebor.*, as above.

DIET must be light. Keep the feet warm, but the head cold, with cloths dipped in ice-water.

It is evident, that in diseases of this kind, medical aid should be obtained as soon as possible.

ASTHMA OF CHILDREN. (*Choking fits. Asthma Millari.*)

If little children seem almost to suffocate, fall into a spasm, and have a bluish face, give *Ipecac.*, one glob. every ten minutes; and when it is characterized more by hard and tight distension of the stomach and around the short ribs, with *shortness of breath, choking*, anxiety, agitation and tossing, cries and retraction of the thighs, give *Chamomile*, one glob. every twenty or thirty minutes, until better.

But if an *asthmatic* attack occurs suddenly and violently in the sleep, with dry, dull cough (resembling croup), the face and extremities become purple, spasms in the hands and feet (*asthma Millari*), give *Sambucus*, every five or ten minutes one glob., until better. Send, however, for a physician directly.

If *Sambucus* should not relieve within two hours, and no physician could be had, *Ipecac.*, *Pulsatilla*, *Arsenic*, *Sulphur*, *Cuprum*, *Spongia*, in succession, in the same manner as *Sambucus* above.

Diet, of the lightest kind. No meats, but gruels.

Remittent Fever of Infants.

Diagnosis.—Languor, irritability, nausea, want of appetite, thirst, slight heat of the skin, and restlessness at night. This is the beginning of the disease above-named. Soon, the symptoms increase; fever; constipation, or diarrhea of a mucous, fetid substance, sometimes mixed with blood; heat in the body and head; extremities cool; tongue coated, dry, and red on the margins; drowsiness, listlessness in the day, restlessness at night; hacking cough.

Treatment.—*Ipecac.* As the first remedy, every three or four hours one glob., for one day; afterward, *Bryonia* and *Rhus*, alternately, every three hours one glob. for two days; then discontinue the medicine for one day; after which, if the patient is better, *Sulphur* may be given once or twice, every three hours one glob.; or, if the head suffers the most, give *Belladonna*, every three or four hours one glob. for one day; or *Chamomile*, if the fever continues, with one flushed cheek, the other is pale; irritability; child does not know what it wants; in the same manner as *Belladonna;* or give

Mercury. If a diarrhea with tenesmus is predominant, and the tongue coated whitish; or

Nux vomica. When constipation is present, with frequent but ineffectual desire.

Lycopodium. When the tongue is dry, yet the patient is

not thirsty; very petulant; does not want to see any one, or talk to any one.

If head symptoms appear, see "Dropsy of the Brain."

APPLICATION OF WATER.—If during the fever the skin is very hot and dry, perspiration may be promoted by packing the patient in a wet napkin or towel, well covered; in this he may remain until perspiration appears, when he is taken out and washed all over in tepid water. This process may be repeated as often as the fever returns. If during the packing the head becomes hot and congested, put cloths, dipped in cold water and well wrung out, on the head; change them frequently.

DIET AND REGIMEN.—Gruels, toasted bread, soaked in milk and water; no meat or broth; no eggs; keep them comfortably warm, always covered, particularly arms and limbs. If perspiration appears, do not check it by exposure, as it frequently breaks the disease and shortens its course.

During convalescence be careful in the diet, as relapses frequently occur from errors in the diet. See what is said about it in "Typhus."

VACCINATION.

It is in accordance with the homœopathic principle, that vaccination can save from an attack of small-pox, the latter being a similar (but not the same) disease to the former. Through vaccination the triumphs of homœopathy have been shown to the world by innumerable blessings, in arresting such a loathsome disease as small-pox.

Vaccination, if salutary and truly protective, must not be negligently applied. The virus, or matter, ought to be taken from the cow itself, or from a healthy child, whose parents are healthy too, and in whose family skin diseases or scrofula are not hereditary.

Persons can be vaccinated at any time, from the first hour

of their existence to any age after that.* The best age for vaccination is from six months to one year; the best time in the year is May or June, when the least sickness generally prevails.

If a child has been vaccinated with bad matter, or scrofulous symptoms develop themselves, give *Sulphur*, every evening one glob., for eight days.

CHOLERA INFANTUM.

DIAGNOSIS.—Violent, copious vomiting, first of food, afterward of sour liquid; diarrhea mostly at the same time; restlessness, child tosses from one side of the bed to the other; nausea; retching on the least movement, or after drinking water, which is soon thrown up again; head hot; extremities cool; thirst great, drinks greedily; very weak; eyes sunken, and half open; eyelids heavy; pulse feeble or none at all.

This disease occurs, usually, in the summer, after errors in diet and other weakening influences on the stomach.

TREATMENT.—In nowise different from *cholera morbus* in adults.

Ipecac. and *Veratrum* (twelve glob. dissolved in half a teacupful of water), give every fifteen or thirty minutes a teaspoonful, until the severest symptoms have diminished, when the intervals ought to be lengthened. If not better after two hours, give

Arsenic (prepared in the same manner) every half hour a teaspoonful until better.

Rhus, in alternation with *Arsenic*, if the child tosses about in the bed, in the same manner.

If the cholera disappears, but drowsiness ensues, child

* I was obliged, once, to vaccinate a child only half an hour old, whose mother, at that time, was seriously ill with the varioloid; the vaccination took well, without rendering the child more sick than common, saving it successfully from an attack of small-pox.

sleeps with eyes half open; head is hot; feet cold; treat as stated under "Hydrocephalus," page 425.

Application of Water, see "Cholera morbus."

Diet and Regimen.—Cold water; gruel; in convalescence great care must be taken in regard to diet.

Summer-complaint.

This disease is well known in the large cities, where it creates a fearful mortality among children, which are yet under allopathic treatment. Teething and the warm weather are its prominent causes; they are sufficient to produce all the subsequent changes, which make up the so-called summer-complaint. In general, careful attention to diet, bathing in cold or salt water, cool, refreshing air, on hills, or mountains, or in the high country, will do much to prevent or cure this disease. But when it has begun, give the following medicines:

Ipecac., for nausea, vomiting of food and bile; fermented stools, with white flocks, tinged with blood; no appetite; great thirst.

Bryonia. Diarrhea in *hot* weather; great thirst; vomiting after eating; stools smell putrid, are white or brownish. (In alternation with *Ipecac.*)

Carbo veg. after *Bryonia*, if the discharges are very thin and offensive, with pain at the time.

Dulcamara. Diarrhea in *cool* weather.

Antimon. crud. Nausea; vomiting; tongue *coated;* stools offensive; urinating frequently.

Tartar emetic. Nausea; gagging; tongue *clean;* stools watery, offensive; child is very weak. (In alternation with *Bryonia* or *Kreosote.*)

Mercury. Stools, with straining (like dysentery), and colic pain, discharges greenish, bloody, slimy. (In alternation with *Nux vom.*)

Veratrum, if the disease assumes the character of cholera infantum. (See this article.)

Administration of the above remedies.—Every six or eight hours, four glob. *Phosphor. acid* and *China,* in alternation, after every evacuation two glob., if great weakness predominates and the stools are frequent, yellowish, watery. (See "Cholerina.")

If the child becomes still weaker, and, finally, a thrush, white sores appear in his mouth, give *Mercury,* every two hours four glob., until better, and in a few days afterward,

Sulphur, two glob. evening and morning.

Diet and Regimen.—Arrow-root, farina, sweet-potatoes, sweet pickled pork, fried smoked herring: if possible, retire with the child to a place in the country high and airy, where the child can be carried out mornings and evenings under the shade of the trees; here it will soon recover.

PART SECOND.

I. ANATOMY AND PHYSIOLOGY.

II. HYGIENE AND HYDROPATHY.

III. MATERIA MEDICA.

I. ANATOMY AND PHYSIOLOGY.

Anatomy describes the mechanism and structure of the parts of the human system, while

Physiology treats of the laws by which the organism is governed, and the various functions in man are performed.

From the above it may be seen how closely these two sciences are related to each other, and that it is almost impossible to treat of them separately, without great disadvantage. They will appear, in this short treatise, interwoven with each other, as the necessity of a clear exposition of their details may require.

The study of anatomy and physiology must be interesting to every one, who wants to know a little more of the wonderful creations and provisions of an allwise Providence, than an outside view of nature around him can give. But it is not alone the thirst for increased knowledge which is satisfied by studying the human system and its laws; this knowledge is often highly beneficial to our physical welfare, and is particularly necessary for those who, from necessity or philanthropy, undertake to minister to the sufferings of their fellow-beings: and to this category not merely the professional physician belongs, in whose hands life and health are trusted, but all men, if possible, should enrich their minds with the treasures of a science whose teachings lighten, to so great an extent, the burden and responsibility of the healing art; particularly as no one knows whether he might not be called upon, in some emergency, to practice medicine to the extent of his knowledge. Viewed in this light, it becomes the duty of every one who prescribes at all in diseases, to make himself acquainted with the human system and the laws of health, as this knowledge only enables him to decide competently where health ceases and disease commences. For a successful and satisfactory use of the prescriptions laid down in a domestic physician, some knowledge of the anatomy and physiology of the human system is indispensable, and we recommend, strongly, a repeated and careful perusal of the following pages.*

Structure of the Human Organism.

The human body consists of fluids and solids, changing constantly from one into the other; their proportion to each other varies in different individuals and at different periods of life. In youth, the fluids are more abundant than in advanced age. The liquids contain, as it were, the whole body in its elementary particles, which by organical attraction, are formed into the different solid parts of the system. These exist in different degrees of solidity, as their different uses require. The simplest form of organized animal substance is a *membrane*, or *tissue*, composed of fibres interwoven like a network; all organs are formed by tissues, which are different, and adapted to their uses.

The *mucous* membranes line all the cavities which communicate with the air, as the mouth, nostrils, intestinal canal, lungs, etc., and are covered with minute cells, which secrete a viscid fluid called *mucus*, to protect the inner surfaces of the cavities from the contact with the air.

The *serous* membranes line cavities which do not communicate with the air, as the skull, chest, abdomen, etc. A *serous* membrane is a shut sac, with one layer opposed to the wall of the cavity, and the other folded around the contents

* If a more extended acquaintance is desired with these necessary branches of practical medicine, it can satisfactorily be found in the work of Calvin Cutter, M. D., on anatomy, physiology, and hygiene, which we mostly followed in its admirable and popular arrangement.

of the cavity; which contents are outside of the sac. A *serous* fluid is secreted between the sides of the sacs, to keep them moist and movable.

Areolar tissue, otherwise called *cellular*, is extensively distributed throughout the system, and is useful in enveloping organs and parts of organs, especially where a considerable degree of motion is required; which motion it never impedes, being abundantly supplied with fluid.

The *adipose* tissue forms distinct bags or cells, filled with *fat*, and is principally located beneath the skin, and around the heart and kidneys.

The *cutaneous* membrane forms the outside covering of the body, called the *skin*, and is similar in its structure (although harder), to the mucous membrane, of which it forms the external continuation. It secretes, constantly, a fluid called perspiration, if it appears in large quantities; it exists mostly, however, in an imperceptible vapor, which, as it were, constitutes the atmosphere of the body.

The *fibrous* tissue forms a thin, dense, strong membrane, and is found where a strong protection is needed, as in the lining of the internal, surface of the skull, around the bones, and at the end of the muscles; here it constitutes the so-called *ligaments* and *tendons*.

The *cartilaginous* tissue covers the ends of the bones, where they concur in forming a joint, and is, on that account, firm, smooth, and elastic.

The *osseous* tissue, which composes the *bones*, varies in different periods of life, as regards solidity and density.

The *muscular* tissue consists of many filaments, which united, form fibres, each of which is inclosed in a fine layer of *areolar* tissue, called *sarcolemma*. *Muscles* are composed of bundles of these fibres.

The *nervous* tissue is composed of two distinct substances, one gray and vascular, the other white and fibrous. The gray forms the external part of the brain, and the internal part of the spinal cord; while the nerves are composed of the white, inclosed in a sheath called *neurilemma*.

ELEMENTS OF THE HUMAN ORGANISM.

These are: first, *inorganic* (*chemical*); or, second, *organic* (elementary products of the system itself).

1. The *inorganic* or *chemical* elements. These are:

a. *Metallic* substances, as Potash, Soda, Lime, Magnesia, Alum, Silex, Manganese, Copper, and Iron.

b. *Non-metallic* substances, as Oxygen, Hydrogen, Carbon, Nitrogen, Phosphor, Sulphur, Prussic acid, etc.

2. The *organic elements* are: Albumen, Fibrin, Gelatin, Mucus, and Osmazome, etc.

ANATOMY OF THE BONES.

The bones, giving strength and solidity to the system, are so united among themselves, and adapted to each other, that they admit of the most numerous and various actions. The elevations or protuberances of the bones are called processes, which generally form the points of attachment for the muscles and ligaments. They are composed of earthy and animal matter; the former giving strength, the latter vitality. At the earliest stage of formation, the bones are cartilaginous, soft, and tender, and become hard and ossified as soon as deposits of phosphate and carbonate of lime commence, at certain points, called *points of ossification*.

The *periosteum* or fibrous membrane investing the bones, except where they are tipped with cartilage, at certain points, gives vitality and nutrition to the bone.

There are two hundred and eight bones in the human body, beside the teeth. They are divided into four parts.

First. The bones of the head.

Second. Of the trunk.

Third. Of the upper extremities.

Fourth. Of the lower extremities.

1. *The bones of the head.* They consist of those of the *skull, ear*, and *face.*

The bones of the *skull*, of which there are eight, consist of two plates or tablets of bony matter, united by a porous portion of bone; the external tablet is fibrous and tough, the internal, dense, hard, and glossy. Thus, the skull is admirably adapted to resist the penetration of sharp instruments, or diminish any vibration occasioned by falls and blows.

The skull is convex externally, and at the base much thicker than at the top or sides; its bones are, as it were, sewed together, united by sutures, whose rugged edges interlock with each other, producing a union, called, by carpenters, *dovetailing.*

In early infancy the bones are not united, leaving interstices of considerable extent, which fill up slowly with bony matter; thus allowing, in the early time of infancy, sufficient room for the expansion of the brain, which, in this time of life, is particularly liable to destructive congestions. No part of the human structure contributes more to the difference existing among the races of mankind than does the skull; in this too are found those eminences and depressions which indicate to the phrenologist the development of the brain.

In each *ear* are four very small bones, which aid in hearing.

In the *face* we count fourteen bones, some of them serving for the attachment of powerful muscles for masticating food, others to retain in place the soft parts of the face. The face forms the most interesting part of the human system, with its rays of intelligence and joy, or its clouds of distress or sorrow; and thus with its wonderful play of passional expression is made the dial-plate of the inner man.

2. The *trunk* has fifty-four bones: viz., twenty-four ribs, twenty-four bones in the spinal column (back-bone), four in the pelvis (forming the hips), the breast-bone (sternum), and the bone at the base of the tongue (os hyoides). They are

so arranged as to form, with the soft parts attached to them, two cavities, called the *thorax* (chest) and *abdomen.*

The *thorax* is formed by the breast-bone in front, the ribs at the sides, and the twelve dorsal bones of the spinal column in the back; this cavity contains the lungs, heart, and large blood-vessels; its natural form is a cone, with its point above, yet fashion often inverts this order boldly, but never without paying the due penalty in diminution of life and happiness.

The *breast-bone* (sternum) consists of eight pieces, in a child, which after uniting, form but three parts in adults; the lower part of the sternum reaching over into the pit of the stomach, remains cartilaginous and flexible until old age, when it is often converted into bone.

The *ribs* are connected with the spinal column, and increase in length as far as the seventh, where they become shorter. The seven upper ribs are fastened to the sternum by cartilages, to facilitate their motions in breathing; they are called the *true ribs.* The next three are united to each other by cartilages, not touching the sternum—therefore called *false ribs;* while the latter two, or lowest ribs, are not connected either with the sternum or the other ribs, therefore, called *floating ribs.*

The *spinal* column contains twenty-four pieces of bone, called *vertebræ.* Each of the vertebræ has seven projections, called *processes,* four of which, called *articulating* processes, join similar ones of the adjacent vertebræ to form the column; two of the remaining processes are called *transverse,* and the other the spinous process; these processes receive the muscles of the back and neck, to allow a firm and elastic motion to the spinal column in all directions.

A canal or tube runs through all the vertebræ in one continuous descent from the round aperture in the skull, to contain the *spinal cord* (medulla spinalis), the immediate continuation of the brain.

Between the vertebræ is a cartilaginous and highly elastic

substance, which facilitates the movements of the spine, and diminishes any shock in walking, running, or leaping, which would otherwise hurt the spine or brain.

The *pelvis*, or the bones forming the *hip*, consists of four parts, two of which are called *innominata* or *nameless* bones; these, in particular, form the hip, having externally, at each side a deep socket like a cup, for the reception of the round head of the thigh bone; internally these bones, in conjunction with the sacrum, form a cavity, which contains those organs called pelvic, as the bladder, rectum, sexual organs, etc. The *sacrum* belongs to the pelvis, forming its posterior part; it is placed between the hip-bones, to which it is bound by ligaments; it is, in reality, the continuation of the vertebra, and forms part of the spinal column, which is terminated, finally, by a small appendix called *coccyx*, in youth, consisting of four pieces, uniting, however, in more advanced age, into one bone, which, in females, is more movable than in males, for a wise purpose.

Fig. 1.

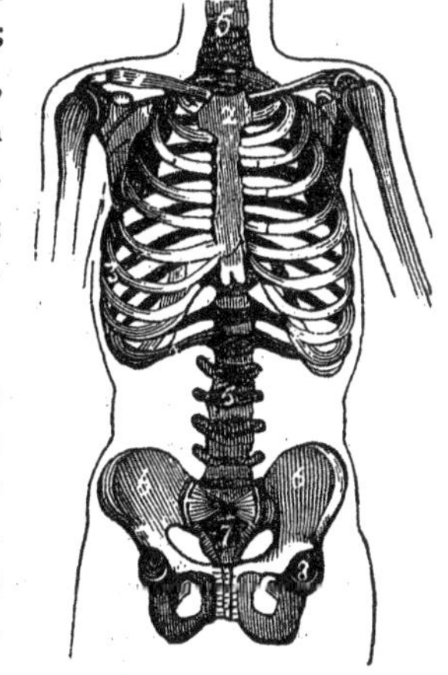

Fig. 1. Representing the bones of the trunk. 1, Clavicula or collar-bone; 2, sternum or breast-bone; 3, last true, or seventh rib; 4, last false, or twelfth rib; 5, spinal column; 6, the innominata (nameless bones); 7, the sacrum; 8, socket for the head of the thigh-bone.

3. The bones of the *upper* and *lower limbs* are enlarged at each extremity, where tendons, muscles, and ligaments are attached. The bones of the extremities are mostly in the form of cylindrical and hollow shafts.

The *upper extremities* contain sixty-four bones, as the shoulder blade (*scapula*), collar-bone (*clavicula*), upper arm-bone (*humerus*), two bones of the fore-arm (*ulna* and *radius*), the wrist (*carpus*), the *metacarpus* (palm of the hand), and the fingers and thumb (*phalanges*).

The *collar-bone* (clavicula, see fig. 1, No. 1), is attached at one end to the breast-bone, at the other to the shoulder bone: it is shaped like the italic *f*, and its use is to prevent the arms from sliding toward the breast; a fracture of this bone requires a more complicated bandage to keep the broken parts together, than any other within the range of surgery.

The shoulder-blade (*scapula*) lies on the upper and back part of the chest, forming the shoulder, where the upper arm bone inserts itself in a shallow (*glenoid*) cavity, surrounded by a strong ligament (*capsular*); the shoulder-blade itself is a thin, flat, and triangular bone, covering the back, and remains in its position, or moves in different directions, by numerous muscles which adhere to its projections.

The *upper arm* (*humerus*) forms a connection, at the elbow, with the ulna of the fore-arm, and at the shoulder, its round head is applied to the glenoid cavity of the scapula, in which it is firmly confined by the capsular ligament, thus forming the most movable joint in the whole system.

The *lower or fore-arm* is composed of two bones, called *ulna* and *radius*: the former articulates with the humerus at the elbow, forming a perfect hinge-joint; this bone is located on the inner side of the fore-arm, while the latter, the *radius*, lies on the outside of the fore-arm (on the side where the thumb is placed), and articulates with the bones of the wrist forming the wrist-joint; the ulna and radius, at their extremities, articulate with each other, so that the hand can rotate, permitting its complicated and varied movements.

The *wrist* (*carpus*) consists of eight bones, ranged in two rows, and firmly bound together, thus allowing only a small amount of movement.

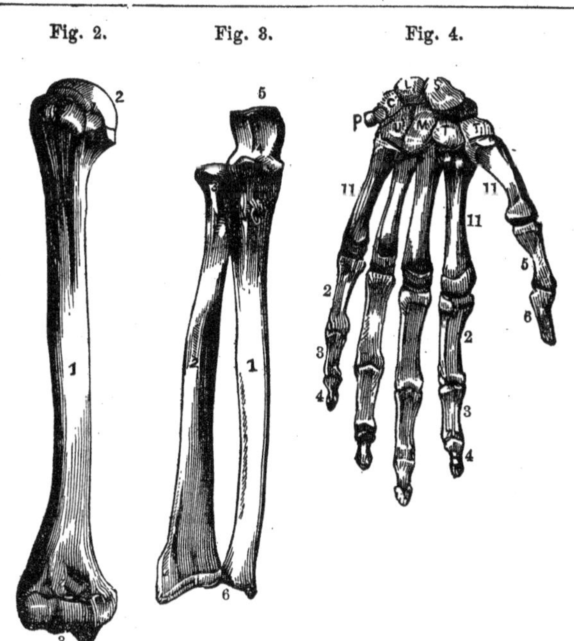

Fig. 2. 1, The shaft of the humerus. 2, The large, round head that is placed in the glenoid cavity. 3, The articulating surface upon which the ulna moves.

Fig. 3. 1, The body of the ulna. 2, The shaft of the radius. 3, The upper articulation of the radius and ulna. 4, Articulating cavity, in which the lower extremity of the humerus is placed. 5, Upper extremity of the ulna, called the olecranon process, which forms the point of the elbow. 6, Surface of the radius and the ulna, where they articulate with the bones of the wrist.

Fig. 4. S, The scaphoid bone. L, The semilunar bone. C, The cuneiform bone. P, The pisiform bone. These four form the first row of carpal bones. T, T, The trapezium and trapezoid bones. M, The os magnum. U, The unciform bone. These four form the second row of carpal bones.

Fig. 4. 11, The metacarpal bones of the hand. 2, 2, First range of finger-bones. 3, 3, Second range of finger-bones. 4, 4, Third range of finger-bones. 5, 6, Bones of the thumb.

The *palm of the hand* (*metacarpus*) contains five bones, four of which are joined with the first range of finger-bones, and the other with the first bone of the thumb.

The *fingers* have three ranges of bones (phalanges), while the *thumb* has but two.

N. B. The mechanism of the hand, with its wonderful adaptation to all the various purposes of life, is one of the many facts which indicate man's superiority over the rest of the animal creation, and must excite in us the deepest interest and astonishment at the Divine wisdom and power.

The *lower extremities* comprise sixty bones, analogous in construction and form to the upper extremities ; the *thigh-bone* (*femur*) ; the cap of the *knee* (patella) ; the *shin-bone* (tibia) ; the *small bone of the leg* on the outside of the tibia (fibula) ; the *instep* (tarsus) ; the middle of the foot (metatarsus) ; and the *toes* (phalanges).

The *thigh-bone* is the longest and *strongest* bone in the system, supporting the weight of the whole body. Its upper part, a large round head, fills a corresponding cavity in the pelvis and forms the so-called *hip-joint,* thus admirably fitted, in its mechanism, for its various offices requiring strength and motion.

The *cap of the knee* (patella) is a small bone in front of the knee, connected with the thigh-bone by a strong ligament ; it acts like a pulley, in the extension of the limb.

The *shin-bone* (*tibia*) is the largest bone of the lower part of the leg, of a triangular shape, and considerably enlarged at each extremity.

The *small-bone* of the leg (*fibula*) is of a similar shape with the former, but smaller, and bound firmly to it at each extremity. It lies on the outside of the leg.

The *instep* (*tarsus*) is formed of seven irregularly-shaped bones, so firmly bound together by ligaments as to allow of but little movement.

The *palm of the foot* (*metatarsus*) consists of five bones, corresponding to the five toes, with which they articulate on the front extremity, while on the hinder one, they articulate with one range of the bones of the instep.

By this arrangement, an arch is formed, convex above and concave below, which gives elasticity to the step, preventing the jarring of the whole frame by any weight thrown upon the feet, in their various uses.

The *toes* are composed of fourteen bones (*phalanges*); each of the small toes has three, while the great toe has but two ranges of bones.

Fig. 5. Fig. 6. Fig. 7.

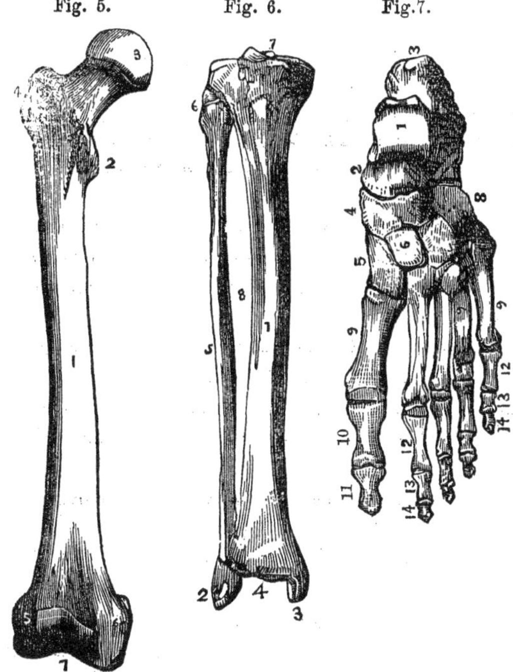

Fig. 5. 1, The shaft of the femur, (thigh-bone). 2. A projection, called the trochanter minor, to which are attached some strong muscles. 3, The head of the femur. 4, The trochanter major, to which the large muscles of the hip are attached. 5, The external projection of the

femur, called the external condyle. 6, The internal projection, called the internal condyle. 7, The surface of the lower extremity of the femur, that articulates with the tibia, and upon which the patella slides.

Fig. 6. 1, The tibia. 5, The fibula. 8, The space between the two, filled with the inter-osseous ligament. 6, The junction of the tibia and fibula at their upper extremity. 2, The external malleolar process, called the external ankle. 3, The internal malleolar process, called the internal ankle. 4, The surface of the lower extremity of the tibia, that unites with one of the tarsal bones to form the ankle-joint. 7, The upper extremity of the tibia, upon which the lower extremity of the femur rests.

Fig. 7. A representation of the upper surface of the bones of the foot. 1, The surface of the astragalus, where it unites with the tibia. 2, The body of the astragalus. 3, The os calcis, (heel-bone). 4, The scaphoid bone. 5, 6, 7, The cuneiform bones. 8, The cuboid. 9, 9, 9, The metatarsal bones. 10, The first bone of the great toe. 11, The second bone. 12, 13, 14, Three ranges of bones forming the small toes.

The *joints*, which have such important functions to perform, are composed of the extremities of two or more bones, lined and surrounded with *cartilages*, *synovial membranes*, and *ligaments*.

The *cartilage* (gristle) is a smooth, solid, elastic substance, of a pearly whiteness. It appears as a thin layer, on the articular surfaces of the bones—thicker in the center upon convex surfaces, while the opposite arrangement exists upon concave surfaces.

The *synovial membrane* forms in a thin layer over the cartilages a closed sack, in the interior of which a constant secretion of a viscous fluid takes place, to facilitate the movements of the joints.

The *ligaments* consist of numerous straight fibres, arranged into short bands of various breadths, or so interwoven as to form a broad layer, which surrounds the joint, forming a capsular ligament. They are white, glistening, and not elastic, and found mostly exterior to the synovial membrane.

Physiology of the Bones.

The bones, by their solidity and form, retain every part of the system in its proper shape. They not only afford points of attachment for the muscles and ligaments, to hold the body together and bring it into motion, but they protect, in strong, bony cavities, all the important organs from external injuries, such as the brain, the eyes, etc.

The bones grow and decay, like any other tissue, by new particles being deposited from out the blood, and old, useless matter removed, by the constant action of the absorbing vessels. This has been tested thoroughly. Some of the inferior animals were fed with food containing madder. After a few days, several of these animals were killed, and their bones exhibited an unusual reddish appearance. The rest of the animals were for a few weeks fed on ordinary food, without containing madder, and when killed their bones had the natural color again.

The extremities of the bones are the best suited to form joints; for which purpose their texture is more porous, consequently more elastic, and the external surface of the parts immediately joining each other in a joint is covered with a cushion of cartilage, to diminish jarring or grinding. The contemplation of each minute particle, its uses and application in the system, its appropriate location, etc., the thousand wonderful machines which can be observed, acting usefully and quietly in our systems, reveal more and more the wisdom and omnipotence of the great Architect. Wonder and adoration fill the heart of the beholder of such creations as the human body, in its detail and in its whole, as a complete and noble machine, to run the errands of the holier part of man, the soul.

The bones serve, in the animal frame, as a proper basis; the ligaments hold the bones in their proper places firmly, as if clasped by steel, yet with room to move. They surround the joints like a hood, or extend from one bone to the other, in the form of side layers. By these ligaments, the lower jaw is bound to the temporal bones, and the head to the neck. They extend the whole length of the spinal column, in strong bands, on the outer surface, as well as within the spinal canal, and from one spinous process to another.

The joints are different as regards movement and complexity of structure. Some permit motions in all directions, as the shoulder; some in two directions, as the elbow, allowing flexion and extension; others in three and more directions; others, again, have no movement at all, as the bones of the skull, in adults.

The Muscles.

A muscle consists of bundles of fibres of different size, each one inclosed in an areolar membranous sheath. Every bundle is composed of small fibres, and each fibre of numerous filaments, each of which is inclosed in a delicate sheath. At the end of the muscle, the fibrous substance ceases, and the *tendon* (cord) commences, by which the muscle is attached to the bone. The union is so firm, that the bone will sooner break than permit the tendon to separate from its attachment.

The form of the muscles varies very much, according to their uses. It is either longitudinal, having a tendon at each extremity, or it diverges in the form of a fan, called a radiate muscle. Others are penniform, converging, like the plumes of a pen, to one side of a tendon; or bi-penniform, where they thus converge on both sides of a tendon.

The color of a muscle is red; each fibre is supplied with arteries, veins, lymphatics, and nerves, both of sensation and motion.

Where a great many muscles congregate around an organ, they are inclosed in a *fascia*, a fibrous membrane, which assists the muscles in their action by keeping up a tonic pressure on their surface. Beside, it protects the parts underneath; as, for instance, in the palms of the hands or feet.

The separate muscles are also inclosed in fasciæ, and arranged in layers, as their use requires it. The interstices between the different muscles are filled with fat, which gives to the body roundness and beauty.

We may arrange the muscles into four parts; those,

1. Of the *head* and *neck*.
2. Of the *trunk*.
3. Of the *upper extremities*.
4. Of the *lower extremities*.

As it is impossible to give an interesting detail of the muscles of the body, their insertions and names, without illustrating them by plates, we content ourselves with the following general remarks.

There are more than five hundred muscles in the human body, forming around the skeleton two layers, a superficial and deep-seated one. Some muscles are voluntary, under the control of the will, such as those on the fingers, limbs, etc.; others are involuntary, as the heart. On the back, the muscles are arranged in six layers, one above the other, for the complicated movements which the back, neck, the upper extremities, and the abdomen require.

The *diaphragm* is a muscle which needs particular explanation. It is located between the chest and abdomen, separating them completely; being penetrated only by the pipe leading to the stomach, and by the great blood-vessels, leading from and to the heart. It may be compared to an inverted basin, its bottom being turned upward into the chest, its edges corresponding to the outline of the edges of the lower ribs and breast-bone. Thus, the cavity of the abdomen is enlarged at the expense of that of the chest. Respiration, however, changes the natural position of the diaphragm constantly, facilitating this process by its own action. During inhalation, the diaphragm descends into the abdomen, enlarging the chest; during exhalation, the reverse takes place; thus a constant and healthy action is given to both the respiratory and digestive organs. In this place we should mention the great benefit which results from inhaling deep, to the full extent of the lungs, which is greatly facilitated by exercising the abdominal muscles, causing them to swell out when inhaling, and drawing them back when in the act of exhaling. A little exercise in this way, will soon show the good results in the ease, and full extent to which the lungs can be filled.

The action of the muscles, in performing their various functions, can be explained only by the supposition of an inherent contractility, as a peculiar characteristic of the muscular fibre, which can shorten its substance, when a sufficient stimulus acts on it. This stimulus is the nervous fluid, directed to the muscles by the will, if voluntary actions shall be performed, or, independently of the will, when the involuntary actions are wanted, such as the beating of the heart, etc. The nature of this nervous influence may be analogous to a galvanic or electrical current; as these agents, when acting on the muscles, produce similar effects.

The rapidity with which the muscles move, is truly astonishing, as any one can observe, in rapid speaking, or playing upon instruments. It is not alone the size of the muscle which determines its strength; but, also, the size of the nerves which lead to it, and the size and activity of the brain, which must supply the nervous fluid necessary as a stimulus to action. Yet a great deal depends on training and exercise, as these enlarge both the muscle and nerve. The blacksmith, wielding the hammer daily and forcibly, will have a stronger arm than the student, who merely exercises his muscles with a pen. From this, it is evident that the muscles ought to be educated or trained for the vigorous and healthful performance of their duty. Strict and systematic rules are given for this purpose, in an art called the gymnastic, which, to understand and practice diligently, we recommend strongly. It is indispensable for the young, and not without advantage foı the middle-aged, to spend part of a day in systematic, healthful exercise of their muscles. The benefits are too great and palpable to bring them forward here, singly. Washing in cold water, also, invigorates the muscles.

The Teeth.

The teeth differ from other bones in composition, nutrition, and growth; while bones, when fractured, generally unite, the teeth never do, when broken. They are divided into two parts, *crown* and *root;* the former, protruding from the jawbone, is covered by the highly polished enamel; the root is placed in the sockets of the jaw, consisting of bony matter, through which several small vessels and nerves pass, giving nutrition and vitality. The teeth, when beginning to grow, are formed within dental capsules, inclosed within the sub stance of the bone, appearing as a fleshy bud or granule, from the surface of which exudes the ivory on the bony part of the tooth. In growing, it rises in the socket, which is formed simultaneously around it, passing, finally, through the fleshy part of the gum.

Fig. 8.

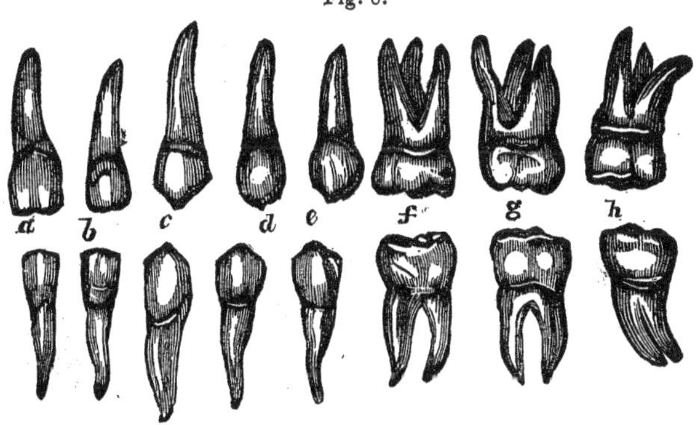

Fig. 8. The permanent teeth of the upper and lower jaw. *a, b* The incisors. *c,* The cuspids. *d, e,* The bicuspids. *f, g,* The molars (double teeth.) *h,* The wisdom teeth.

The first teeth, called milk-teeth, are twenty in number; they are temporary, and disappear from the seventh year upward; the last, or wisdom-teeth, do not appear until a person is twenty years of age.

The four front teeth are called *incisors*; the next one on each side is the *eye-tooth* (cuspid); the next two are *bicuspids* (small grinders); and the next two are grinders (molars); and the last one is called the *wisdom-tooth*. The incisors, cuspids, and bicuspids have each but one root. The molars of the upper jaw have three roots, while those of the lower jaw have but two.

Alimentary Organs.

These comprise the mouth and teeth, salivary glands, pharynx, œsophagus (stomach-pipe), stomach, intestines, lacteals (milk, or chyle vessels), thoracic duct, liver, and pancreas.

The *mouth* contains the instruments of mastication and the organs of taste. The preparation of food for digestion commences already in the mouth, where it is masticated and mixed with saliva from the *salivary glands*, of which there are six, three on each side of the jaw. Their names and positions are:

The *parotid gland* lies in front of the external ear, and behind the angle of the jaw; its duct opens into the mouth, opposite the second molar tooth of the upper jaw; this gland is swollen and inflamed when children have the *mumps*.

The *submaxillary gland* lies within the lower jaw, anterior to its angle. Its duct opens into the mouth by the side of the string or bridle of the tongue (frænum linguæ), on each side of which lies

The *sublingual gland*, of an elongated and flattened form, beneath the tongue; it empties its saliva through seven or eight small ducts, into the mouth, by the side of the string of the tongue; a disease called the "frog" consists in the swelling of this gland.

The *pharynx* or *throat* is the continuation of the mouth, and forms that cavity immediately below the palate where four passages unite, two coming from the nose and mouth, the other two going to the stomach and lungs.

The *stomach-pipe* (œsophagus) is a large membranous tube, descending behind the windpipe, the heart and lungs, through the diaphragm into the stomach; it has two membranes, an internal, or mucous, and an external, or muscular coat; the latter consists of two sets of fibres, one circular, the other longitudinal.

The *stomach* lies on the left side of the abdomen, immediately below the diaphragm, where the stomach-pipe enters its upper part at an opening called the *cardia;* from this point it enlarges into a sack, which lies with its larger end on the left side, while its smaller end contracts gradually toward the pit of the stomach, where it empties into the intestines; this opening in the stomach is called the *pylorus.* The stomach has, beside the mucous and muscular coats, an outer or serous coat, which is very tough and strong, of a smooth and highly polished appearance, and confines the stomach in its proper location. The stomach has a great number of glands, to secrete the gastric juice.

The *intestines*, or alimentary canal, are divided into two parts, the *small* and *large.* The former, commencing at the stomach, measures about twenty-five feet, while the large intestine, ending at the rectum, is about five feet in length. The latter is divided into three parts, the *cœcum,* (the beginning of the large intestine), which lies near the right upper hip-bone; the *colon,* which, from this point on the right side, ascends to the region below the liver, then transversely crosses the upper part of the abdomen, from below the liver, to the lower part of the stomach on the left side, where it bends again, descending to the left hip-bone, and entering the cavity of the pelvis, being called here the *rectum.*

The *small* intestine, commencing at the stomach and ending

at the *cœcum,* is also divided into three parts; the *duodenum,* called so from being generally twelve fingers long, commences at the stomach, ascends obliquely to the under surface of the liver, then descends perpendicularly (where it receives the ducts from the liver and pancreas), and passes transversely across the lower portion of the spinal column behind the colon, terminating in the *jejunum,* its continuation; and this, in its turn, is continued by the *ileum,* which empties itself into the *cœcum* at the right hip, after the small intestines have made numerous windings. While the stomach and intestines receive the food for digestion, and assimilate it, various other secretions from the liver, pancreas, etc., enter the alimentary canal to foster this process, and still other vessels are ready to absorb the assimilated juice and carry it into the circulation of the blood. Of the latter are the *lacteals* or minute vessels, which commence on the mucous membrane of the small intestines; from these they pass between the membranes of the *mesentery* to small glands, out of a collection of which larger vessels run to another range of glands, and so on, through several ranges of these glandular bodies, until they all empty themselves into one large duct, called the left *thoracic* duct, which ascends from the abdomen upward, lying in front of the spinal column, and passes through the diaphragm to the lower part of the neck; here it makes a sudden turn downward and forward, emptying itself into a large vein, which passes into the heart; its diameter is equal to a goose-quill.

The *liver* is a gland, which lies under the short-ribs of the right side, below the diaphragm, and is composed of several lobes; its upper surface is convex, its lower concave; it is the largest organ in the system, weighing about four pounds; its use is to secrete the bile, a fluid so necessary for chylification. The *gall-bladder,* containing the surplus of bile not immediately necessary for the system, being, as it were, a reservoir, lies on the under surface of the liver, and empties into the gall duct, which carries the bilious fluid to its destination in the duodenum.

The *pancreas* is a long, flattened gland, similar to the salivary glands on the neck; it is about six inches long, weighs three or four ounces, and lies transversely across the posterior wall of the abdomen, behind the stomach; its product, a saliva or *pancreatic juice* (necessary for digestion), is carried by a duct into the intestines in the duodenum, just where the gall duct opens into the intestines.

The spleen (*milt*), of an oblong, flattened form, lies in the left side below and touching the diaphragm, stomach, and pancreas. It is a reservoir capable of containing a great quantity of blood, ready for the purpose of the liver, to secrete the bile. The blood, in passing through the spleen, loses a portion of its red globules and thus becomes less stimulating.

The *omentum* (caul) descending in four layers of serous membrane from the stomach and transverse colon, contains fatty matter, deposited around the vessels, which ramify through its structure. Its functions are: to protect the intestines from cold, and to facilitate their movements.

The whole digestive apparatus is supplied with arteries, veins, lymphatics, and nerves; the latter chiefly from the *ganglionic* system. (See this.)

One of the most wonderful processes in the animal economy is that of the assimilation of food.

During its mastication (chewing) a considerable quantity of saliva (spittle) is mixed with it, the object of which is, to soften and moisten the food, preparing it for easy deglutition. When it reaches the stomach, it is subjected to the powerful action of the so-called stomach-juice (gastric juice), which is secreted by the glands, immediately located in the substance of the stomach. Beside, it is constantly in motion by the action of the muscles of the stomach, which brings the food into contact with the mucous membrane, and thus it becomes completely saturated with gastric juice, and at length dis-

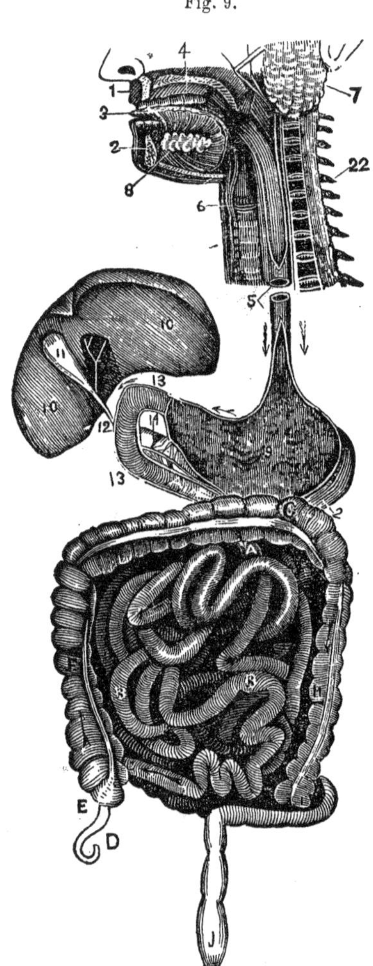

solved into a pulpy, homogeneous mass of a creamy consistence, called *chyme,* which passes, as fast as it is made, through the pylorus into the duodenum.

Fig. 9. An ideal view of the organs of digestion. 1, The upper jaw; 2, the lower jaw; 3, the tongue; 4, the roof of the mouth; 5, the œsophagus; 6, the trachea; 7, the parotid gland; 8, the sublingual gland; 9, the stomach; 10, the liver; 11, the gall-cyst; 12, the duct that conveys the bile to the duodenum 13, 13, 14, the pancreas; A, A, the duodenum; C, the junction of the small intestine with the colon; D, the appendix vermiformis; E, the cœcum; F, the ascending colon; G, the transverse colon; H, the descending colon; I, the sigmoid flexure of the colon; J, the rectum.

In the duodenum, the bile and pancreatic fluid mix with the chyme, which, by their action, is separated into a creamy fluid (chyle) which is nutritious, and a reddish sediment, which is excrementitious; at this point, the formation of the fecal matter commences.

From the above it is seen that the bile has no agency in the change through which the food passes in the stomach. The common belief, that bile is in the stomach, is erroneous. If bile is ejected in vomiting, it merely shows that not only the action of the stomach is inverted, but also that of the duodenum. Emetics will, generally, bring bile from the most healthy stomach, by inverting the action of the stomach and duodenum; the expression being bilious, having a bilious attack, etc., is generally wrong, the bile having nothing to do with these disorders, for which a better expression would be; the stomach is out of order; if persons, generally, would know this fact, a great deal of wrong and disastrous treatment would be avoided, as they would not force the stomach to eject bile continually, where there is none located.

The Urinary System.

This system, whose duty it is to secrete and carry out of the system the urine, is composed of the *kidneys*, the *ureters*, and the *bladder*, with the *urethra* attached to it.

The *kidneys*, between four and five inches long, and two and a half broad, lie in the lumbar region, behind the peritoneum, on each side of the vertebræ. Their texture is dense and fragile, presenting, in its interior, two structures, an external (cortical), and an internal (medullary) substance. The former contains the blood-vessels, which carry the blood from which the urine shall be separated; the latter consists of tubes, which conduct the urine away from the secreting vessels. It is then received in the pelvis of the kidney, from which it runs into the *ureter*, the excretory duct of the kidney, a membranous tube of the size of a goose-quill, about eighteen inches in length; this runs down along the posterior wall of the abdomen, behind the peritoneum and crossed by the spermatic vessels, to the bladder in front, in which it empties from behind and on the side.

The *bladder* is of an oblong, ovoid shape, situated behind the os pubis and in front of the rectum. It is the reservoir for the urine, which is carried there by the two ureters from the kidneys. It is retained in its position by eleven ligaments, supporting it on all sides. The bladder is composed of three coats, an external, or serous, a muscular, and a mucous, or internal coat.

The *urethra* is the membranous canal issuing from the neck of the bladder. It is curved in its course, composed of two layers, a mucous and an elastic fibrous coat. Through it passes the urine out of the body.

The Respiratory and Circulatory Organs.

These organs are closely connected with each other. All the blood must pass through the lungs, to receive there new life and energy, by being exposed to the oxygen of the air. For this and other reasons, we will treat of these organs, here in connection.

After the nutrient portion of the food (the *chyle*—see page 454) is discharged by the thoracic duct into the left subclavian vein, at the lower part of the neck, it is carried to the right cavity of the heart, where it mixes with a large quantity of venous blood. This mixture of fluid, as such, would not be suitable to restore the lost powers of the body, unless subjected to a process, by which the chyle is converted into blood, and the venous blood freed of its carbonic acid and water.

The *respiratory* organs consist of the *windpipe* (*trachea*), the *bronchia* (continuations of the *trachea*), and the *air-cells* (the extreme points of the bronchia). The *lungs* are composed of innumerable ramifications of the bronchial tubes, ending in air-cells, lymphatic vessels, and the pulmonary arteries and veins; their connections by cellular tissue, forms the *parenchyma* of the lungs, or its substance. The lungs are divided into two large parts, the left and right, each one of which is inclosed in a layer of the serous sac, called the *pleura*. Between the right and left lung, more to the left side, lies the heart, separated from either by a serous membrane.

Fig. 10.

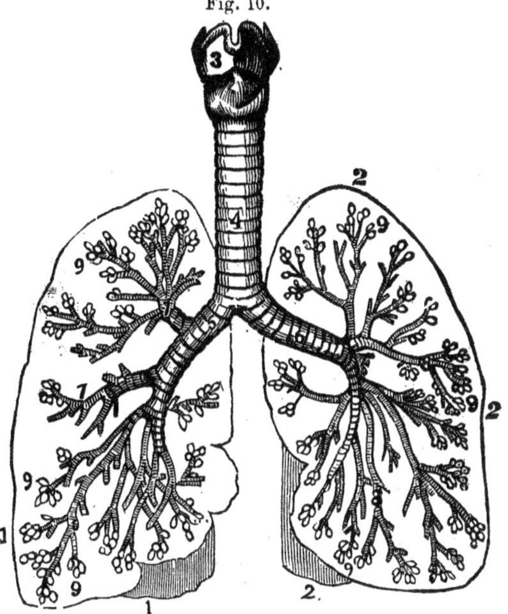

Fig. 10. A representation of the larynx, trachea, bronchia, and air-cells. 1, 1, 1, An outline of the right lung. 2, 2, 2, An outline of the left lung. 3, The larynx. 4, The trachea. 5, The right bronchial tube. 6, The left bronchial tube. 7, 7, 7, 8, 8, 8, The subdivisions of the right and left bronchial tubes. 9, 9, 9, 9, 9, 9, Air-cells.

The *trachea* proceeds from the larynx, descending to the pit of the neck, where it divides into two parts, assuming the name of

Bronchia, which descend in numerous ramifications, into the lungs, and form altogether a surface of twenty thousand square inches, or about thirty times the surface of the human body.

The *air-cells* are small bronchial tubes, and form the ends of these ramifications, retaining the air, when once inflated, except pressed out by force.

The trachea, bronchia, and air-cells are lined with the mucous membrane, and supplied with arteries, veins, and nerves.

The object of respiration is to free the system of carbon and hydrogen, which accumulate in the system, and would make an end to its existence, if not removed. For its removal, an allwise Providence has used the inhaling of air, which contains oxygen, in sufficient quantity to form a combination with the carbon and hydrogen, which then is exhaled, in the form of carbonic acid and water. In this process, another wonderful provision was contained, which gives life and motion to the whole system. It is the generation of heat. The blood, in passing through the lungs, receives oxygen from the atmosphere. The oxygen thus obtained is carried to the minute vessels, called capillaries, where it unites with the carbon and hydrogen of the decaying organs, as well as with the same elements furnished by the food, and thus maintains the heat throughout the entire system.

The *circulatory* organs are the *heart, arteries, veins,* and *capillaries.*

The *heart,* placed obliquely, in the left cavity of the chest, has the form of an inverted cone, the base of which lies upward and backward in the direction of the right shoulder and its apex points forward to the left side, about three inches, to a space between the fifth and sixth ribs; below, it rests on the tendinous part of the diaphragm. The sac, by which the heart is surrounded, is called *pericardium.* This is lined by a serous membrane, one layer of which invests the heart.

Between the lining and investing layer a serous fluid is secreted, to facilitate the action of the heart. The dropsy of the heart has its seat in this place.

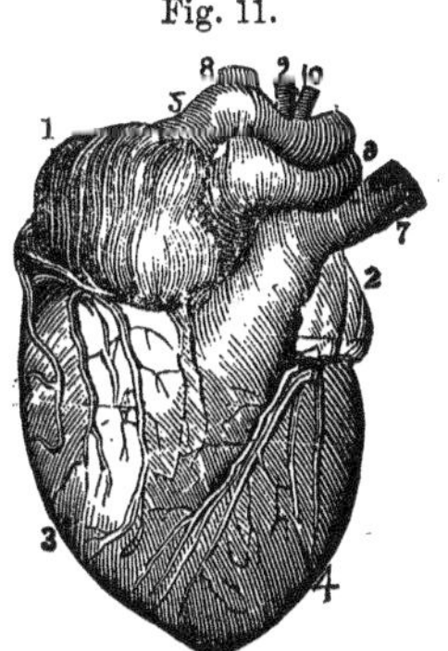

Fig. 11.

Fig. 11. A front view of the heart. 1, The right auricle of the heart. 2, The left auricle. 3, The right ventricle. 4, The left ventricle. 5, 6, 7, 8, 9, 10, The vessels through which the blood passes to and from the heart.

The heart itself is a muscle, whose fibres run in different directions, but mostly in a spiral direction. It is divided into four distinct compartments, the right and left auricle and the right and left ventricle. Before the birth the auricles are united by an opening. After birth, this opening closes, preventing the venous blood of the right auricle from passing directly into the left. If this opening, by a fault of nature, remains unclosed, a disease ensues, called the *blue disease*, because the child looks bluish, on account of the venous blood of the right heart entering the circulation of the arterial blood of the left auricle. All vessels leading from the heart are called *arteries;* those leading to the heart, *veins*. The right heart sends a *pulmonary artery*, filled with venous blood, to the lungs, and the left heart receives *pulmonary veins*, filled with arterial blood, from the lungs; in this case only, such an exception exists. Otherwise, all the arteries in the body carry red or arterial blood, and all veins, dark or venous blood.

The venous blood, together with the chyle, is propelled through the pulmonary arteries, by the right heart into the lungs. Here it receives the oxygen of the air, is converted into red blood, and carried by the pulmonary veins into the left heart, which sends it through the great artery, called the *aorta*, in innumerable divisions, into all parts of the body.

In this way, two systems of circulation are formed; one called the *lesser* or *pulmonic circulation*, where the blood rushes from the right heart, through the lungs, and returns, changed into red blood, to the left; the other, called the *greater*, or *systemic circulation*, where the blood rushes through all parts, and to the very confines of the body; and returns, changed into dark blood, to the right heart. This double circulation may be illustrated easily by the figure 8, the center of which is the place where the heart is located.

Fig. 12.

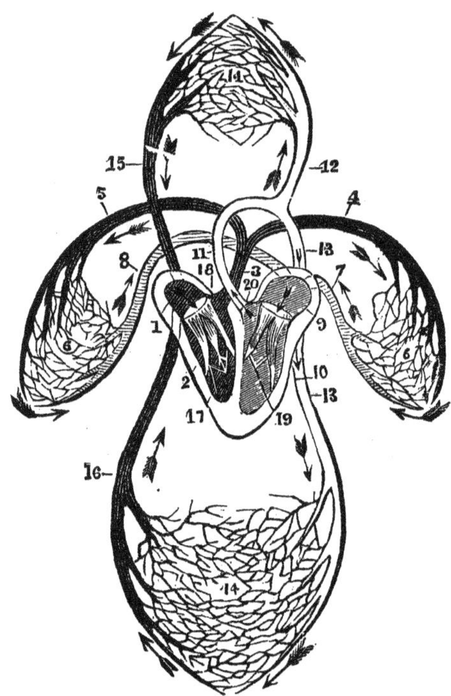

Fig. 12. An ideal view of the circulation in the lungs and system. From the right ventricle of the heart (2), the dark, or venous, blood is

forced into the pulmonary artery (3), and its branches (4, 5) carry the blood to the left and right lung. In the capillary vessels (6, 6) of the lungs, the blood becomes arterial, or of a red color, and is returned to the left auricle of the heart (9) by the veins (7, 8). From the left auricle the arterial blood passes into the left ventricle (10). By a forcible contraction of the left ventricle of the heart the blood is thrown into the aorta (11). Its branches (12, 13, 13) carry it to every organ or part of the body. The divisions and subdivisions of the aorta terminate in capillary vessels, represented by 14, 14. In these hair-like vessels the blood becomes dark-colored, and is returned to the right auricle of the heart (1) by the vena cava descendens (15) and vena cava ascendens (16). The tricuspid valves (17) prevent the reflow of the blood from the right ventricle to the right auricle. The semilunar valves (18) prevent the blood passing from the pulmonary artery to the right ventricle. The mitral valves (19) prevent the reflow of blood from the left ventricle to the left auricle. The semilunar valves (20) prevent the reflow of blood from the aorta to the left ventricle.

The *arteries*, which convey the blood from the heart to every part of the system, are composed of three coats. The external or fibrous, is firm and strong; the middle or musculo-fibrous, is contractile and elastic; the internal is a thin, serous membrane, which gives the artery inside a smooth polish. Communications between arteries are numerous.

The *veins*, which return the blood to the heart, are thinner, and more delicate in structure than the arteries. They are composed, like these, of the same three coats, but each one is more delicate and fine.

The *capillaries* form an extremely fine network of vessels, between the ends of the arterial and the beginning of the venous system. Through these, all the blood must pass; and in this point, the capillary system resembles the fine ramifications in the parenchyma of the lungs, where the blood passes through infinitely small vessels.

The *pulse* is caused by the periodical action of the heart, projecting the blood in jets. In infants, it beats in a minute more than a hundred times; in adults, about seventy times; in old persons, less than that, sometimes only sixty times.

The quantity of blood in a healthy individual varies very much; fat persons have generally less. On an average, a healthy adult has from twenty-five to thirty pounds.

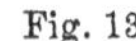
Fig. 13.

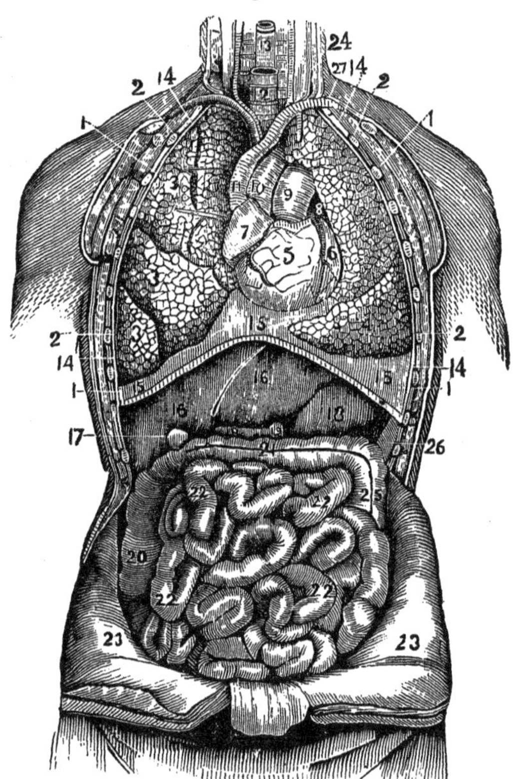

Fig. 13. A front view of the organs within the chest and abdomen. 1, 1, 1, 1, The muscles of the chest. 2, 2, 2, 2, The ribs. 3, 3, 3, The upper, middle, and lower lobes of the right lung. 4, 4, The lobes of the left lung. 5, The right ventricle of the heart. 6, The left ventricle. 7, The right auricle of the heart. 8, The left auricle. 9, The

pulmonary artery. 10, The aorta. 11, The vena cava descendens. 12, The trachea. 13, The œsophagus. 14, 14, 14, 14, The pleura. 15, 15, 15, The diaphragm. 16, 16, The right and left lobes of the liver. 17, The gall-cyst. 18, The stomach. 26, The spleen. 19, 19, The duodenum. 20, The ascending colon. 21, The transverse colon. 25, The descending colon. 22, 22, 22, 22, The small intestines. 23, 23, The abdominal walls turned down. 24, The thoracic duct, opening into the left subclavian vein (27).

The *lymphatics* are the vessels by which the process of *absorption* is carried on, to remove particles of useless or injurious matter. They are extremely minute at their origin, and are distributed upon the skin and other membranes as well as upon the surface and in the substance of organs. As they increase in size, they diminish in numbers. At certain points, they pass through soft bodies, called *lymphatic glands*, which are mostly located in the groins, armpits, on the neck, in the chest, and the abdomen. Sometimes these glands swell, producing lumps known as *kernels*, etc.

The *lacteals* are vessels similar to the former, but designed to absorb the chyle from the small intestines, where they are located in great numbers. They transfer their contents to the thoracic duct, and this conveys the chyle to the left subclavian vein, at the lower part of the neck.

The Nervous System.

This system, by which life is distributed and sensation imparted, consists of two distinct parts, the *brain*, with its spinal appendix, together with all the nerves leading from these great nervous centers to all parts of the body, and the *ganglionic* system of nerves, called, also, the sympathetic nerve, located chiefly on each side of the spinal column, but having its principal plexuses around the abdominal organs.

We give here a short anatomical synopsis of these most interesting parts of the body; requesting our readers, at the same time, to peruse larger works on this subject, if their time and inclination will permit.

The *brain* is located within the skull-bones (cranium), and is divided into two hemispheres, the right and left. This is the case in the upper part of the brain; below, the two hemispheres are connected by a dense layer of transverse fibres, called the *corpus callosum*. In the interior of the brain, there are several cavities, two of which are of considerable size, called the lateral ventricles. Water collects in these cavities, in that disease called "Dropsy of the Brain."

Fig. 14.

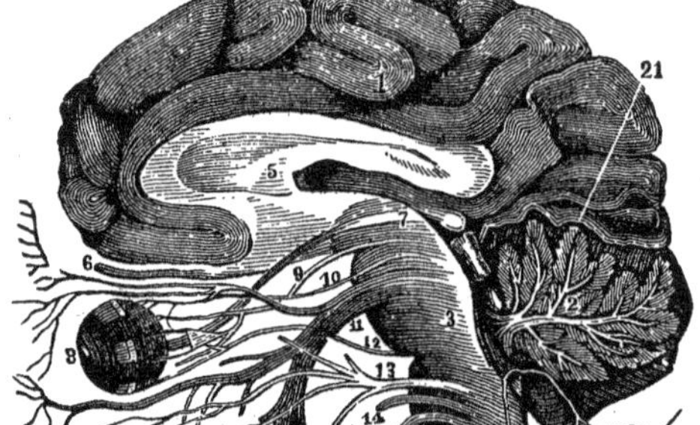

Fig. 14. A vertical section of the cerebrum, cerebellum, and medulla oblongata, showing the relation of the cranial nerves at their origin. 1. Cerebrum; 2. Cerebellum, with its arbor vitæ represented; 3. The medulla oblongata; 4. The spinal cord; 5. The corpus callosum; 6. The first, or olfactory nerve; 7. The second, or optic nerve; 8. The eye; 9. The third, or motor oculi; 10. The fourth, or patheticus; 11. The fifth, or tri-facial; 12. The sixth, or abducens; 13. The seventh, or facial; 14. The eighth, or auditory; 15. The ninth, or glosso-pharyngeal; 16. The tenth, or pneumo-gastric; 17. The eleventh, or spinal accessory; 18. The twelfth, or hypo-glossal; 20. Spinal nerves.

The substance of the brain is of a pulpy character, quite soft in infancy and childhood; it gradually becomes more consistent in advanced years.

It is divided into three parts, the large brain (cerebrum), the small brain (cerebellum), and the medulla oblongata, or that part of the spinal cord which lies within the skull together with the pons Varolii.

These three parts of the brain within the skull are invested and protected by the three membranes of the brain; the *dura mater*, a firm and fibrous membrane next to the skull; the *arachnoid*, a serous membrane, which envelops the brain and spine, and is like the serous membranes of the heart and lungs, a closed sac: this is the middle membrane of the three; the *pia mater*, a vascular membrane, composed of innumerable vessels, held together by areolar tissue; this is the nutrient membrane of the brain.

From the brain issue the *cranial nerves*, in twelve pairs, to supply the organs of sense and motion with life and vitality. They are arranged, as regards local origin, as follows: 1. The olfactory; 2. The optic; 3. The motor oculi; 4. The patheticus; 5. The tri-facial; 6. The abducen; 7. The facial; 8. The auditory; 9. The glosso-pharyngeal; 10. The pneumogastric; 11. The spinal accessory; 12. The hypo-glossal.

The *spinal cord*, its membranes, and the roots of the *spinal nerves*, are contained within the spinal column. The cord is continuous with the brain, or its lowest part, the medulla oblongata, and is divided into two lateral halves by an anterior and posterior fissure. Each of the lateral halves is divided by furrows into three distinct sets of fibres, called the anterior, lateral, and posterior columns; the posterior are the columns of sensation; the anterior, those of motion, and the lateral are divided in their functions between motion and sensation.

From these divisions issue the *spinal nerves*, thirty-one pairs in number, each one from two roots, an anterior and posterior, combining the functions of motion and sensation. After the two roots have united, which constitute the spinal nerve, it passes through the opening between the vertebræ on the sides of the spinal column, and distributes itself to its re-respective organs in innumerable ramifications.

Fig. 15.

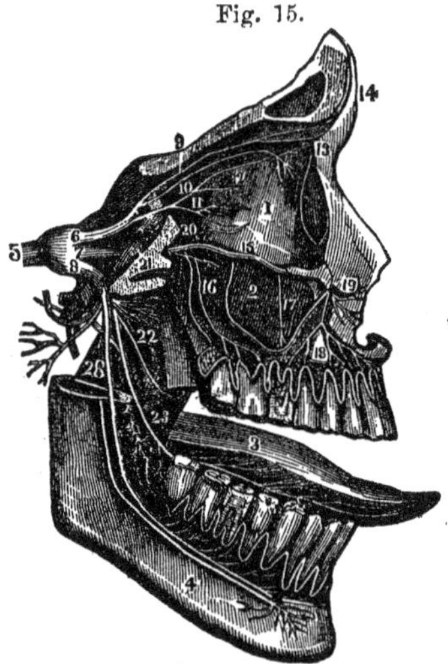

Fig. 15. The distribution of the fifth pair of nerves. 1, The orbit for the eye; 2, The upper jaw; 3, The tongue; 4, The lower jaw; 5, The fifth pair of nerves; 6, The first branch of this nerve, that passes to the eye; 9, 10, 11, 12, 13, 14, Divisions of this branch; 7, The second branch of the fifth pair of nerves distributed to the teeth of the upper jaw; 15, 16, 17, 18, 19, 20, Divisions of this branch; 8, The third branch of the fifth pair, that passes to the tongue and teeth of the lower jaw; 23, The division of this branch that passes to the tongue; 28, The division that is distributed to the teeth of the lower jaw.

The spinal nerves are divided from the head downward, into eight cervical pairs, twelve dorsal, five lumbar, and six sacral pairs.

The *ganglionic system*, or *sympathetic nerve*, consists of a series of knots, or ganglia, lying on each side of the spinal column, united with each other by nervous threads. It connects itself with the brain and spinal nerves. Each ganglion or knot, may be considered as a distinct center, from which branches issue in four directions, some for communication with other ganglia, some for distribution. The latter accom pany the arteries to the different organs, and form a network around them, called plexuses, and named after the artery which they accompany ; for instance, the mesenteric plexus, hepatic plexus, etc. In this way all the internal organs of the head and trunk receive branches from the sympathetic nerve, which, therefore, is considered a nerve of organic life.

THE SKIN.

The skin covers the exterior of the body, and appears, to the naked eye, as composed of one membrane only. By closer examination, however, it is found to consist of two distinct layers of membrane, the upper or scarf-skin (epidermis), and the real skin (cutis vera), which lies underneath the former.

The upper-skin (epidermis) is thin, semi-transparent, like a fine shaving of horn ; it has no nerves or blood-vessels, and is without sensation. The hair and the nails are of the same nature.

The real skin, (cutis vera, or corion) consists of minute fibres, interwoven with each other to a firm, strong and flexible web. This manner of composition permits innumerable interstices or pores, which are finer or closer on the superficial part of the skin than on its lower surface. The upper surface of the skin contains blood-vessels and nerves, looks, therefore, more red or pinkish, and is sensitive ; while the lower strata of the skin connects with the fibrous web, in which the subcutaneous fat of the body is deposited.

Beside, the skin is supplied with nerves; lymphatics also exist in great numbers. The oil-glands are contained in some parts of the true skin, in great abundance, as on the face and nose, the head. etc. ; they communicate with the surface of the skin through small tubes, which penetrate the skin, and open mostly at the roots of hairs. These glands deserve our particular notice, as their usefulness is so great, that neglect in cultivating their healthy action is felt very severely. They appear in great distinction on the eyelids, where their disease causes the so-called sty; they produce in the ear-passages the so-called ear-wax: they impart oil to the hair by infusing it into the sheath of each hair.

In some persons these oil-glands cannot discharge their contents on the surface of the skin, on account of some diseased state, when it becomes dry and dense, appearing in round, dark spots, produced by the presence of a minute worm.

The *perspiratory glands* are oval-shaped, or globular balls, lying in the deeper meshes of the real skin, from whence they communicate with the surface through minute cylindrical tubes, called "pores." The quantity of these pores is truly astonishing; they average about twenty-eight hundred in the square inch of surface; and if an ordinary sized man has twenty-five hundred square inches of surface, the whole number of pores in the skin amounts to seven millions. How important must be, therefore, the culture of the skin, as an organ for secretion and exhalation.

II. HYGIENE AND HYDROPATHY.

Hygiene.

Hygiene comprises the knowledge of instituting such a mode of living as is best calculated to preserve health. The clearer this knowledge is, and the closer we follow the rules of health, the surer the prevention of diseases will be. It is certain, beyond doubt, that less misery, disease, and death, would mar the happiness of this fair world, if its inhabitants would live more in accordance with the laws of nature, and less after their own often mistaken notions and passions.

Reform, in this respect, has already commenced; and, with a more rational method of healing, and the application of a more efficient and salutary tonic agent (the water), invalid and enfeebled mankind can look forward to a happier, because a healthier future.

In the following pages, we will notice briefly the most important subjects affecting the physical well-being of an individual. These are: *food* and *drink*, *sleep*, *air*, and *exercise*, *clothing* and *occupation*.

In all our wishes and necessities of physical and mental things, we must never forget two important principles: first, to inquire whether they are really beneficial or useful, and if so, to use them in moderation.*

---

* For more minute details on this subject, see Dr Tarbell's Sources of Health

FOOD AND DRINK.

The waste of bodily strength must be supplied by suitable food and drink. This is the greatest necessity of nature: and if errors are committed in this respect, our injured system must suffer the bad consequences. It is, therefore, of the utmost importance to pay particular regard to the selection of our daily food and drink, in order to escape disease, and often premature death.

Suitable food must have two paramount qualities: it must be *nutritious* and *digestible*. Not all nutritious food is digestible, and *vice versa*. A great many experiments have been made, to test the relative digestibility of food, and from these and the experiments on the sick bed, valuable knowledge in regard to the choice of food has been collected. According to these investigations, boiled rice is the most digestible, and roasted pork, fat and lean, the most indigestible substance.

In order to give the reader a more comprehensive view of the relative digestibility of food, we insert Dr. Beaumont's results, as related in Dr. Tarbell's "Sources of Health."

			H.	M.
Rice	Boiled	Digested in	1	
Pigs' Feet, soused	"		1	
Tripe, soused	"		1	
Eggs, Whipped	Raw		1	30
Trout, Salmon, fresh	Boiled		1	30
" " "	Fried		1	30
Apples, sweet	Raw		1	30
Venison steak	Broiled		1	35
Brains	Boiled		1	45
Sago	"		1	45
Tapioca	"		2	
Barley	"		2	
Milk	"		2	
Liver, beef's, fresh	Broiled		2	
Eggs, fresh	Raw		2	
Codfish, cured, dry	Boiled		2	
Apples, sour	Raw		2	
Cabbage, with vinegar	"		2	

		H.	M.
Milk	Raw......Digested in	2	15
Eggs, fresh	Roasted	2	15
Turkey, wild	"	2	18
" domestic	Boiled	2	25
" "	Roasted	2	30
Gelatine	Boiled	2	30
Goose	Roasted	2	30
Pig, sucking	"	2	30
Lamb, fresh	Broiled	2	30
Beans, pod	Boiled	2	30
Cake, sponge	Baked	2	30
Parsnips	Boiled	2	30
Potatoes, Irish	Roasted	2	30
" "	Baked	2	30
Cabbage, head	Raw	2	30
Spinal Marrow	Boiled	2	40
Chicken	Fricassee	2	45
Custard	Baked	2	45
Beef	Boiled	2	45
Oysters	Raw	2	55
Eggs	Soft Boiled	3	
Beef, fresh, lean, rare,	Roasted	3	
Beefsteak	Broiled	3	
Pork, salted	Raw	3	
" "	Stewed	3	
Mutton, fresh	Broiled	3	
" "	Boiled	3	
Chicken soup	"	3	
Dumpling, apple	"	3	
Oysters	Roasted	3	15
Pork-steak	Broiled	3	15
Pork, salted	Broiled	3	15
Mutton	Roasted	3	15
Bread, corn	Baked	3	15
Carrot	Boiled	3	15
Sausage	Broiled	3	20
Flounder	Fried	3	30
Oysters	Stewed	3	30
Beef	Boiled	3	30
Butter	Melted	3	30
Cheese, old	Raw	3	30

			H.	M
Bread, wheaten, fresh	Baked	Digested in	3	30
Turnips	Boiled		3	30
Potatoes, Irish	"		3	30
Eggs	Hard Boiled		3	30
"	Fried		3	30
Green Corn and Beans	Boiled		3	45
Beets	"		3	45
Salmon, salted	"		4	
Beef	Fried		4	
Veal	Broiled		4	
Fowls, domestic	Boiled		4	
" "	Roasted		4	
Ducks, domestic	"		4	
Heart, animal	Fried		4	
Beef, old, salted	Boiled		4	15
Pork, salted	Fried		4	15
" "	Boiled		4	30
Veal	Fried		4	30
Ducks, wild	Roasted		4	30
Suet, mutton	Boiled		4	30
Cabbage, with vinegar	"		4	30
Suet, beef	"		5	3
Pork, fat and lean	Roasted		5	15

The above table is very explicit, as regards the digestibility of certain substances, and we can ask its particulars with confidence, whenever we wish to decide this point in the choice of food; but, in relation to its nutritious qualities, whether highly nutritious or less nutritious food is necessary, we must follow the researches of Prof. Liebig, who first explained satisfactorily the connection of digestion and respiration. He showed that the lungs receive a greater quantity of oxygen in cold than in warm climates and seasons. A corresponding amount of carbon, which is contained in the food, is necessary to mix with the blood, and unite in the lungs with this oxygen, to produce such a degree of animal heat, as is required by the external circumstances of the individual. The colder the climate, therefore, the more carbon (or food containing carbon) is necessary, to produce animal heat; the warmer the season or climate, the less of it is necessary. For this reason, is fish-oil the staff of life for the Greenlander; because it contains the greatest amount of carbon, for producing a great quantity of animal heat, which he needs in those regions; while persons under the equator live principally upon watery, vegetable productions, affording but little support to animal heat; as nature supplies this by the hot climate itself. Animal food, in general, is more nutritious than vegetable; but the structure of our digestive organs, from the teeth to the lowest part of the intestines, shows conclusively that man was destined to partake of both kinds, animal as well as vegetable. The latter must preponderate, however, on account of the reasons above given, in warm seasons and climates, while the animal food takes precedence in cold regions and seasons: in the highest latitudes, even to the exclusion of all vegetable diet. In temperate regions, a judicious combination of both kinds of food is necessary to sustain life harmoniously.

The digestibility of food varies according to individual strength and habit. Pork may be completely indigestible to the invalid and student, although it is highly nutritious, while it is perfectly digestible for the woodcutter and hunter in wild regions.

Animal food contains, principally, *fibrine, albumen, gelatine, oil, casseine,* and *osmazome.*

Fibrine is digestible and nutritious.

Albumen is nutritious, but becomes indigestible when hardened too much by heat.

Gelatine, the substance which forms the so-called jelly, is nutritious and readily digested; but its digestibility is frequently impeded by improper ingredients mixed with it, particularly in the form of acids.

Oil sustains heat but is difficult of digestion; it requires the action of bile in the intestines to assimilate it properly.

Casseïne is both nutritious and digestible. It is contained in the cheesy part of milk.

Osmazome is that substance which imparts flavor to the meat and the soups. Its presence shows the nutritious and digestible quality of the meat.

According to the predominance of one of the above-named substances, animal food has been divided into three classes :

1. *Fibrinous* class ; comprising mutton, beef, pork, ducks, geese, and venison.

2. *Gelatinous* class ; to which belong veal, lamb, young poultry, and most kinds of fish.

3. *Albuminous* class ; containing oysters, eggs, brain, and liver, the sweetbread in calves.

The digestibility of meat varies according to the mixture of oil, or osmazome ; for instance, ducks and geese, although belonging to the fibrinous, or best digestible class, are more indigestible than beef; because they are of an oleaginous nature.

Mutton and *beef* are among the most nutritious and digestible of meats. The former is rather better for invalids, dyspeptics in particular. *Venison*, also, is very nutritious and digestible.

Pork is difficult of digestion ; because it is united to so much oily or fat substance. Beside, its continual use causes diseases of the skin and lymphatic system.

Veal and *lamb* belong to the gelatinous class ; very nutritious, but not so easily digested, because they are not sufficiently matured or ripened, as it were.

Poultry differs, also, according to its age ; the young containing more gelatine, and requiring, in consequence, not so much roasting or baking ; the older ones containing more fibrine, and requiring, therefore, more cooking and roasting.

Among the fowls, there are none more suitable for invalids than the wild fowls, such as partridges, pheasants, etc.

Eggs and *oysters*, are very nutritious, and very digestible, in their natural state ; but to harden their albumen, by cooking or stewing too much, renders them very objectionable for the sick. Clams are not so digestible.

Fish, in general, differ as regards their digestibility, in the same proportion as they contain more oily substance. Marine fish generally contain more oil than fresh water fish. Fish without scales contain more oil, and are, therefore, more indigestible than other fish.

Vegetable food contains, principally, *starch* (fecula), *gluten, mucilage, oil*, and *sugar*.

Starch, like oil, furnishes carbon, and abounds in the grains, in potatoes and other roots, as well as in arrowroot, sago, tapioca, etc.

Gluten, the nutritious part of grain also, enables it to form a tenacious paste, by the mixture of flour with water ; it is similar to the animal fibrine.

Mucilage, or gum, is innutritious, but useful, by furnishing carbon and hydrogen to the oxygen of the blood.

Sugar and *oil* serve the same purpose.

Rice is a digestible and nutritious vegetable, wholesome for healthy and debilitated persons.

The *potato* ranks next, if roasted or baked, while it is less digestible when boiled ; the sweet-potato is less digestible than the common potato.

Arrowroot, sago, tapioca, farina, are both digestible and nutritious.

Beets contain a good deal of sugar, and on that account, furnish considerable carbon and hydrogen ; but, as the fibrous part of the beet is entirely indigestible, invalids must abstain from its use.

Onion, cabbage, asparagus, and tomato, contain but very little nutriment, and must not be indulged in by persons having, or being disposed to the diseases of the abdomen.

Fruits, in general, are refreshing and wholesome, but not very nutritious. This latter quality makes them very desirable in diseases, where a nutritious diet otherwise would be detrimental. In the convalescence from fevers, apples, baked or roasted, dried prunes stewed, etc., form a refreshing and grateful diet for the recovering patient; in the green state, fruit produces flatulency, and must be avoided by patients, although a moderate use of ripe fruit for a well person, is very good, except in seasons when bowel complaints predominate.

In order to enable the reader to distinguish between substances, as regards their nutritious quality, we subjoin here a list of some of those most in use, as given in Carpenter's Physiology. In this table *human milk* is taken as the standard of comparison=100.

NUTRITION TABLE.

Vegetable.

Rice	81	Wheat	119-144
Potatoes	84	Carrots	150
Turnips	106	Brown bread	166
Rye	106	Peas	239
Maize	100-125	Lentils	276
Barley	125	Mushroom	289
Oats	138	Beans	320
White bread	142		

Animal.

Human milk	100	Portable Soup	764
Cow's milk	237	White of egg	845
Oyster	305	Crab, boiled	859
Yolk of eggs	305	Skate, raw	859
Cheese	331-447	——boiled	859
Eel, raw	434	Herring, raw	910
—— boiled	428	—— boiled	808
Mussel, raw	528	——milt of	924
—— boiled	660	Haddock, raw	920
Ox liver, raw	570	—— boiled	816

Pork-ham, raw	539	Flounder, raw	898
——— boiled	807	——— boiled	954
Salmon, raw	776	Pigeon, raw	756
——— boiled	610	——— boiled	827
Lamb, raw	833	Veal, boiled	911
Mutton, raw	773	Beef, raw	880
——— boiled	852	—— boiled	941
Veal, raw	873	Ox lung	931

Water is the only liquid which nature has furnished in abundance for drink; without it, all living beings and organized forms would perish. How important it is, therefore, to procure an article, so indispensable and necessary, in as pure a state as possible. The best water for drink is, without doubt, rain water, as it is free from admixtures of earthy substances; yet, even rain-water frequently becomes impure by falling through an impure atmosphere, particularly that hanging over large towns, or by running on roofs of houses, through unclean spouts before it reaches the cistern.

Equal to rain-water, in purity and taste, is the water procured by the melting of snow and ice, if the latter has been formed in clean ponds or rivers.

But where rain water cannot be obtained in sufficient quantity or purity, it is generally taken from the rivers and lakes, which furnish a better water than wells. The latter contains more or less lime, salts, or other earthy impurities, which render it neither palatable nor healthy.

Water, coming from marshy regions, is entirely unfit for drinking; at least, not until, by boiling, the inherent organic matter is destroyed.

A healthy person ought to habituate himself to a free use of cold water. Beside using it externally in baths, he should drink morning, noon, and evening, with his meals, a sufficient quantity to dilute the food. But the water he drinks must be cold, as it is this latter quality which offers to the stomach a natural and strengthening stimulus for digestion; in summer, and in southern latitudes, ice is necessary to render the water fit for hygienic purposes. If a person is once used to drink plenty of cold or ice-water at or after his meals, he seldom suffers from indigestion, and needs not the use of stimulating drinks; and every one can easily habituate himself to this practice. It is a wrong idea, which seems yet to prevail to a great extent, that it is unwholesome to drink water at the meals; but experience has the advantage, and one can soon test the matter for himself. The trial must only be continued for some time, in order to allow the system to accommodate itself to the new habit. Health and good spirits will be the consequence of such a change in a person's living.

It is also very proper to drink a tumbler of fresh water when retiring in the evening, or on rising in the morning. In doing this, the want of other drinks or beverages of a stimulating nature, such as coffee, or tea, is not felt so much, and can be dispensed with easier by degrees.

Coffee, especially, is one of those enticing, palatable beverages which have laid the majority of the civilized world under contribution; it is made nutritious by the addition of cream and sugar; but the greatest part of its contents is medicinal, and consequently, not fit for daily consumption, without creating artificial alterations in a person's healthy condition. Hahnemann, the illustrious founder of Homœopathy, was the first who drew the attention of the coffee-drinking community to the destructive tendency their favored article had on the constitution. He distinguished well between a moderate use of this drink and an immoderate consumption in large quantities and strong decoctions. We recommend our readers to read his admirable article on this subject. It exhausts all that can be said in regard to it, and is capable to cure the most inveterate coffee-drinker. Homœopathy forbids its use in most all diseases, and insists on a more natural diet; in this important undertaking, she is supported by the rigorous system of hydropathy, which demands the abolition of all stimulating drink, and allows nothing but water.

But, if coffee cannot be abstained from, or if a person is only using it moderately, without experiencing bad consequences, it would be well to recommend a good preparation of the bean, by roasting it but slightly, grinding it never long before it is used, and adding to the decoction one-half of boiled milk. In this way, coffee may be drank with comparative impunity.

Tea, as a daily drink, meets with the same objections as coffee, and is only tolerated in its use for the sick, because these have not been sufficiently estranged from such stimulants to do without it.

To healthy persons we would recommend to abstain from its use entirely, as tea is neither nutritious, nor capable of fostering the digestion.

If any tea shall be used, let it be black tea, as this contains less of the tannin, or the astringent principle, which forms an ingredient of all kinds of teas.

Chocolate, or *cocoa*, is decidedly preferable to coffee or tea as a daily drink, although it is, to some extent, an indigestible article, which needs good digestive powers and exercise to render it wholesome. It is frequently allowed to patients who have no abdominal diseases, or do not suffer from weakness of the stomach.

Milk is very nutritious, but not always digestible. Although nature designed infants to subsist for some time on milk, it is no stronger proof, on that account, of its greater digestibility; as it is well known that an infant's stomach is not yet weakened by stimulating food or drink, and is better prepared for the digestion of milk than that of adults.

The practice of drinking milk at dinner is very injurious; it is more wholesome toward evening, particularly in the summer, and in the morning, when bread-and-milk forms a good diet for healthy persons.

The reason why country people can eat and drink milk with impunity, while persons living in cities dare not do the same, lies simply in the constant exercise of the former, combined with less care and hasty pursuits of life.

After drinking milk, no sour articles must be drank or eaten, as an undue coagulation will ensue in the stomach, with all its morbific consequences.

Buttermilk is a healthy beverage, but it must be used with care, not allowing any acids or fruits to follow after it.

Spiritous liquors, wine, brandy, etc., must be considered as medicines, never as drinks, which might be adopted for daily consumption with impunity. And, in a medicinal capacity, they are truly beneficial, while, in the other, they have proved to be the greatest curses of mankind.

But enough has been said and argued on this point, and it would be useless here to repeat the proofs, that the habitual use of spiritous liquors ruins both body and soul.

As medicines they are prescribed by the physician; for instance, brandy, after having eaten indigestible articles, or as a stimulus in Asiatic cholera; wine after debilitating diseases, or after great loss of blood; and ale or porter for nursing women, etc. We advise strictly to adhere to the principle, "Touch not, taste not, handle not."

Sleep.

This interruption of the voluntary activity of the bodily powers is as necessary for their renovation and strength as food and drink; in sleep reparation is not counteracted by waste as it is during the period of wakefulness. If we would eat and fill our blood with nourishment, yet have not sufficient bodily exercise to exhaust strength, we would soon produce a disturbance of the equilibrium, which must exist in our system between loss and supply. In the following order we should regulate the hours of life; first, *work* (mental and bodily exercise for every healthy individual, without exception); second, *eating* (the principal meal ought to be had toward evening, after the labor is done); third, *sleep* (soon after eating, in order to permit the nourishment in the blood to crystallize into the different solids of the system).

The time which should be passed in sleep varies according to age, occupation, and constitution. Children need more sleep than those of a maturer age, where the growing, or solidification of the system is not so much required. Vigorous, mental activity needs longer sleep to recruit than mere bodily labor; because the nervous energy, which facilitates solidification, becomes more exhausted by mental than bodily fatigue. The lymphatic constitution needs more sleep than the nervous and bilious, because the former having less nervous energy, requires longer time to convert, during the sleep, the blood into muscle, nerve, sinew, etc.

There is no normal quantity of hours to repose in sleep; as a general rule, it may range from six to seven hours in twenty-four; circumstances alter these, however, frequently; every one must try to find out which number of hours will suit for him.

The best time for sleep is, without doubt, from nine or ten o'clock, before midnight, until three or four o'clock in the morning. Early rising has so many advantages in point of health and happiness, that it hardly needs a further recommendation here.

The place of sleep ought to be chosen from among the best in a house. The lower floors are never fit to contain bedrooms, as the confined air, during the night, in the lower part of a house, is unfit for respiration. The sleeping apartment should be the best located and the largest room in a house; an eastern and southern exposure is the best; during the day, its windows must be kept open, and the bed-clothing aired; the best surface to repose on is the hair mattress, which combines all the necessary requisites for this purpose. During the sleep, the cover ought to be sufficient; if possible, let it consist of quilts, whose number is regulated as to comfort.

Some persons have the erroneous idea that, to lie on the back during sleep, is the most healthy position one can assume; the most natural and healthy position is to lie on the side, the very best is the right side. But this varies as to habit, and, if so, does not signify disease. By lying on the back, the spine is pressed and heated, beyond what may be good for it. Lie with the head supported, by one pillow, slightly elevated above the rest of the body.

Air and Exercise.

The quality of the air which fills our lungs has the greatest influence on the healthy state of our system; as on it depends the thorough change which the blood must undergo, from the venous to the arterial. The atmospheric air consists of one-fifth part of oxygen and nearly four-fifths nitrogen, and a small quantity of carbonic acid gas. The first, or oxygen, is the only life-sustaining fluid, while the nitrogen and carbonic acid gas, each by itself, are life-destroying; but, in the above mixture of the three, the air becomes just adapted to the wants of our physical existence. Alter this proportion in the least, and sickness and death must be the inevitable consequence. It is of the highest importance, therefore, to have the air which we breathe as nearly like that which nature has prepared for us as possible. This, however, we can only accomplish by a thorough system of ventilation, which carries of the vitiated air, and permits fresh air to enter our apartments freely. The rooms for the sick are no exception to this most necessary rule. The more air a patient can have, the sooner he will recover. The only precaution necessary in such cases, is to prevent a draught from passing over the patient.

We direct the attention of our readers particularly to this subject, and invite them to make themselves acquainted with works treating extensively on the necessity and the art of ventilation; as in many a situation in life, it will be of the utmost importance for them to carry the theories of ventilation into practical execution; for instance, in building dwelling-houses, churches, halls for meetings, etc. We would here make one remark in regard to churches, which receive their ventilation at the sides, by opening the windows at the time of meeting. This seems to me a practice fulfilling well enough its immediate object—the ventilation—but doing harm in another direction, namely, creating a draught, which passes over part of the assemblage, thereby rendering their seats very uncomfortable, and dangerous for health and life. An edifice with high ceilings ought to be always ventilated from the top of the ceiling, where the heated air will sooner be found than at the side or below.

In short, we would advise everybody to try always to breathe as pure and fresh air as possible; may he be in health or in sickness.

Everything which has a tendency to deteriorate the air must be avoided and removed. Exhalations from marshy grounds, damp cellars, or any place where animal or vegetable decomposition is going on, are frequent sources of disease and death. Everything must be avoided which renders the air moist and damp, or prevents a free circulation all around the places where we dwell. The more air, the better; particularly in childhood, where the healthy development of the system depends so much on the lively stimulus which the plentiful consumption of the oxygen gives to the energies of the system. An infant, instinctively wants to be carried in the open air, where it delights to breathe the invigorating fluid. Parents should send their children in the free, open air as often as possible; as nothing more contributes to health and a good constitution than exercise in the open air.

Activity, motion, exercise, is a principal object and fundamental condition of organic life. Without it, there is no energetic expressions of the functions of the organs, which become torpid, and act sluggishly. Without exercise, the muscle will never swell and become strong and well-formed; the joint never will become supple. Without exercise, the appetite never will be stimulated, the nerves invigorated, and the blood system put in vigorous motion. Exercise, however, brings life and energy to every part of the system. Look at the blacksmith's arm—how muscular, strong, and healthy. Bodily exercise and labor is required of every one, may he be rich or poor, learned or ignorant, to keep healthy, and become strong.

It should be the particular care of parents, beside mental culture, not to neglect the bodily education of their children. The training in all the arts of life must have reference to the wants and necessities of the present and future well-being of those dear ones, placed under our especial guardianship. Gymnastic exercises now form a branch of the education of our youth, and should be practiced regularly and constantly, commencing with the lighter exertions, until the severer feats can be performed with ease. Walking, and running at a moderate gait, is perhaps the best and most suitable exercise for adults, beside that exercise which the daily occupations offer. It ought to be borne in mind, however, that no severe exercise must be undertaken directly after meals; as a full stomach, for digestion, requires suspension of muscular activity.

Clothing and Occupation.

In no department of civilized life has the fancy of man committed so many errors, leading to destruction of health and life, as in that which relates to the external covering of the body. In choosing a garment, one must always first remember its purpose and use, before he follows the dictates of fashion. If fashion was directed more by the utility than by the oddity and fancifulness of clothing, its reign might be tolerated; but this is, unfortunately not the case. It is, for instance, fashionable among ladies to wear thin-soled shoes; yet there is no greater destroyer of human life than a thin-soled shoe—not even pestilence and vice.

The object of clothing the body, beside for decency, is to shield it from the heat and cold of weather. To this purpose all other considerations, as of beauty, convenience, etc., ought to yield the preference; and even healthy persons should not easily depart from a rule so imperative and necessary.

Cotton, linen, and wool, manufactured into different kinds of stuff, are the articles mostly used for clothing. Linen is the best article for summer, and should not be laid aside in winter, except by persons subject to rheumatism and frequent colds.

Cotton has won its way almost into universal use, and its applicability for summer and winter wear is generally admitted. Yet it is not a sufficient substitute for the woolen goods, particularly flannel, when persons liable to rheumatic attacks need, beside protection from cold, a covering which stimulates the skin to a higher degree of action, and absorbs at the same time, its perspiration. This the woolen fabrics, especially flannel, etc., do, better than any other, and are, therefore indispensable to persons of a tender skin, and to those liable to great exposure to the extremes of cold and heat. Wool is a bad conductor of caloric, and, therefore, the best calculated to retain the heat generated within the body upon the surface, as well as to protect it from external heat.

The quantity of clothing must be regulated according to the seasons; but in such a manner that its change should never be in advance of the coming season, but only after it has fully set in. A change of under-clothes before June is seldom without serious consequences; while the summer dress may be retained until late in the fall and winter, without great inconvenience and detriment.

Clothing must be made so that it does not incommode the body either in motion or rest.

The human system is so admirably constructed in all its parts, that none presses or weighs heavily upon the other; and in this way, only, the perfect harmony and healthy condition of all its functions is rendered possible; for the same reason, however, does it not permit any external pressure, by clothing, etc., without serious injury. If the boots or shoes are too tight, painful corns appear, and imbitter the hours of the sufferer; if the waist is laced too tight, lung complaints are its fearful and destructive consequences. It would be unnecessary to enlarge upon this subject; it is known too well by every one, at the present time.

In general, keep the head and breast cool; the feet and stomach, however, warm. If the dress has become wet, hasten to change it. Be not careless in this respect; as frequently negligence in undressing, after having become wet, has been the cause of lingering diseases, or even death; particularly the feet require our whole attention in this respect. Young girls, at the age of change, must be especially watched well as regards the protection for their feet and abdomen.

After violent exercise, we must cool off by degrees, covering ourselves more, as we become cooler.

The *occupation* of a person has a great and increasing effect on his health, mentally as well as bodily. That this is undoubtedly the case, has been clearly proved by the statistical tables, carefully made for the purpose of showing the relative longevity of persons pursuing different avocations of life.

The following statistical table, made at Berlin, in 1834, and taken from Dr. Tarbell's "Sources of Health," is very instructive in this respect:

Of 100	Clergymen, attained the age of 70 years and upward,	42
" "	Farmers,	40
" "	Commercial men,	35

Of 100 Military men, attained the age of 70 years and upward,		33
"	" Lawyers,	29
"	" Artists,	28
"	" Teachers,	27
"	" Physicians,	24

It is evident, from the above, that the quiet pursuits of life, which require a constant and certain amount of mental and corporeal activity, of not too exciting a character, such as the professional labors of a minister of the Gospel, or the occupation of a farmer, are the most favorable to the attainment of a high age; while the physician, the very opposite of these two, as regards regularity and uniformity of action, is the lowest in the scale of his years of life. There is no doubt that the above table is correct; and if so, it teaches volumes to every one who has either already chosen a pursuit of life, or who has yet to do it. The former must adhere the more to the strictest rules of health, if he has chosen a less favorable profession; the latter may benefit himself infinitely by selecting the more healthy pursuit of life, if he has to choose between two.

A greater sense of duty, and a lesser degree of unchecked ambition, might have saved many a valuable life from an early grave. It is our duty to live as long and as usefully as possible.

Hydropathy.

Hydropathy is the name for a method of curing diseases by the application of cold water, in various ways, internally and externally, as circumstances may require. Although the advantage of cold water in disease was known in the earlier times, yet its systematic use for that purpose was never looked upon as an essential part of the healing art, and, therefore, no decided results were elicited. To Prissnitz, a simple farmer in Germany, belongs the honor of having first boldly proclaimed, and sustained by facts, the high qualities of cold water, as a remedy for diseases. And so rapid was the progress of this new and startling doctrine, that while its propounder was still enjoying his fame and fortune, his discovery had already been adopted in almost every part of the world.

The appearance of Hydropathy, as an auxiliary branch of medicine and hygiene, seems to have been providential in our time; as it was never before more needed, and never would have been appreciated as much. Our generation, so weakened, physically and morally, by a thousand influences which we could hardly enumerate here, needed, with the change of medicine which was consummated in the discovery and cultivation of Homœopathy, a system of dietetic rules and strengthening appliances, which should be as much *according* to nature as those formerly prescribed had been *against* nature. In this hygienic or preventive feature of the cold water lies one of its greatest blessings; another one, however, presents itself in its healing powers, for a number of diseases. Although its healing effects are wonderful, and entitled to all consideration and praise, yet its universal application, as the only curative agent, superseding direct medication, is impossible; because its principle is more negative in its effects upon disease in general. The cold water, in strengthening the powers of nature, prepares them to throw off disease, or, in other words, to produce a crisis, which enables nature, in a struggle with the disease, to throw it off. This principle of Hydropathy is true in chronic as well as acute diseases; but in the latter, its application is more limited, and this in proportion to the acuteness and severity of the diseases. To treat Asiatic cholera, for instance, or cholera infantum, with cold water alone, might be, to say the least, a questionable and hazardous undertaking. Neither would it be necessary or right to trust, in the thousands of medical cases, to one healing agent alone, which at best only assists in keeping up sinking nature, when we have the knowledge of other agents which have a direct annihilating effect upon the disease itself. And this is Homœopathy, whose application in diseases does not prevent the use of cold water; but, in most cases, prescribes its use, to strengthen nature, that the remedies may destroy the disease in a direct or specific manner. These two systems, properly combined and practiced together, will form the most complete code of medical rule and action which has existed, as yet. Allopathy and Hydropathy can never act together; because the principle of the former, to break down the natural strength, is too antagonistic to the objects of the latter, which tries to elevate, and not to destroy the strength of nature. There is no other alliance left, neither could any other be conceived, as natural, harmonious, and effective as that of Homœopathy and Hydropathy, each one supporting and strengthening the doings of the other. Providence was evidently at work in permitting the former to be discovered by the most learned and philosophic mind of the age, the illustrious Hahnemann; and the latter to be practiced first by an unlearned, but unsophisticated peasant; the first being the result of deep reasoning and research in matters of nature, the latter of simple and clear observation. The power of this double lesson, given to the medical world almost at the same time, was too overwhelming not to arouse it from perversion and affectation.

Hahnemann at first broke down, with a giant's strength, the learned fetters which for ages had encompassed the best minds among the medical profession. He opened and showed the true way; a new era had begun, and men, liberated from old prejudices, were willing to try anything offered with some degree of plausibility, reserving for themselves the final judgment.

After such changes were wrought in the mode of thinking, it was possible that Mesmer could succeed and find followers, and that Oertel and Prissnitz could draw the attention of sufferers to the remedial powers of water.

The pretensions of Hydropathy to constitute a perfect medical system, in which light some of its most modern practitioners have tried to establish it, must and will be abandoned, as they have neither a theoretical basis nor practical demonstration. In fact, efforts of this kind, if persisted in obstinately, must finally result in detriment to the good cause itself, diminishing the reputation of the cold water, in those spheres where its application is deservedly of the greatest benefit. And this range of action is by no means so small or so inferior as to make the exclusive friends of Hydropathy seek for a larger dominion, even beyond the reach of its principle or easy application. It needs but a slight acquaintance with the workings of Homœopathy, in comparison with Hydropathy, to come to the conclusion that the former could sooner dispense with the assistance of the latter, than *vice versa,* but that a judicious union of both insures the most blessed results.

In a great many cases, the cold water may be applied alone, without giving any medicines. This is particularly the case in those chronic forms of diseases, which have been treated or produced by allopathic medicines; such as chronic rheumatism and gout, syphilis, mercurial diseases, dyspepsias, chronic diarrheas, constipation, etc. But even in such cases a recourse to a full use of Hydropathy is not necessary, if the patient seems to possess yet a sufficient amount of natural strength to produce a reaction. Homœopathic medicine, rightly administered, will be found efficacious in a majority of such cases, as the practice of thousands of homœopathic physicians proves daily.

But where the patient's constitution has been weakened by the disease, strength and material power are necessary to overcome the disease. In such cases, the cold water is the only agent which can safely and quickly accomplish that.

In many acute diseases, the cold water can be used to mitigate the intensity of the symptoms, in subduing local irritation and fever, in softening hardened surfaces, and repelling congestions. In other acute diseases, it may be applied as an accessory remedy, without interfering in the least with the specific action of the homœopathic medicines, as in sore throat, inflammation of the brain and other organs. In acute diseases of the skin, such as measles, scarlatina, etc., the application of cold water on the diseased surfaces must not be attempted, except prescribed and attended to by a physician, as repressions of these eruptions on internal organs may take place, followed by dangerous consequences.

We will mention here those diseases, in the treatment of which cold water may be applied, as an accessory, without hesitation. The mode of application for each disease is explained further, below.

Inflammation of Internal Organs.

If there is inflammation of the brain, eye, throat, bowels, liver, spleen, or kidneys, apply, beside giving the necessary homœopathic remedies for these diseases internally, cold bandages externally, as near the organs affected as possible. Their application is described below. In the commencement of those diseases, the cold bandage applied in the evening is very beneficial in its results. If applied after the disease has taken too deep a hold on the system, it is of less benefit.

Congestions of the Head, Breast, and Abdomen. (Piles.)

Are frequently mitigated by the application of the cold-water bandages, often changed, and foot-baths; the sitz-baths, if the abdomen is the seat of the disease.

Rheumatism in its various forms, Gout, Tic Douloureux, and Sciatica,

Are diseases, where hydropathic applications may be used beneficially with the homœopathic treatment. The mode of applying the water varies in these diseases according to the constitutionality of the patient and the severity of the case. The cold-water bandage, wet sheet, and local baths are mostly necessary, although sometimes warm or lukewarm applications of water may be found more serviceable.

Constipation and Chronic Diarrhea.

Allows of mitigation by hydropathy; the former by the wet sheet, drinking of cold water, and a good deal of exercise; the latter by drinking cold water and using sitz-baths, with exercise and a suitable diet.

Different Modes of applying the Cold Water

In regard to this subject we prefer to lay before our readers what one of the most experienced hydropathists, Dr. Weiss, of Freywaldau, has communicated in his Handbook of Hydropathy:

1. *Ablutions.*

These may be local or general; they are performed in the following manner: The naked hands, or, better, a large sponge or woolen cloth is dipped into a vessel containing cold water, placed upon a chair. The sponge is to be gently pressed, and then conveyed, for some few minutes, rapidly over the whole surface of the body; water may also, at the same time, be poured over the head; but not every one is able to bear the latter application, especially in the winter. Another method of performing ablutions with cold water, consists in wrapping a linen sheet, dipped into cold water, around the body, and thus washing all the parts; this process is more powerful, abstracting more heat from the body. In pursuing this, or any other mode of ablution, it is advisable to stand in a spacious vessel, so that the water which runs off may not wet or soil the room in which the operation is conducted.

The best time, undoubtedly, for these ablutions, is the morning. They are to be performed immediately after rising from bed, when the temperature of the body is raised by the heat of the bed. The sudden change favors, in a great measure, the reaction which ensues, and excites the skin, rendered more sensitive by the perspiration during the night, to renewed activity. In some cases, and under certain conditions, more than one of these ablutions becomes necessary the same operation may then be repeated at different intervals. In most cases a second ablution, before going to bed, will suffice. Local ablutions will have to be repeated most frequently, where we wish to produce increased reaction; even in these cases, the temperature of the body, or its natural warmth, should be restored before proceeding to a second ablution. To increase the beneficial effects of this washing, it should be accompanied by friction during the process; this is also essential immediately after it. Quite as necessary is exercise in the open air, if circumstances will in any way permit it. Very great invalids only may be allowed, after washing, to retire to bed.

Ablutions are, for the most part, preparations for a more powerful system of treatment, in order to accustom the body, by degrees, to water which is absolutely cold; tepid ablutions are, therefore, to be recommended at first, especially to irritable and weakly individuals, or such as have never brought cold water in contact with their bodies.

Ablutions continued for a quarter of an hour, or longer, act as a stimulant and refrigerant; those of a shorter duration have a strengthening and exhilarating effect, and also the property of equalizing the circulation of blood, as may readily be perceived after general ablution of the whole body.

Cold ablutions are fitted for all constitutions; they are best adapted for purifying and strengthening the body; for women, weak subjects, children, and old age. Even in pulmonary complaints they produce alleviation, and even perfect amendment, where these diseases have not made too great a progress.

The room in which the ablution is performed, may be slightly heated, for debilitated patients, in winter, to prevent colds, in consequence of too low a temperature of the apartment; this exception is, however, only admissible for very weakly persons. Generally speaking, ablution may be performed in a cold room, especially where persons get through the operation quickly, and can, immediately afterward, take exercise in the open air. After ablutions, as regards mildness of operation, follow

2. *Shower-Baths.*

These baths are taken in a machine, or box (Schneider's bath), constructed for the purpose. The internal arrangement of this machine, or bath, is such, that, on opening the cock closing the pipes which communicate with a reservoir, the water is brought in contact with different parts of the body at the same time, in the form of many fine streams. Very weakly or irritable people may begin with tepid water, and they will soon accustom themselves to cold water, as these baths produce a very grateful impression. Those who cannot obtain a proper machine, may stand in an empty bathing vat, or other vessel, sufficiently large, while an assistant, standing on a chair, pours water over them from a common watering-pot, which answers the purpose perfectly.

The action of these baths consists in a general shock to the nervous system, and to the skin; in consequence of which, the secretion and excretion are promoted, and the whole economy benefited. They are to be recommended, chiefly, in the diseases requiring repeated sweatings for their cure; for patients who, in consequence of congestions, and diseases of the chest, cannot bear the full baths after the process of sweating. These baths deserve recommendation to families. Children may be best accustomed to cold water in these machines, where the temperature can at first be raised. and then gradually decreased.

3. *Partial, or Half-Baths.*

All baths, where the common bathing vats are half, or three parts filled with water, are thus denominated. The half-baths, serve, frequently, as a preparation for the full-baths (Vollbäder), or for a more active system of treatment; they have, therefore, a higher temperature, between fifty-nine and seventy-seven degrees of Fahrenheit. They should be continued from five minutes to an hour, or more, according to the purposes we have in view. If these baths be intended as a preparation for more active treatment, they must be of short duration, as also for persons who cannot bear cold baths, or full-baths. If our object be to produce a derivative effect, to remove congestions from other organs, the duration of these baths must be regulated by their effects. The patient must remain in them until revulsion is produced. Neither the temperature, nor the length of time can be determined beforehand ; this must be regulated always by the constitution, the nature of the disease, or the obstinacy of the case : generally speaking, a quarter, half, or a whole hour will suffice.

If our intention be to call forth a higher degree of reaction, or even fever, by these baths, the temperature must be lower, their duration extend from one to three hours. Baths continued for so great a length of time must only be used by the advice of a practical hydropathist, as they not only considerably derange the organs of digestion, but produce sufferings with which the patient was unacquainted before.

The whole time the patient is in these baths, he should continually rub himself with the water contained in the vat, extending the friction to the parts above and under the water, that he may not take cold. If this mode of application be intended as preparatory to the use of cold baths, or to produce increased reaction, it is advisable to pour a few buckets of cold water over the patient before he rises from the bath.

Neither half-baths, nor any other kind of bath, are to be taken on a full stomach. Exercise, further, is especially to be taken after long-continued half-baths; it must not, however, be neglected after the use of cold water in any form.

4. *Full-Baths.*

For these baths, spacious and deep receptacles are necessary; they should admit of freedom of motion, and fresh water (if possible) should uninterruptedly flow into them.

That the body must be, in a certain measure, prepared for their use, I have already mentioned; and even after a proper preparation, as caution, it is desirable to wash the head, or pour cold water over it before entering the bath. This rule is to be strictly observed where the patient has perspired for a length of time, or where he is suffering from congestions of the head and chest. The latter circumstance requires our especial consideration, where these attacks are increased after the first baths, notwithstanding the necessary preparation. Such patients must be spared the further use of them, to prevent dilatation, or rupture of blood-vessels. Only young, robust persons may, without injury, venture, after protracted sweating, to plunge suddenly into the bath without washing the head. It is, moreover, necessary that every patient should enter the bath as soon as possible after gently and quickly cooling his head and chest; for all unnecessary delay is attended with pernicious consequences.

The length of time the patient should remain in the bath varies in different cases; half a minute, or one minute, is generally sufficient; an experienced hydropathist only may prescribe full-baths for a lengthened period. During the bath, the patient must exercise the members of the body. Immediately after leaving the bath, he should quickly dry the whole body, using friction to promote reaction. If possible, he should perform the rubbing himself; and, where this is impracticable, he should be aided by an assistant. Exercise, after dressing, is next required, where circumstances will allow it, in the open air, to further reaction also.

Cold full-baths are indicated in all those diseases where augmented reaction, invigoration, or a shock to the nervous system is to be produced, where the warmth of the whole body is to be equalized ; where all secreting and secerning vessels are to be invigorated ; where the circulation of the blood is to be determined to the skin for the elimination of morbid matter.

These baths are to be avoided, or used, at least, with caution, in all congestions, in inflammations of internal vital organs, in diseases of the chest without exception, in certain head affections, in cases where a very active crisis ensues, and in all those where violent excitements or shocks would prove injurious.

5. *General Plunging-Baths.*

The plunging-bath should be taken like the former bath, in a large reservoir, or trough, filled with water. The patients, generally, such as cannot of themselves enter the bath, are placed upon a chair above it, arranged by means of ropes and pullies to move upward and downward, so that the patients in the sitting posture may be plunged into the water as deeply and as often as is necessary. As a substitute for an apparatus of this kind, the patient may be laid upon a sheet, held by several persons, which is quickly plunged into the water, and again withdrawn. The intention of these plunging-baths is pretty much the same as that of the former ; but their action is more stimulating, and the shock severer than in those cases where the patient can enter the bath unassisted, and use exercise while bathing. Hence one, for the most, five plunges, suffice to cool the body ; in obstinate nervous fevers, however, they are occasionally to be repeated several times in the course of the day.

6. *Local-Baths.*

By this term, we understand baths of tepid or cold water, into which a portion of the body is immersed for a certain period. Their action is more powerful than that of local ablutions. We will commence with

7. *Head-Baths.*

They are applied, according to the object we may have in view, to different parts of the head, in the form of eye-baths, ear-baths, or derivative-baths. The use of these baths is attended with some inconvenience. A large dish or basin is to be filled with water, and placed on the floor at the upper end of a mattress. The patient lays himself at full length upon the mattress, and immerses the part of the head to be bathed into the water; *e. g.*, if it be an eye-bath, the whole face is to be introduced into the vessel filled with water. In this case, it is necessary, moreover, to open and shut the eye-lids frequently, in order to bring the water in contact with the eye-ball. The duration of these cooling and strengthening baths is from two to six minutes, but both their duration and temperature are subject to variations. In some diseases of the eye, as we shall hereafter show, cold baths are not only inefficient, but they even augment the affection and sufferings considerably. Under these circumstances, we must endeavor to discover the temperature best adapted to the case, and make use of other detersive baths as auxiliaries. These and all other varieties of topical baths are to be repeated, according to circumstances, three to five times a day.

We use for these purposes, also, boat-shaped eye-baths resembling liquor-glasses, and adapted to the shape of the eye; but baths in these vessels are less worthy of recommendation than the former bath, inasmuch as they contain a less quantity of water, and press, moreover, on the appendages of the eye.

The ear-bath is taken in a similar manner; the side affected, or, where both ears are diseased, both sides are to be alternately immersed into the water, so that it may enter the meatus. These baths should, with few exceptions, be cold; their duration should extend from six to ten minutes. A more protracted use of them is not advisable, because it would produce more injury than benefit. The same applies to all head-baths.

Where head-baths are used as derivatives for violent and local pains of the head, the side of the head opposite to that affected is immersed in the water for three or four minutes. This may be repeated several times during the day, if necessary.

If the head-baths are to have an anodyne or soothing effect in gouty or rheumatic affections, they should be used at a temperature of fifty-nine degrees to seventy-two degrees of Fahrenheit. One side, of the head, and then the occiput, afterward the other side is to be plunged into the water, and this proceeding is to be repeated several times, until the desired alleviation ensues. In cases of necessity, this process may be repeated several times in the course of the day.

8. *Sitting-baths.* (Sitz-baths.)

For these baths we use water of various degrees of temperature. The vessel for this purpose is rather inconvenient, but so constructed that the patient can remain for the necessary time in it in the sitting posture. The dimensions of the vessel should be the following; height of the pedestal, four to five inches; the inner depth of the vessel, nine to ten inches; height of the back, six to eight inches; whole breadth of the vessel, twenty-two to twenty-four inches. These baths are made of wood or tin; the latter, however, deserve the preference. The vessel in which the bath is taken should be filled with water, until it reaches the navel of the patient when in the sitting posture. In especial cases, a greater or less height of water may be requisite. During the bath, the upper part of the body is to remain covered, the shirt should be turned up, and the legs and feet are to be enveloped in a woolen coverlet. While the person is in the bath, he should rub the abdomen with a woolen cloth, to increase the action of the skin, and to facilitate the passage of flatulent collections. The action of sitting-baths varies, partly according to the length of their duration, partly according to the temperature of the water. Where they are desired to have a tonic action, the temperature should be from fifty to fifty-nine degrees of Fahrenheit, and they should be continued from ten to fifteen minutes. Of course, they are to be repeated frequently during the day. To act as a stimulant, and to produce more powerful reaction, they must be continued for the same length of time ; but their temperature must not exceed forty-one degrees to forty-four degrees of Fahrenheit. In summer, this temperature may be obtained by the aid of ice.

Where the sitting-baths are to act as derivatives, determining the blood from parts which suffer from congestion, the patient must remain twenty minutes to half an hour in the bath. It is sometimes necessary, during the bath, to adapt cold applications (umschläge) to the parts affected ; this is the more necessary, if the congestions increase during the bath.

If the sitting-baths be intended to produce a solvent effect, a moderate temperature of fifty-nine degrees to sixty-eight degrees of Fahrenheit, and rather a lengthened continuation of them, say from half an hour to an hour or more, will be required. It is, moreover, advisable, that patients suffering from obstructions or hemorrhoids, should sit in deeper water ; it may, in this case, extend beyond the umbilicus.

For sitting-baths in rivers, a peculiar apparatus is necessary. A board with a round hole, about eight inches in diameter, is fixed about five or six inches below the level of the water ; on this aperture the patient is to sit. At a distance of more than one fathom from this board the water is to be confined by means of any suitable contrivance, so that it may be made to flow with force against the abdomen during eight, at the most, fifteen minutes. In all abdominal diseases, and in debility of the organs of generation, these baths are of extraordinary benefit.

Whatever object we may aim at in the use of these varieties of sitting-baths, we must not lose sight of the rule, that they are never to be taken immediately after eating (unless especial cases call for an exception), as they will otherwise derange the digestion, and produce irregularities in the evacuations. The best time for the use of these baths, is an hour before dinner, or before going to bed. In the latter case, they offer the advantage of securing a night's rest to the patient. Generally speaking, two sitting-baths a day will suffice; in particular cases, especially, if not persevered in for a long time, five to six may be taken during the day. Exercise in the open air is to be strictly recommended both before and after these baths.

9. *Foot-Baths*

Are taken in a small tub, or in the same vessel as the sitting-baths. The temperature and volume of water must depend on the action we wish to produce. If these baths are to act as stimulants, they must be very cold, not exceeding forty-one degrees of Fahrenheit. The water should have a depth of one, at the most, two inches, and the bath must not be continued longer than five minutes. They may be repeated several times during the day, according to circumstances. Rubbing, immediately after the baths, to promote speedy reaction, and also exercise after them, are indispensable. If the object of the foot-bath be to determine from the head or chest, the vessel must not be too large, in order that the water may become somewhat warm during the bath, which may be continued, in that case, from twenty minutes to one hour. In this case, also, the water must not be as cold as for the former purpose, and should cover the ankles. If congestion increase during the bath, cold applications should be at the same time applied to the parts affected. Friction and motion of the feet are absolutely necessary during and after the bath.

A variety of other partial baths, adapted to the different members of the body, are brought into operation in a general course of treatment by cold water. The effect desired is obtained partly by the duration of the bath, partly by the temperature of the water, as I have before mentioned in speaking of local baths in general. Where the baths are to act as stimulants, the water must be very cold, not exceeding forty-one degrees of Fahrenheit; they may, however, be repeated several times in the course of the day, if requisite. They are to be continued from five to eight minutes. By friction, immediately after the bath, we arrive more speedily at the desired end.

If the intention of these baths be to produce a soothing effect, their temperature must not be below fifty-nine degrees of Fahrenheit; they may, however, be continued for a longer period of time; fifteen to thirty minutes will, in most cases, suffice; they may also be repeated on the return of the attacks of pain. Where their action is to be derivative, the temperature should be from forty-six to fifty-nine degrees of Fahrenheit, and they should be continued for half an hour to one hour or longer. If they are to produce this effect gradually, and not rapidly, we frequently resort, at the same time, to applications (umschlage) to the part affected. Cooling applications, frequently repeated, will often lead to the desired result, and, at other times, applications producing warmth, will be most serviceable; we should, therefore, consider whether the object be to produce cold or heat.

10. *The Drop-Bath.*

This term is applied to single drops of water falling from a height of several fathoms. For this forrr of bath, a vessel is used, filled with very cold water, and furnished with a very small aperture, through which the water passes in the form of drops. The small aperture should be partly closed by a plug, to prevent the drops from following each other in rapid succession. By these means, their operation is considerably increased, and it becomes yet more potent if we allow the drops to fall upon a particular part at certain periods, and rub the part during the intervals. The reaction about to commence, will, indeed, be thus interrupted, but will afterward make its appearance in a more powerful and energetic form.

The violent excitement and irritation of the nervous system produced by these baths, render it necessary to restrict the use of them to half an hour; nor are they, indeed, adapted for vital parts, or such as are abundantly supplied with nerves.

They are often used with more effect in obstinate and chronic cases of paralysis, than the douche or affusion, with which they may alternate. Powerful and continued friction with a horse-hair glove, is never, in this case, to be neglected after the baths.

11. *The Douche.*

This description of bath is prepared with the aid of mechanical contrivances, by means of which a stream of water is made to fall upon the body with more or less force. In many respects it is most advantageous to make use of a natural fall of water for this purpose; we can then conduct the water simply into a channel, giving it a fall of twelve to twenty feet, and to the stream a caliber of half an inch to five inches. These simple douches are far less disagreeable to the sensations of the patient than those of artificial construction. In the former, the patient can turn himself freely and alter his position so as to expose any part of the body to the stream. Douche rooms, admitting, by their construction, of the access of the air from above, produce an agreeable sensation, especially in summer, and are very beneficial in their action. After the first time of using these baths, the dreadful ideas which many patients preconceive of them quickly disappear.

Our chief consideration, in the use of the douche, should be to guard against applying it to the body when quite cold, or when in a state of perspiration after active exercise. The patient, after undressing in a moderate temperature, steps below the falling stream, attempting to receive it in the palms of his hands, that the whole force and volume of the water may not fall upon his body immediately, which is not, to say the least, at all times agreeable. After having thus prepared himself for the more potent shock, he must expose himself to the full stream, and in such a manner that the whole column of water will fall chiefly on the neck and spine. From time to time, he must equably expose the other members of the body to the stream; but the affected parts chiefly, and for a greater length of time. He should be careful not to allow the stream to fall perpendicularly on the head, chest, or on the region of the liver, especially if these parts be weak or affected with disease.

The duration of the douche must be regulated by the constitution of the patient, and the effect we wish to produce; it should never be continued for less than one, nor more than twelve minutes.

Where a natural douche is not to be obtained, we make use of the well known machines resembling a fire engine in shape and construction. By means of these contrivances, we may bring one or more streams of any given force into operation. Our care must be directed to the selection of cold and fresh water for this purpose; finally, the same rules are to be observed which we laid down for the use of the former douche.

The period of the day at which these different douches (excepting those for the eye and ear) are used, varies. They are only to be taken, as an exception, fasting, or immediately after sweating, and never on a full stomach, nor oftener than once or twice daily.

Rather active exercise should be taken after the douche, until the peculiar sensation of reaction has totally disappeared, or an uncomfortable sensation of cold, accompanied by headaches, fainting, etc., will be experienced, instead of an agreeable and beneficial glow. It is, moreover, not advisable to drink cold water immediately after the douche, because a rapid generation of heat is thus impeded, and inflammations of the stomach and bowels might be caused.

The douche, the most powerful stimulant known in hydropathy, is always applicable where excitement is necessary, but attention must be paid in every case, to age, constitution, and to the vital powers. Cases are not unfrequent, where the nature of the diseases calls for this stimulant to complete the cure, but where it must be avoided in consequence of pregnancy, pulmonic affections, etc. No mode of applying cold water is more abused than the douche; in most hydropathic establishments, even at the present day, this is, unfortunately, too often the case. But very few experienced hydropathists regard it as a stimulant requiring caution. For the most part, it is looked upon as a remedy indispensable to every cure, is brought into use injudiciously, and without mature deliberation, and continued to the detriment of all organs; the beneficial results, therefore, which a judicious use of it would produce, are, necessarily, oftentimes frustrated.

12. *Local Applications* (*Umschläge*). *Wet Bandages.*

By these applications, two different effects may be produced, viz., that of cooling the part to which they are applied, or that of raising its temperature. Where they are intended as refrigerants or derivatives, the cloths must be of a size suited to the part inflamed; they should be folded six or eight times, dipped into very cold water, gently pressed before application, and are to be renewed every four or ten minutes, according to the degrees of inflammation. If we cannot obtain water sufficiently cold in summer-time, ice must be added to it until its temperature sinks to forty-one or forty-four degrees of Fahrenheit. This low temperature is especially necessary in dangerous inflammations of important organs; *e. g.*, of the brain. The bandages must then be continued without intermission, day and night, until danger is averted. Neglect in changing the wet clothes (umschlãge), at the proper time, will cause fatal results. One omission of the change is sufficient to frustrate their beneficial operation; for violent reaction is only to be subdued by continual cold.

The warming applications of cold water consist of pieces of linen folded two or three times, and dipped into cold water; they must be well pressed out before application, and not changed until they begin to dry—this is the indication for their repetition. This variety of application must be not only well adapted to the part, but it is to be further secured against the access of the air by a dry bandage, in order that the reaction it produces may generate a degree of heat in the part covered exceeding the temperature of the body. The combined action of the moisture and heat thus produced is that of a solvent or morbid matter, dispersing swellings and indurations, which are thus rendered more fit for absorption and elimination. These applications are not only well adapted for the removal of tumors, but may be applied also, with great benefit, in various cases of affections of the abdomen. Their efficacy, in all derangements of the digestive organs, and diseases of the liver, etc., is proved.

The applications to the abdomen vary somewhat in form from the former bandages. A piece of linen, two yards in length, and rather more than one foot in breadth, is to be doubled, sewn together, and furnished with strings, to enable us to adapt it closely to the body, and secure it in its situation. In using the bandage thus arranged, about one foot of it in length should be wetted with fresh water, well wrung out, and applied round the body; thus, the wet portion will extend once, the dry part twice round the body. These abdominal belts are to be worn according to the urgency of the case, sometimes for several hours in the day, or through the whole night; in some instances, again, for weeks, both by day and night.

13. *Applications around one-half of the body, or around the whole body. Wet linen sheets.*

For this purpose, the bed must be prepared in the same manner as for the process of sweating. The wet sheet is laid upon the extended blanket, the patient lays himself at full length upon the former, whereupon it is folded around him, so as to come in close contact with every portion of the body. The patient is now to be enveloped in the blanket and the bed-covering (feather beds).

The wet sheets are of remarkable utility in all febrile diseases. In acute fevers they must be changed according to the degree of heat, every quarter or half hour, until the dry, hot skin of the patient becomes softer, and more prone to perspiration. When this symptom is observed, the renewal of the wet cloths may be delayed for a longer period, until perspiration actually ensues. The patient must then remain for several hours in this state, until uneasy sensations, and other inconveniences, render it necessary to extricate him; but it is more advisable to keep him in the loosened envelopment until perspiration ceases spontaneously, when a tepid ablution, or half-bath, should follow. In acute eruptions of the skin, measles, scarlatina, small-pox, etc., the wet sheets are not less serviceable, when the eruption cannot make its way to the surface in consequence of the dry state and heat of the skin, and of the violence of the fever; or where the rash has receded suddenly, owing to other disturbances. In both cases, the wet sheets are of essential service; one application of them suffices, sometimes to re-establish the eruption. If the rash fail to make its appearance after the first or second envelopment, cold affusion is to be preferred. There are cases in which the use of this remedy may be deemed objectionable, and a continuance of the wet sheets may appear more proper; we must, then, examine the skin carefully before every change, to see whether the eruption be nearer the surface, the skin softer, and the heat abated. In the latter case, the applications are to be discontinued, that the reaction of the skin may not be disturbed. The wet sheets, followed by tepid ablutions, cannot be sufficiently recommended, in all diseases of children. Many severe complications are averted, or relieved, at least, by them; or, where this is not the case, the disease itself is brought more speedily to a favorable termination.

The envelopment in wet sheets is not only of great advantage in acute diseases, but is, also, an admirable remedy in a variety of chronic cases, attended with an irritable, rough, and inactive skin, and in a multitude of skin-diseases; but in all those cases, a frequent change of the sheets is seldom necessary. In using the envelopment, we generally raise the temperature of the patient, and occasionally allow him to perspire, according to the circumstances of the case. Determination to the head, during the process, must be removed by cold applications to that part. If the feet remain cold for a long time in the wet cloths, and show no disposition to become warm, they are to be extricated and wrapped in the dry blanket only.

14. *Sweating.*

In the treatment by water, perspiration is brought about in the following manner: The patient is undressed and laid upon a woolen coverlet or blanket, extended on the bed. A servant wraps first the one side of the blanket round the body of the patient, drawing it close in all directions; grasping now firmly with the one hand the portion in which the patient is enveloped, he draws, with the other hand, the blanket round the patient, and tucks this portion also closely under him. Care must be taken that the coverings be in close contact with the body, especially at the neck, that the heat given off by the body may be well retained, and not suffered to escape. It is the excess of caloric, thus confined, which induces exhalation from the skin. Individuals who are to perspire for several hours, and cannot retain their urine long, may be furnished with a urinal, placed between the legs at the time of wrapping them up. The head may be included in the covering, or enveloped even in the pillow, so that the face alone is free, provided the patients do not suffer from congestions. The head must remain uncovered, on the other hand, if a disposition to congest be observed. Slight excitement of the vessels, before the outbreak of perspiration, generally passes off spontaneously; but where this favorable termination does not ensue, a cooling bandage (umschläge) is to be laid on the head of the patient, who must, at the same time, drink a little cold water. Warming applications (umschläge) are to be wrapped around all parts affected with nodes, gouty swellings, etc., before enveloping the patient. The use of these auxiliaries is to allay pain, which is generally more violent before the appearance of perspiration, and to excite a more copious exhalation from the parts to which they are applied.

Patients who are very restless in the blanket, and thus loosen it, should be confined more closely in the encasement by additional cloths and girths, as they would otherwise have to remain wrapped up during half a day or longer. Persons thus enveloped being totally helpless, an assistant should be always in attendance to open the windows as soon as perspiration ensues, and to administer, every ten or fifteen minutes, as much cold water as is necessary to promote perspiration. The action of the skin must be kept up uninterruptedly, and the perspiration should pass off in form of vapor, or in drops, as long as the case requires it.

The result of this mode of treatment is pretty certain, but the time necessary for the production of perspiration is not the same in all cases; for some individuals perspire sooner than others. The season, and many other inevitable circumstances, exert, moreover, a considerable influence on the skin; thus, some patients, especially in summer, will perspire in a quarter of an hour, while others require three to five hours for that purpose. In febrile and inflammatory diseases, we frequently cannot produce perspiration in less than twelve or twenty-four hours, although we change the wet sheets often, and resort to other auxiliary means.

The best time for exciting perspiration, in chronic cases, is in the early hours of the morning, from four to five o'clock at the latest. In acute diseases, the time depends on the fever itself, or on renewed exacerbations; it must be produced, therefore, when required, without reference to time. A repetition of the process twice on the same day, is only admissible and advisable as an exception. The indication for such practice would occur more frequently in chronic than in acute diseases; because in the latter perspiration should be kept up until it ceases spontaneously, or is interrupted by other circumstances. Two sweats daily can only be recommended to the robust, and even these persons will not be able to endure the protracted sweating required in some few troublesome cases, without injuring the skin and other important organs.

We cannot determine, *a priori*, how long each patient should sweat. The ordinary duration, in chronic cases, is from half an hour to three hours, daily; but moderate perspiration is to be encouraged for a longer time in acute diseases. Critical perspiration requires the longest duration, and should not be disturbed; we should rather, in this case, do everything in our power to aid and promote it, until it ceases spontaneously.

When the patient has remained in a state of perspiration long enough, the woolen covering should be loosened about his feet and legs, to enable him to walk. The attendant then raises him in bed, and leads him to the place where he is to bathe or wash. Sedan chairs or other contrivances, will be necessary to convey patients quickly to the bath, in serious cases. No danger is to be dreaded from the transition from heat to cold (as experience in many thousand cases has proved), if the necessary precautionary rules laid down for the use of full-baths be duly observed; for, in this mode of producing perspiration, important internal organs are not excited.

After the bath, the patients who can walk, or take other exercise, must not return to bed; but should dress quickly, go into the open air, drink the quantity of water prescribed, and afterward take their breakfast. Those patients, on the other hand, who can take no corporeal exercise, must be rubbed, after the bath, for some time, the friction extending over the whole surface of the body. This peculiar mode of inducing perspiration is to be brought into use in all diseases where morbid matter is to be eliminated from the system, because the skin, as daily experience teaches us, is the organ best adapted for this purpose. At the commencement of the treatment, the perspiration is clear and aqueous for some time; at a later period it becomes more viscid, then varies in color, and assumes a powerful odor. The urine, at the same time, or later, in the course of treatment, assumes the same properties in color and odor; open sores and the breath participate in this change. These symptoms usually make their appearance at different intervals, in a protracted case. Critical excretions seldom continue without intermission from their first commencement, until all extraneous substances are removed from the body; it is true, that this phenomenon is observed sometimes, but it is always a rare occurrence, and the critical discharges will not then unfrequently continue two to four months.

There can be no doubt that an incalculable quantity of morbid matter is removed from the body in the act of perspiring; for it is often to be recognized by the organs of sense, by its color and odor during the process. Most striking is, at times, the odor of valerian, turpentine, iodine, musk, asafœtida, sulphur, and mercury. The colors observed, are generally confined to red and yellow; brown and blue are less frequently met with: the latter occurs often in the deposits in the urine, which may assume, also, all other colors.

III. MATERIA MEDICA.

1. Aconite.

Acute local inflammations; active, sanguineous congestions; evil consequences of a chill in a dry, cold air; affections in consequence of fright or of anger; measles; erysipelatous inflammations; inflammatory fevers, even with bilious or nervous symptoms; mental alienations, with fixed ideas of approaching death; cerebral congestion, with dizziness; croup, first period; hooping-cough, first period.

General Symptoms.—Shooting pains, or rheumatic, which are renewed by wine, or other heating articles; sufferings which, particularly at night, seem insupportable; attacks of pain, with thirst and redness of the cheeks; uneasiness, as if in consequence of suppressed perspiration, or in consequence of a chill.

Skin. Skin dry and burning; scarlet rash; measles; nettle-rash.

Sleep. Sleeplessness from anxiety, with constant agitation and tossing; starting in sleep.

Fever. Dry, burning heat, with extreme thirst, sometimes, especially at the beginning of the disease, preceded by shiverings with trembling; heat, chiefly of the head and face, with redness of the cheeks, shuddering over the entire body; shivering, for the short time that they may be uncovered during the heat; pulse hard, frequent, and accelerated.

Moral Symptoms. — Great agitation and boasting, with anguish, discouragement that cannot be consoled, cries, tears, groans, complaints and reproaches; apprehensions and fear of approaching death; a great disposition to be angry, to be frightened; alternate paroxysms of laughter and tears; inquietude under disease, and despair respecting a cure; delirium, chiefly at night.

Head. Weight and fullness in the forehead and temples, with pressing outward, as if everything was going to issue through them; congestion of blood to the head; aggravation of the pains in the head by movement, by speaking, by rising from a recumbent position, and by drinking; amendment in the open air.

Eyes. Eyes red and inflamed, with deep redness of the vessels, and intolerable pains.

Ears. Buzzing in the ears.

Nose. Bleeding from the nose.

Face. Red spots on both cheeks.

Throat. Pain in the throat, with deep redness of the parts affected, and difficult deglutition; burning and pricking in the throat, chiefly when swallowing.

Stomach. Sensation of swelling tension and pressure, as from a weight in the pericordial region and in the stomach.

Abdomen. Tension and pressure in the hypochondriac region; pressure in the hepatic region; painful sensitiveness of the abdomen to the touch, and to the least movement.

Fæces. Loose, watery stools; white stools, with red urine.

Urine. Urine scanty, burning, dark red, and with a brick-colored sediment.

Larynx. A constant desire to cough, produced by an irritation or a tickling in the larynx; short and dry cough, principally at night; spitting of blood, with the cough; shootings and pains in the chest when coughing.

Chest. Short breathing, chiefly during sleep, and on getting up; breathing difficult, anxious, and attended with groans; painful stitches in the chest, chiefly when breathing, coughing, and moving; stitches in the side; palpitation of the heart, with great anxiety.

Trunk. Painful stiffness in the nape of the neck.

2. Arnica.

Affections in consequence of mechanical injuries (falls, commotion, blows, etc.), wounds, principally those inflicted by blunt instruments; bites; excoriation of bed-ridden patients; bruises, dislocations, sprains, and fractures; accidents resulting from a strain; stings of insects; corns, by an external application of it, after having pared them.

General Symptoms.—Pains, as from dislocation; fainting fit, with loss of consciousness, in consequence of mechanical injuries; paralytic state, on the left side, in consequence of apoplexy.

Skin. Red, bluish, and yellowish spots, as if from contusions.

Head. Whirling giddiness, with obscuration of the eyes, chiefly when getting up, moving the head, or walking.

Eyes. Pain like excoriation in the eyes and eyelids, with difficulty of moving them.

Face. Face pale and hollow.

Mouth. Tongue dry, or loaded with a white coating; putrid smell from the mouth in the morning.

Stomach. Vomiting of dark, coagulated blood.

Abdomen. Pain, as from contusion in the sides.

Anus. Involuntary stools, chiefly in the night.

Urinary Passages. Involuntary emission of urine; urine of a brownish red, with brick-colored sediment.

Respiratory Organs. Cough, with expectoration of blood; even without cough, expectoration of black, coagulated blood after every corporeal effort.

Chest. Respiration short, panting, difficult, and anxious; shootings in the chest and sides, with difficulty of respiration, aggravated by coughing, breathing deeply, and by movement; pain as of a bruise, and of compression of the chest.

Trunk. Pains, as from a bruise, and dislocation in the back, in the chest, and in the loins.

Arms. Pain, as of dislocation in the joints of the arms and hands; want of strength in the hands, on seizing anything.

Legs. Pains, as if from fatigue or from dislocation; tension in the knee, as if from contraction of the tendons; inflammatory, erysipelatous swelling of the feet with pain, and aggravation of the pain by movement; hot, painful, hard, and shining swelling of the great toes.

3. Arsenic.

General Symptoms.—Burning, chiefly in the interior of the parts affected, or sharp and drawing pains; nocturnal pains, so unbearable that they excite to despair and fury; aggravation of suffering in the evening in bed, on lying on the part affected, or during repose; mitigation by external heat and movement of the body; want of strength, excessive weakness, and complete asthenia, even to prostration.

Skin. Skin dry as parchment, or cold and bluish; ulcers with raised and hard edges; fetid smell, ichorous suppuration, ready bleeding, putridity, and bluish or greenish coloı of the ulcers.

Sleep. Nocturnal sleeplessness, with agitation and constant tossing.

Fever. Coldness over the whole body, sometimes with cold and clammy sweat; pulse irregular, or quick, weak, small and frequent, or suppressed and trembling.

Moral Symptoms. Anxiety, inquietude, and excessive anguish, principally in the evening in bed.

Face. Face pale, hollow, and cadaverous; lips bluish or black, dry, and chapped.

Mouth. Offensive smell from the mouth; tongue brownish or blackish, dry, cracked, and trembling; ulceration of the tongue on the anterior edge; thrush of the mouth.

Throat. Inflammation and gangrene of the throat.

Appetite. Violent burning, choking, and unquenchable

thirst, with inclination to drink constantly, but little at a time; want of appetite.

Stomach. Vomitings after drinking and eating; vomiting of mucous, bilious, or serous matter, of a yellowish, greenish, brownish, or blackish color; burning internal heat, diarrhoa, and fear of death; excessive pain in the epigastrium, chiefly when touched; insupportable heat and burning in the pericordial region, and in the stomach.

Abdominal Region. Swelling of the abdomen, as in ascites; violent cutting pains, cramp-like pains in the abdomen; colic, chiefly after eating and drinking, or in the night, and often accompanied with vomiting or diarrhea, with coldness, internal heat, or cold sweat.

Fœces. Violent diarrhea, of greenish, yellowish, whitish color, or brownish and blackish; burning in the rectum and in the anus.

Larynx. Dry cough, in the evening after lying down, with a wish to rise; also, after drinking, with difficulty of respiration.

Chest. Breathing short; difficult, stifling dyspnœa, and attacks of suffocation, sometimes with cold sweat, spasmodic constriction of the chest or of the larynx, anguish, great weakness, coldness of the body, pain in the pit of the stomach, and paroxysms of cough; oppression of the chest when coughing, when walking, and when going up stairs; violent and insupportable throbbings of the heart, chiefly when lying on the back, and especially at night.

4. Belladonna.

Scarlatina; sleeplessness; inflammatory fevers, with nervous, gastric, or rheumatic affections; erysipelas.

General Symptoms.—The least contact, and sometimes, also, the slightest movement, aggravates the sufferings; dread of every movement, and of all exertion; over-excitement, and too great sensibility of all the organs.

Skin. Swelling, with heat and scarlet redness of the whole body, or of several parts, chiefly the face, the neck, the abdomen, and the hands; red, hot, and shining swelling of the diseased parts.

Sleep. Constant desire to sleep; nocturnal sleeplessness, in consequence of excessive anguish or great agitation; when sleeping, frequent starts, with fright, groans, cries; on waking, headache, and aggravation of sufferings.

Fever. Dry, burning heat; pulse strong and quick, or full and slow, or small and slow, or small and quick, or hard and tense; sweat of the parts that are covered only.

Head. Fullness, heaviness, and violent pressure on the head, as if going to burst, with desire to lie down; dartings into the head, as if from knives; strong pulsation of the arteries of the head; bending the head backward; boring with the head into the pillow while sleeping.

Eyes. Aching pains in the eyes and the sockets, extending into the head; inflammation of the eyes, with injection of the vessels; dread of light.

Ears. Piercing pressure, sharp pain, pinching, squeezing, and shooting in the ears; swelling of the parotids.

Face. Face pale, sometimes suddenly alternating with red; burning heat of the face; dark, or scarlet, or bluish redness of the face; swelling of the submaxillary glands, and those of the neck.

Teeth. Sharp and drawing pains, at night or in the evening; the touch and the open air aggravate the toothache.

Mouth. Sensation of great dryness, or actual and excessive dryness and choking in the mouth; tongue red, hot, shining, dry, and cracked, or loaded with whitish mucus; redness of the edges of the tongue; paralytic weakness of the tongue, with difficult and stammering speech.

Throat. Excoriating, scraping, and shooting pains in the throat and in the tonsils, principally when swallowing; inflammation and swelling of the throat, of the velum palati, of the uvula, and of the tonsils; suppuration of the tonsils; complete inability to swallow, even the least liquid, which frequently is forced out through the nostrils; sensation of choking, and spasmodic constriction in the throat.

Appetite. Burning, excessive, and intolerable thirst, often with dread of all drink; drinking with trembling precipitation.

Stomach. Spasmodic hiccough.

Abdominal Region. Cramp-like, contractive and constrictive pains in the abdomen, and especially around the navel, with a sensation as if the parts were squeezed or seized with the nails; the pains force one to bend himself, and are accompanied by vomiting or by inflation and protrusion of the transverse colon in the form of a pad; soreness of the whole abdomen, as if everything in it were excoriated.

Urine. Frequent discharges of urine, copious, pale, and watery; difficulty of retention and involuntary emission of urine.

Genital Organs. Violent pressure toward the genital parts, as if all were going to fall downward, principally when walking or sitting upright; menses too copious and too early.

Larynx. Loss of voice; cough chiefly at night, or in the afternoon, in the evening in bed, mostly dry, short, and sometimes convulsive; when coughing, cutting in the abdomen; the least movement, when in bed at night, renews the cough.

Chest. Oppression of the chest, difficult respiration, dyspnœa, and short breath, sometimes with anxiety; respiration short, anxious, and rapid; pressure on the chest.

Trunk. Painful swelling, and stiffness of the neck and the nape.

5. Bryonia.

Rheumatic and arthritic affections, even with inflammatory fever and swelling; local inflammations; inflammatory fevers, with nervous, gastric, or bilious affection, and strong excitement of the sanguineous and nervous system; typhoid fevers, in the inflammatory period.

General Symptoms.—Tension, drawing pains, acute drawings, and stinging, especially in the limbs, and chiefly during movement, with insupportable pains on being touched; red, shining swelling of some parts of the body; aggravation of the pains and sufferings at night, and from movement; amelioration during repose; desire to remain in a recumbent posture.

Sleep. Restlessness, especially before midnight, caused by heat, agitation of blood, and anxiety; sleep, disturbed by thirst, with bitter taste in the mouth when waking; inability to remain lying on the right side.

Fever. Cold and shivering of the body, even in bed, accompanied by pains in all the limbs; shiverings; with trembling, often with heat in the head, redness of the face, and thirst; before the shiverings, vertigo and headache; universal dry heat, external and internal, almost always with a great desire for cold drinks.

Moral Symptoms. Irascibility and passion; delirium, with ravings about the transactions of the day.

Head. Great fullness and heaviness of the head, with raking pressure toward the forehead, and when stooping, a sensation as if everything were going to fall out through the forehead; headache, aggravated by movement.

Nose. Swelling of the nose; frequent bleeding of the nose, sometimes in the morning, or when the menses are suppressed, or even when sleeping.

Face. Face red and burning; swelling of the face, sometimes on one side only, or under the eyes, and at the root of the nose; lips swollen and cracked, with bleeding.

Teeth. Toothache, with desire to lie down; mitigated by lying on the parts affected; jerking, drawing toothache, with a sensation as if the teeth were too long or loose.

Mouth. Dryness of the mouth, with burning thirst; tongue dry, loaded with a white, dirty, or yellow coating.

Throat. Sensation of dryness, and great dryness in the throat.

Appetite. Bitter taste in the morning; repugnance and disgust for food.

Stomach. Nausea and desire to vomit, especially after eating; vomiting, as soon as one has drank, and especially on drinking after a meal; shootings in the stomach during movement; burning in the pit of the stomach.

Abdominal Region. Pains in the liver, when touched, on breathing or coughing; cramp-like pains, or cuttings and shootings in the abdomen.

Fæces, Constipation; diarrhea in the summer.

Urine. Urine scanty, reddish, brownish, and hot.

Genital Organs. Menses suppressed; metrorrhagia of a deep-red blood, with pain in the loins and in the head; swelling of the labium, with a black and hard pustule.

Larynx. Cough, mostly dry, excited by a tickling in the throat; cramp-like, suffocating cough, after having eaten or drank, and often with vomiting of food; cough, with stinging in the sides of the chest, or with aching pains in the head, as if it were going to split; cough, with expectoration of mucus of a dirty-reddish color.

Chest. Respiration impeded by stinging in the chest; stingings in the chest and in the sides, especially when coughing or breathing deeply, allowing one to lie only on the back, and aggravated by any movement whatever; heat and burning pain in the chest, with anxiety and tightness; beatings of the heart, frequently very violent, with oppression.

Trunk. Pains in the loins, like a painful weight; shootings in the loins and in the back, aggravated by cough and respiration; rheumatic heaviness and tension in the nape of the neck, and in the neck.

Arms. Tractive pains in the joints of the shoulders and the arms, with tension, stinging, and shining, red swelling; pain of dislocation in the joints of the hands on moving them.

Legs. Drawing pains in the thighs; swelling of the legs, extending to the feet; pain, as of dislocation, in the foot, when walking.

6. Calcarea Carbonica.

Muscular weakness, difficulty of learning to walk, atrophy and other sufferings of scrofulous children; rickety affections, polypus; fistulous ulcers; delirium tremens; difficult dentition in children, with convulsions.

General Symptoms.—Agitation of blood, mostly in plethoric individuals, often in the head and in the chest; epileptic convulsions, with cries; the symptoms are aggravated after washing and laboring in the water, in the evening, after a meal, and every second day.

Skin. Nettle-rash, chiefly disappearing in the fresh air; swelling and induration of the glands, with or without pain.

Sleep. Restlessness from flow of ideas, or in consequence of frightful images, which appear as soon as the eyes are shut; dreams, frequent, vivid, anxious, fantastic, frightful.

Fever. Excessive internal coldness; frequent attacks of transient heat, with anguish and beating of the heart.

Moral Symptoms. Melancholy and disposition to weep and to be frightened.

Head. Piercing in the forehead as if the head were going to burst, hammering pains in the head after a walk in the open air; icy coldness in and on the head; falling off of the hair; tumors in the hairy scalp.

Eyes. Ulcers, spots, and opacity of cornea; red and thick swelling of the eyelids.

Ears. Purulent discharge from the ears ; polypus in the ears ; cracking in the ears, when swallowing and chewing ; hardness of hearing ; inflammatory swelling of the parotids.

Face. Swelling of the upper lip ; painful swelling of the submaxillary glands.

Stomach. Regurgitation of sour substances ; sour vomitings.

Abdominal Region. Swelling and induration of the mesenteric glands ; enlargement and hardness of the abdomen.

Fœces. Evacuations like clay ; diarrhea during dentition, of a sour smell, fetid, or yellowish, in infants.

Genital Organs. Menses premature and too copious.

Larynx. Cough at night, violent and dry, sometimes even spasmodic.

Chest. Pain as from excoriation in the chest, especially on breathing and being touched ; palpitation of the heart.

Trunk. Hard and painful swelling of the glands of the neck.

Arms. Drawing pains in the arms, also at night ; boils on the hands and the fingers.

Legs. Drawing lancinations, or cutting, acute pains in them ; swelling of the knees ; corns on the feet, with burning pain as of excoriation.

7. Carbo Vegetabilis.

Evil effects from the abuse of mercury, or of cinchona ; sufferings caused by warm and damp weather ; sensibility to changes of weather ; intermittent fevers, even those which the abuse of cinchona has rendered obstinate ; Asiatic cholera, with total absence of pulse.

General Symptoms.—Burning pains in the limbs and in the back ; the majority of symptoms appear while walking in the open air ; soreness of all the limbs, especially in the morn ing, when one has just risen; sudden prostration of the physical powers; liability to take cold.

Fever. Shivering and coldness in the body; cold sweat on the limbs and face.

Moral Symptoms. Inquietude and anxiety, especially in the evening.

Head. Heaviness of the head.

Nose. Violent coryza, with hoarseness and raucity of the chest.

Teeth. Opening, retraction, excoriation, and ulceration of the gums; bleeding of the teeth and gums.

Mouth. Dryness, or accumulation of water in the mouth.

Throat. Scraping and burning pain in the throat, the palate, and the gullet.

Appetite. Salt taste in the mouth and of food; after a meal, great inflation of the abdomen.

Stomach. Rising of fat food; sour risings after a meal.

Fæces. Evacuations liquid, pale, or mucous; involuntary evacuation.

Urine. Diminution of the secretion of urine.

Larynx. In the morning and in the evening, hoarseness, aggravated by prolonged conversation, and chiefly in cold and damp weather.

Chest. Dyspnœa on walking; pain as from excoriation of the chest.

Trunk. Rheumatic, drawing pains, acute pulling and shootings in the back, the nape of the neck, and the muscles of the neck.

Arms. Pullings, and acute drawing pains in the fore-arms, the wrist, and the fingers: paralytic weakness of the wrists and of the fingers.

Legs. Drawing, and paralytic pains in the legs; cramps in the legs, and in the soles of the feet.

8. Chamomile.

Different affections of women and of children, chiefly lying-in women and new-born infants; bad effects from the abuse of coffee and of narcotic palliatives; suffering in consequence of a chill; affections arising from sudden grief, or a fit of passion; convulsive and spasmodic attacks; excoriation of the skin; disposition for every wound to ulcerate; bilious and gastric affections; excoriation of the nipples; erysipelas on the breasts; catarrhal cough, with hoarseness, chiefly in children.

General Symptoms.— Rheumatic, drawing pains, chiefly at night in bed; pains with thirst, heat and redness of one of the cheeks; over-excitement, and excessive sensibility of the nervous system, with great sensibility to pain.

Sleep. Nocturnal sleeplessness; when sleeping, starts with fright, cries, tossing, tears, talking.

Fever. Burning heat and redness (often only in one) of the cheeks, chiefly at night, with groaning, tossing.

Moral Symptoms. Disposition to weep and to be angry, with great sensibility to offense; quarrelsome and choleric humor.

Head. Headache on waking in the morning, or while asleep.

Eyes. Eyes inflamed and red, with pressive pains, chiefly on moving the eyes, and on shaking the head; bleareduess in the eyes, and nocturnal agglutination.

Ears. Shootings extending into the ears, with disposition to be angry at trifles; buzzing in the ears; inflammatory swelling of the parotids, as well as of the sub-maxillary glands and of those of the neck.

Face. Face hot, red, burning, or redness and heat of one cheek, with coldness and paleness of the other.

Teeth. Toothache, mostly of one side, and chiefly at night, in the heat of the bed, with insupportable pains which almost drive one to despair, frequently after eating anything hot (or cold), and chiefly after having taken coffee.

Throat. Sore throat; deep redness of the parts affected.

Appetite. Bitter taste in the mouth and of food; excessive thirst for cold drinks.

Stomach. Bitter, bilious vomiting.

Abdominal Region. Flatulent colic, with inflation of the abdomen; excessively painful colic, pullings and cuttings in the abdomen.

Anus and Fæces. Diarrhea at night, with slimy or greenish fæces, or mucus.

Urine. Menstrual colic, before the catamenia; pressure toward the uterus, as if from the pains of childbirth; metrorrhagia, with discharge of deep-red blood and of clots, and accompanied with labor-pains.

Larynx. Dry cough, produced by constant titillation in the larynx; anger excites cough (in children).

Chest. Attacks of flatulent asthma, with anxiety and fullness in the pericordial region.

Legs. Cramps in the calves of the legs, chiefly at night.

9. China.—Cinchona.

General Symptoms.—Pains or sufferings, excited or aggravated by touch, at night, or after a meal; great general weakness, with trembling; great tendency to perspiration when moving and sleeping.

Skin. Yellow color of the skin.

Sleep. Painful, frightful dreams, which continue to produce agitation after waking.

Fever. Shiverings, with shuddering, or feverish trembling, commonly without thirst; the thirst generally takes place only before or after the shiverings; easy perspiration during sleep; nocturnal debilitating sweats.

Moral Symptoms. Hypochondriacal dejection; excessive irascibility, with pusillanimity.

Head. Headache as if from suppressed coryza; pain as from a bruise in the brain; pressive headache; acute jerking or pressive pains in the head; headache as if the head were going to burst; congestion to the head; sensibility of the exterior of the head, and even of the roots of the hair, when touched.

Eyes. Sparkling, black, dancing spots, and obscuration before the eyes.

Nose. Bleeding of the nose and of the mouth.

Face. Complexion pale, earth-like, sometimes of a blackish yellow.

Teeth. Dull and distressing pains in the carious teeth.

Mouth. Tongue with a yellow or white coating.

Appetite. Bitter taste of food and drink; desire for a variety of food and for dainties, without knowing exactly which; great weakness of digestion.

Stomach. Eructations, with taste of food; pressure in the stomach, with cramp-like pains, especially after having eaten.

Abdominal Region. Hardness and swelling of the liver; swelling and hardness of the spleen; piercing in the spleen; dropsical swelling of the abdomen, with asthmatic sufferings and fatiguing cough.

Fæces. Slimy, watery, yellowish diarrhea; loose evacuations, with excretion of undigested food; loose evacuations, chiefly after a meal or at night; crawling in the anus, as if from worms.

Urine. Urine deep-colored, with sediment like brick-dust.

Genital Organs. Congestion to the uterus; leucorrhea, with cramp-like contraction.

Larynx. Violent, convulsive cough, sometimes even with inclination to vomit; cough, with expectoration streaked with blood.

Chest. Shooting in the chest, when coughing and breathing; stitches in the side; violent congestion to the chest.

Arms. Paralytic, jerking, tearings in the muscles and bones of the upper and lower extremities, excited by touch.

10. CINA.

Scrofulous affections; acute hydrocephalus of children; wetting the bed; hooping-cough; chiefly in scrofulous children or in those suffering from worms.

GENERAL SYMPTOMS. — Convulsions and distortion of the limbs; epileptic convulsions, with cries, turning on the back, and violent movements of the hands and feet; external pressure aggravates or renews the sufferings.

Sleep. Nocturnal sleeplessness, with agitation, tears, cries, heat and anguish.

Moral Symptoms. Child cries when it is touched.

Eyes. Pupils dilated.

Nose. Desire to put the fingers into the nose; stoppage of the nose.

Teeth. Grinding of the teeth.

Appetite. Hunger a short time after a meal.

Fæces. Loose evacuations, of the consistence of pap; discharge of ascarides and of worms by the anus; loose, involuntary, whitish evacuations.

Urine. Wetting the bed, urine soon becomes turbid.

Larynx. Cough, with sudden starts and loss of consciousness.

Extremities. Contraction and jerking of the hand and of the fingers; cramp-like extension of the legs.

11. COFFEA.

Excessive nervous excitability; excessively painful neuralgia; sleeplessness from nervous excitement; evil consequences of unexpected or excessive joy.

GENERAL SYMPTOMS. — Painful susceptibility of parts affected; mental and physical excitability; sleeplessness from excitement of the imagination, flow of ideas, and fantastic visions; desire to lie down and to shut the eyes, without being able to sleep.

Head and Throat. Pains in the head, as if the brain were bruised; sore throat, with great and painful sensibility.

Stomach and Fæces. Cramps in the stomach; abdominal pains, which even drive one to despair, especially in women; diarrhea, also, during teething.

12. Colocynthis.

Evil effects from mental emotions, with indignation and mortification.

General Symptoms. — Painful cramps and cramp-like contractions, in the internal or external parts.

Skin. Troublesome itching, with great restlessness in the whole body, especially in the evening in bed, followed by perspiration.

Head. Attacks of semi-lateral headache.

Stomach. Colic and diarrhea, however little is eaten.

Abdominal Region. Inflammation of the abdomen, as if from tympanitis: cramp-like pain and constriction in the intestines, especially after a fit of passion; excessively violent colic, with cutting, cramp-like, or contractive pains, which compel one to bend double, with restlessness in the whole body, and with a sensation of shuddering in the face, which seems to proceed from the abdomen; coffee and tobacco smoke diminish the colic.

Fæces. Loose evacuations of a greenish yellow; dysenterical evacuations, with colic.

Urine. Diminished secretion of urine.

13. Cuprum.

Spasmodic affections and convulsions; encephalitis; Asiatic cholera; hooping-cough; spasmodic asthma.

General Symptoms.—Tonic spasms, with loss of consciousness, throwing of the head backward; the convulsions generally begin in the fingers and in the toes; convulsive startings at night when sleeping; violent convulsions, with great display of strength; symptoms which appear periodically, and in groups.

Head. Whirling vertigo, as if the head were going to fall forward; stupefying depression in the head, with crawling in the vertex; pains in the occiput and nape of the neck, on moving the head.

Eyes. Convulsions and restless movements of the eyes.

Face. Spasmodic distortion of the face; lips bluish.

Teeth and Mouth. Foam in the mouth.

Stomach. Violent vomitings, with cramps in the abdomen, aggravated by touch and by movement.

Abdominal Region. Spasmodic colic.

Fæces. Violent diarrhea.

Chest. Respiration accelerated; short, difficult respiration, with spasmodic cough and rattling in the chest; suffocating fits; cramps in the chest, which interrupt the respiration and the voice.

Trunk and Arms. Cramps of the fingers and of the toes.

14. Drosera.

Catarrh and hoarseness; hooping-cough; affections of the respiratory organs, in consequence of croup.

Larynx. Crawling in the larynx, which excites a short cough and shootings as far as the throat; sensation of dryness or roughness, and of scraping in the bottom of the gullet, with inclination to cough; hoarseness and very low voice; dry, spasmodic cough, with inclination to vomit; fatiguing cough, like hooping-cough, with bluish face, wheezing respiration, attacks of suffocation, bleeding from the nose and mouth, and anxiety; vomiting of food during the cough and afterward.

Chest. Difficulty of respiration when coughing or speaking.

15. Dulcamara.

Affections, in consequence of taking cold in general; tetters of different kinds; nettle-rash.

General Symptoms. — Aggravation of sufferings, chiefly in the evening or at night, and during repose, mitigated by movement; swelling and induration of the glands; dropsical swelling of the whole body, limbs, and face.

Skin. Dry, furfuraceous, humid, scaling, or suppurating tetters; reddish tetters, bleeding after being scratched, with painful sensibility to the touch, and to cold water.

Fæces. Diarrhea, as if after a chill, of greenish or brownish mucus; nocturnal, watery diarrhea with colic.

Larynx. Catarrh and hoarseness, as if from having taken cold; moist cough.

Arms. Tettery eruption on the hands.

16. Graphites.

Tetters of several kinds especially on the face; **wens.**

General Symptoms. — Great disposition to take cold, and fear of the open air and of currents of air.

Skin. Tetters, and other humid or scabby eruptions, sometimes with secretion of corrosive serum, or with itching in the evening and at night; unhealthy skin, every injury tends to ulceration; deformity and thickness of the nails.

Eyes. Inflammation of the eyes, injection of the veins, swelling and abundant mucous secretion from the eyelids.

Ears. Dryness of the internal ear; scabs, tetters, running and excoriation behind the ears; hardness of hearing mitigated by the motion of a carriage.

Nose. Dry scabs on the nose; nostrils excoriated, cracked, and ulcerated, fetid smell from the nose.

Face. Flushes of heat in the face; erysipelatous inflammation and swelling of the face, with eruption of vesicles;

one-sided paralysis and distortion of the muscles of the face, with difficult articulation; ulcers on the internal surface of the lips; scabby eruption on the chin and around the mouth.

Throat. Sore throat, even at night, as if there were a plug within it.

Appetite. Weakness of digestion; inflation of the abdomen after a meal.

Abdominal Region. Immoderate expulsion of fetid wind, preceded by pinchings.

Fæces. Obstinate constipation, with hard fæces; large hemorrhoidal excrescences in the anus.

Urine. Wetting the bed.

Menses. Suppression of menses; in place of menses, flow of blood from the anus.

Arms. Arthritic nodosities on the fingers; tettery excoriation between the fingers; thickness of the nails of the fingers.

Legs. Tetters on the thighs, hams, and tibia; cold feet, even in the evening in bed; tettery excoriation between the toes; thickness and deformity of the toe-nails.

17. Helleborus.

Dropsical affections, especially some kinds of anasarca, and chiefly those which proceed from the repercussion of eruptions, such as measles; scald-head, with obstruction of the glands of the neck; acute hydrocephalus.

General Symptoms.— Convulsions.

Sleep. Sleepiness, with eyes half open and pupils turned upward.

Moral Symptoms. Dullness of the internal senses

Head. Stupefying pain and sensation of a bruise in the head; painful heaviness of the head; disposition to bury the head in the pillow, when sleeping.

Fæces. Watery and frequent evacuations.

Chest. Difficult respiration, as if from hydrothorax; constriction of the chest.

18. Hepar Sulphuris.

Evil consequences of the abuse of mercury; scrofulous affections icterus; scald-head; eruptions and tetters on the face; scrofulous catarrhal ophthalmia; ulcers on the cornea.

General Symptoms.—Pains as if from excoriation or a bruise on different parts when touched; swelling, inflammation, and ulceration of the glands; aggravation of the pains at night.

Skin. Eruption of pimples and tubercles, painful when touched; unhealthy skin, every injury tends to ulceration; suppurations.

Sleep. Jerking at night, as if from want of air.

Fever. Dry heat at night; great disposition to perspire in the day-time.

Head. Pain in the head, as if a nail were driven into it; pain, as if from ulceration in the head, directly above the eyes; tuberosities on the head, with pain as if from excoriation when touched.

Eyes. Stinging in the eyes; inflammation of the eyes and eyelids, with pain as from a bruise and excoriation when touched; specks and ulcers on the cornea; spasmodic closing of the eyelids.

Ears. Heat, redness, and itching in the ears; scabs behind and on the ears.

Nose. Pain as from a bruise and excoriation in the nose when touched.

Face. Face burning and of a deep red; erysipelatous inflammation and swelling of the face; pains in the bones of the face when touched.

Teeth. Toothache, with jerking and drawing pains, aggravated by closing the teeth, by eating, and in a hot room;

swelling and inflammation of the gums, which are painful to the touch.

Mouth. Salivation; sore throat, as if there were a plug in it.

Appetite. Desire only for acid or pungent things.

Stomach. Eructations, with burning sensation in the throat.

Fœces. Whitish diarrhea, of an acid odor, especially in children; dysenteric evacuations, greenish, or of a clay-color, with evacuation of sanguineous mucus.

Urine. Wetting the bed; discharge of mucus from the urethra.

Genital Organs. Flow of prostatic fluid, especially after making water, and during a difficult evacuation; excoriation between the thighs; leucorrhea, with smarting.

Larynx. Hoarseness; dry cough in the evening, from any part of the body becoming cold, or when lying on the bed; attacks of dry, rough, and hollow cough, with anguish and suffocation, often causing one to weep.

Chest. Anxious, hoarse, wheezing respiration, with danger of suffocation when lying down.

Arms. Pain, as from a bruise, in the bones of the arm; arthritic swelling of the hand, fingers, and joints of the fingers, with heat, redness and pain, as from dislocation, during movement; skin of the hands cracked, rough, and dry; panaris.

Legs. Swelling of the knees; cracks in the feet.

19. Hyoscyamus.

Convulsions and other spasmodic affections, chiefly in pregnant or parturient women, as well as in children, and in consequence of worms; excessive nervous excitement, with sleeplessness; encephalitis; acute hydrocephalus.

General Symptoms.— Convulsions, with cries, great anguish.

Fever. Burning heat of the body, especially of the head.

Moral Symptoms. Desire to run away ; loss of consciousness, with eyes closed, and raving about business ; delirium ; perversion of all actions.

Head. Headache, as if from concussion of the brain; pressive and benumbing pain in the forehead.

Eyes. Eyes red, fixed, convulsed, spasmodic closing of the eyelids ; nocturnal blindness, weakness of sight, as if from incipient amaurosis.

Mouth and Throat. Redness of the tongue ; constriction in the throat and inability to swallow liquids.

Appetite and Stomach. Vomiting of food and drinks immediately after a meal.

Fœces. Involuntary evacuations.

Genital Organs. Metrorrhagia, of a bright-colored blood.

Larynx. Cramp-like cough at night, especially when lying down, sometimes with redness of the face and vomiting of mucus.

Chest. Pressure on the right side of the chest, with great anxiety and shortness of breath when ascending stairs ; spasms in the chest, with short breathing.

Arms. Hands clenched, with retraction of the thumbs (in the convulsive fits).

Legs. Painful cramps in the thighs and calves of the legs.

20. Ignatia.

Spasmodic affections, especially in consequence of fright or contradiction, and chiefly in hysterical women, or in children ; melancholy and other mental affections caused by affliction ; difficult teething of children, with convulsions ; prolapsus recti also, in children.

General Symptoms. — Violent pain, merely on being touched, in different parts ; attacks of cramp and of convulsions ; hysterical debility and fainting-fits ; the pains are removed always by change of position.

Skin. Excoriation of the skin; itching, when becoming warm in the open air.

Sleep. Violent spasmodic yawnings, especially in the morning.

Fever. Absence of thirst during the heat and perspiration.

Moral Symptoms. Tenderness of character, and delicacy of conscience; love of solitude.

Head. Pressive headache, especially above the root of the nose; aggravated or relieved by stooping; the headaches are aggravated by coffee, brandy, tobacco-smoke, noise, and strong smell; headache, as if a nail were driven into the brain.

Eyes. Convulsive movements of the eyes and eyelids.

Face. Convulsive jerkings, and distortion of the muscles of the face; convulsive twitchings of the corners of the mouth.

Throat. Sore throat, as if there were a plug in it; shootings in the throat, extending sometimes to the ear, chiefly when not swallowing; inflammation, swelling and induration of the tonsils, with small ulcers; impeded deglutition (of drinks).

Appetite. Dislike to milk and tobacco-smoke; painful inflation of the abdomen after a meal.

Stomach. Hiccough every time after eating and drinking; periodical attacks of cramp in the stomach, aggravated by pressing on the part affected.

Abdomen. Shootings and pinchings in the abdomen, especially in the sides; flatulent colic, especially at night.

Fæces. Hard evacuations, with frequent ineffectual efforts; prolapsus of the rectum during evacuation; itching and crawling in the anus.

Catamenia. Cramp-like and compressive pains in the region of the uterus, with attacks of choking.

Larynx. Short cough, as if from a feather in the throat, becoming more violent the more one coughs.

Chest. Difficult respiration, as if hindered by a weight upon the chest; choking with running; palpitation of the heart at night.

Arms. Insupportable pains in the bones and joints of the arms, as if the flesh were being loosened; convulsive jerkings in the arms and in the fingers.

Legs. Convulsive jerkings of the legs.

21. Iodium.

Scrofulous and lymphatic affections; abdominal phthisis; inflammatory swelling of the knee.

General Symptoms. — Swelling and induration of the glands; atrophy and emaciation until reduced to a skeleton.

Fever. Pulse quick, small, and hard.

Head. Congestion to the head, with beating in the brain.

Face. Complexion pale, yellowish; swelling of the submaxillary glands.

Teeth. Softening of the gums.

Stomach. Eructations, generally acid, with burning sensation.

Abdominal Region. Abdominal pains, which return after every meal; enlargement of the abdomen, which renders it impossible to lie down without danger of suffocation.

Fæces. Loose, soft evacuations, alternating with constipation; violent, frothy diarrhea.

Catamenia. Catamenia, at one time too late, at another too soon.

Larynx. Inflammation of the throat and trachea, with contractive sore pain; copious secretion of mucus in the trachea, with frequent hawking; dry cough; cough in the morning.

Chest. Difficulty of respiration when going up stairs.

Trunk. Swelling of the exterior of the neck; swelling of the glands of the neck, nape, and armpits; hard and large goitre.

22. Ipecacuanha.

Gastric and bilious fevers; intermittent fevers; gastric uneasiness, especially when caused by indigestion; Asiatic and sporadic cholera; gastric affections, with vomiting and diarrhea, asthmatic affections.

General Symptoms.—Attacks of uneasiness, with dislike to all food, and excessive and sudden debility.

Fever. Coldness, especially of the hands and feet; thirst only during the shivering or chill.

Head. Attacks of headache, with nausea and vomiting.

Appetite. Great repugnance and dislike to all food.

Stomach. Nausea; vomiting of drink and undigested food, of bilious, greenish, or acrid matter, and sometimes immediately after a meal; vomiting, with diarrhea.

Fæces. Loose evacuations like matter in a state of fermentation; diarrhea, with nausea, colic, and vomiting; dysenteric evacuations, with white flocks, and followed by tenesmus.

Genital Organs. Metrorrhagia, with discharge of bright-red and coagulated blood.

Larynx. Cough, especially at night, with painful shocks in the head and stomach, with disgust and inclination to vomit, and vomiting, or with fits of suffocation, stiffness of the body, and bluish face.

Chest. Spasmodic asthma, with contraction of the larynx.

23 Lachesis.

Sufferings of drunkards, from the abuse of mercury; fainting fits; erysipelas.

General Symptoms.—Great weakness of body and mind.

Skin. Skin yellow, green, lead-colored, or bluish, or blackish, chiefly around the wounds and ulcers.

Head. Vertigo, chiefly on waking in the morning; apoplectic fits, with blue face, convulsive movements of the limbs; headache, with congestion of blood, sparkling before the eyes; headache every morning on waking, or after dinner, or else from every change of weather.

Mouth. Tongue shining, red, and cracked; painful excoriation and inflammatory swelling of the throat; constant desire to swallow, and a sensation on swallowing as if there were a tumor, some foreign body, or a plug in the throat; ulcers on the palate, back of the mouth and throat.

Appetite. Desire for wine.

Stomach. Excessive sensibility of the precordial region to the slightest touch.

Abdominal Region. Inflammation and softening of the liver; pain and stitches in the region of the spleen; abdomen hard and distended, with flatulent colic.

Fæces. Obstinate constipation, with hard and difficult evacuation; loose evacuations, principally at night, or after a meal, or in warm (and damp) weather, or from having taken fruits and acids.

24. Lycopodium.

Obstruction of the glands; typhus fever; inertia of the intestines and obstinate constipation; chronic pneumonia; tuberculous phthisis.

General Symptoms.—Excessive sensibility to fresh air; great tendency to take cold.

Skin. Excoriation of the skin of children.

Moral Symptoms. Melancholy and disposition to weep, aversion to speaking.

Face. Frequent flushes of transient heat in the face; swelling of the submaxillary glands.

Mouth. Dryness of the mouth without thirst.

Throat. Dryness of the throat; inflammation of the throat and palate, with shooting pain.

Stomach. Pressure in the stomach after every meal;

swelling of the epigastrium, with painful sensibility to the touch.

Abdominal Region. Tension around the hypochondria, as if caused by a hoop; induration of the liver; fullness and distension of the stomach and abdomen; obstructed flatulency.

Fœces. Obstruction of the abdomen.

Genital Organs. Leucorrhea, milky, yellowish, reddish and corrosive; excoriation and running sores of the nipples.

Larynx. Nocturnal cough, which affects the head, diaphragm, and stomach.

Chest. Short respiration during almost every exertion; palpitation of the heart, especially during digestion; painful eruption and liver spots on the chest.

Trunk. Swelling of the glands of the neck and shoulder, with shooting pain.

Arms. Nocturnal aching pains in the arms; dryness of the skin of the hands.

Legs. Swelling of the knees; ulcers on the legs; pain in the soles of the feet when walking.

25. Mercurius Vivus.

Swelling and inflammation of the glands; inflammatory fevers, with disposition to perspire profusely; rheumatic or catarrhal headache; scrofulous, rheumatic, catarrhal (and arthritic) ophthalmia; syphilitic ophthalmia; rheumatic and catarrhal otalgia; rheumatic prosopalgia and toothache; dysentery; mucous or bilious diarrhea; influenza.

General Symptoms. — Rending or drawing, or stinging pains in the limbs, principally at night, in the heat of the bed, which renders the pain insupportable; nocturnal aching pains; rheumatic pains, with profuse sweat, which affords no relief; the whole body feels as if it had been bruised, with soreness in all the bones; emaciation and atrophy of the whole body; excitability and sensibility of all the organs.

Skin. Enlargement, inflammation, and ulceration of the glands, with pulsative and shooting pains, hard, red, and shining swelling; violent and voluptuous itching over the whole body, principally in the evening, or at night, augmented by the heat of the bed, and sometimes with burning after being scratched.

Fever. Copious, excessive, and colliquative sweats, both day and night, in the morning; sweat, with nausea and desire to vomit; great fatigue.

Head. Vertigo, principally on getting up, or on raising up the head; fullness and pressure in the head, as if the forehead were squeezed by a band, or that the cranium would split; heat and burning, or tearing and drawing pains, or stinging in the head, often only one-sided and extending to the ears, teeth, and neck.

Eyes. Itching, tickling, and burning in the eyes; eyes red and inflamed; eyelids red, inflamed, swollen, ulcerated on the margins, and covered with scabs.

Ears. Tearing, stinging, and drawing pains in the ears, increased by the heat of the bed; purulent otorrhea, with tearing in the affected side of the head and in the face.

Face. Bloatedness and swelling of the face; tearing in the bones and muscles (of one side) of the face; obstruction and inflammatory swelling of the submaxillary glands, with stinging or pulsative pains.

Teeth. Tearing, stinging, or pulsative pains in the carious teeth, or in the roots of the teeth, often spreading as far as the ears, and in the entire cheek of the side affected, sometimes, also, with painful swelling of the cheek or of the sub maxillary glands, with salivation and shivering; appearance or aggravation of toothache, principally in the evening or at night, in the heat of the bed, where it is insupportable; renewed by the fresh air, as well as by eating, and taking anything hot or cold into the mouth; retraction and swelling of the gums, principally at night, with burning pain and sensation of excoriation on touching them and on eating; gums livid, discolored, and very sensitive; ulceration of the gums.

Mouth. Putrid smell from the mouth; inflammatory swelling of the inside of the mouth; burning pain, vesicles, blisters, aphthæ, and ulcers in the mouth; accumulation of tenacious mucus; profuse discharge of excessively fetid saliva; tongue moist, with white and thick coating; inflammatory swelling and ulceration of the tongue, with stinging pains; entire loss of speech.

Throat. Stinging pains in the throat and tonsils, principally when swallowing; inflammatory swelling and redness of all the back parts of the mouth and throat; constant desire to swallow; inability to swallow the least liquid, which escapes through the nostrils; the pains in the throat commonly extend as far as the ears, the parotids, the submaxillary glands and those of the neck: they are aggravated, for the most part, by empty deglutition, as well as at night, in the fresh air and when speaking, and they are accompanied with salivation.

Appetite. Acid and mucous taste; dislike to all food, principally solid nutriment, meat.

Stomach. Violent, empty eructations; excessive tenderness of the stomach and precordial region; pressure as if from a stone in the pit of the stomach.

Abdominal Region. Painful sensibility of the hepatic region, with stinging, burning pain; complete icterus; obstruction and inflammatory swelling of the inguinal glands.

Fæces. Loose and dysenteric evacuations, principally at night, with colic and cuttings; tenesmus and burning in the anus; nausea and eructations; shivering and shuddering, exhaustion and tremor of all the limbs; scanty evacuations of sanguinolent mucus; evacuations which are mucous, or bilious, or putrid, or acid, or of a greenish or brownish color; evacuation of acrid and burning fecal matter; discharge of blood or of mucus from the rectum; discharge of ascarides and lumbrici.

Urine. Frequent, copious emission of urine, like diabetes; corrosive and burning urine.

Larynx. Catarrh, with febrile shivering; continued hoarseness and loss of voice; pains in the head and chest when coughing, as if these parts were about to burst.

Chest. Difficulty of respiration, with attacks of suffocation at night, or in bed, in the evening when lying (on the left side) shootings in the chest and side, or extending as far as the back, principally when breathing, sneezing, and coughing; pain as from excoriation and of ulceration in the chest.

Trunk. Obstructions and inflammatory swelling of the glands of the neck.

Arms. Sharp pains in the shoulders and arms, principally at night and when moving these parts.

Legs. Sharp and piercing pains in the hip-joints, as well as the thighs, principally at night, and when moving; œdematous, transparent swelling of the thighs and legs.

26. Nux Vomica.

Sufferings from the abuse of coffee, wine, or other spiritous or narcotic drugs; bad effects from passion or excessive study, prolonged watching, or a sedentary life; periodical and intermittent affections; gastralgia; gastritis; gastrico-mucous or bilious affections; dyspepsia, also with vomiting of food; vomiting of drunkards, of pregnant women; incarcerated hernia; obstinate constipation; blind and bleeding hemorrhoides.

General Symptoms.—Repugnance to the open air; great desire to remain lying down or sitting.

Sleep. Too short sleep, with difficulty in going to sleep again after midnight, and inability to remain in bed after three o'clock in the morning; on waking in the morning, pain in the limbs as if they were bruised, great lassitude, with desire to remain lying down, and fits of stretching and of convulsive yawning.

Fever. During the shivering, skin, hands and feet, face or nails are cold and bluish; during the heat, vertigo, headache, shivering when moving in the least, or when uncovered in the slightest degree, thirst.

Moral Symptoms. Hypochondriacal, sorrowful, and sad humor; ill-humor, vexation, and anger; dislike to, and unfitness for, bodily and mental labor.

Head. Vertigo, with sensation of turning and of wavering of the brain; heaviness, pressure, and sensation of expansion in the head, as if the forehead were about to burst, especially above the eyes.

Eyes. Eyes inflamed, with redness and swelling, also the eyelids.

Nose. Obstruction of the nose, sometimes on one side only, and often with itching in the nostrils and discharge of mucus; obstruction in the head, principally in the morning, or at night, and dry coryza with heat and heaviness in the forehead, and obstruction of the nostrils.

Teeth. Putrid and painful swelling of the gums.

Mouth. Fetid, putrid, and cadaverous smell from the mouth; tongue loaded with a white coating, or dry, cracked, brownish or blackish.

Throat. Swelling of the uvula; bitter taste of the mouth; desire for brandy.

Stomach. Frequent, bitter, and acid eructations; violent hiccough; vomituritition and violent vomiting of mucous and sour matter, after drinking or eating, or in the morning; pressure in the stomach as if by a stone; tension and fullness in the epigastrium; tight clothes are insupportable.

Abdominal Region. Flatulent colic, sometimes in the morning, after eating or drinking, with pressing pains, as if by stones.

Fæces. Frequent but ineffectual and anxious desire to evacuate; obstinate constipation, as if from inactivity of the intestines; incomplete evacuations; small, loose, aqueous or mucous and sanguinolent evacuations; hemorrhoides, with excoriating, stinging, burning pain, and pressure in the anus and rectum.

Urine. Ineffectual desire to urinate; frequent emission of watery and pale urine; burning pain in the neck of the bladder when making water.

Larynx. Catarrhal hoarseness and painful roughness of the larynx and chest; accumulation of tenacious mucus, which it is impossible to detach; pains, as from excoriation in the larynx when coughing.

Chest. Asthmatic constriction of the chest at night, in bed, when going up stairs, choking, anxiety.

Trunk. Pains, like those caused by a bruise in the back and loins; rheumatic, drawing, and burning pains in the back.

27. Opium.

Recent affections rather than those of long standing; nervous torpor, and want of vital reaction against the medicines that have been administered; sufferings of drunkards; affections of old men; bad effects of fright, with continued fear, or of sudden joy; typhus; delirium tremens; ileus; constipation, principally that caused by torpor of the intestinal canal, after frequent diarrhea, or from want of exercise, and especially in the case of vigorous persons, or those who are plethoric, or well fed, as well as in the case of children and pregnant women; tympanitis; suppressed or false and spasmodic labor-pains.

General Symptoms. — General insensibility of the whole nervous system.

Sleep. Lethargy, with snoring and mouth open; excessive desire to sleep, with absolute inability to go to sleep.

Fever. Pulse generally full, slow; fever, with lethargic sleep, snoring.

Face. Face dark red, sometimes brownish, hot, and bloated.

Stomach. Vomiting of fecal matter and of urine.

Abdominal Region. Abdomen hard and distended, as in tympanitis.

Fæces. Constipation, long-continued; involuntary evacuations.

Chest. Noisy, stertorous, and rattling respiration; attacks of suffocation on making an effort to cough.

28. Phosphorus.

Physical and nervous weakness caused by protracted influences injurious to the vital economy; hemorrhage and congestion of blood; cholerine; chronic and colliquative diarrhea; chronic laryngitis; disposition to croup.

General Symptoms.—The majority of the symptoms manifest themselves morning and evening, in bed, as well as after dinner, while several others appear at the beginning of a meal and disappear after it.

Skin. Lymphatic abscesses, with fistulous ulcers, which have callous margins, and secrete a fetid and colorless pus, with hectic fever; copious bleeding from small wounds.

Sleep. Unrefreshing sleep; in the morning it appears as if one had not slept enough; nocturnal heat; hectic fever, with dry heat toward evening, especially in the palms of the hands, sweat and colliquative diarrhea, circumscribed redness of the cheeks, etc.

Morul Symptoms. Anguish and uneasiness, especially when alone.

Head. Vertigo, with nausea and pressing pains in the head; congestion to the head, with beating; falling off of the hair.

Eyes. Inflammation of the eyes; nocturnal agglutination of the eyes; black spots before the sight.

Nose. Unpleasant dryness of the nose; continual discharge of yellow mucus from the nose.

Face. Face pale, wan, dirty, earthy, with hollow eyes, surrounded by a blue circle.

Stomach. Sour regurgitations of food; nausea of various kinds, especially in the morning; spasmodic pain and contraction in the stomach.

Abdominal Region. Spasmodic colic; sensation of coldness, with heat and burning in the abdomen; flatulent colic, with grumbling.

Fæces. Prolonged looseness of the bowels.

Larynx. Aphonia; cough excited by a tickling and itching in the chest, or with hoarseness and sensation as if the chest were raw; cough, with purulent and saltish expectoration, or of blood.

Chest. Obstructed respiration of various kinds; congestion to the chest; palpitation of the heart.

Arms. Trembling in the arms and hands.

Legs. Drawing and tearing in the knees; swelling of the feet.

29. Pulsatilla.

Affections of persons of mild character, inclined to pleasantry, and to laughter or weeping, with a mild countenance, and of phlegmatic temperament, inclining to melancholy, lymphatic constitution, with pale complexion, blue eyes, and light hair, freckles, disposition to take a cold in the head, or to other mucous discharges, etc.; bad consequences from the abuse of sulphur-waters, of mercury, cinchona, chamomilla, or from the fat of pork; rheumatic and arthritic affections, with swellings; inflammatory otalgia; dyspepsia, with vomiting of food; mucous or bilious diarrhea; inflammatory swelling of the testes; organic affections of the heart; inflammatory swelling of the legs and feet.

General Symptoms. — Sharp, drawing, and jerking pains in the muscles, aggravated at night, or in bed in the evening, as well as by the heat of the room, mitigated in the open air, and often accompanied by torpor, with paralytic weakness or hard swelling of the parts affected; shifting pains which pass rapidly from one part to the other, often with swelling and redness of the joints.

Skin. Red spots like measles or nettle-rash; chilblains, with bluish-red swellings, heat and burning, or pulsative pains.

Head. Vertigo, as during intoxication; headaches in the evening after lying down, or at night, compression sometimes mitigates them.

Eyes. Pressive, or sharp, shooting pain in the eyes, with inflammation; sties on the eyelids.

Ears. Shootings, with itching, or sharp, jerking pains and contraction in and around the ears; the pains sometimes come on by fits, attack the whole head, appear almost insupportable, and almost cause the loss of reason; inflammatory swelling, heat, and erysipelatous redness of the ear and auditory duct, as well as the surrounding external parts; tingling, roaring, and humming in the ears; hardness of hearing.

Nose. Obstruction of the nose and dry coryza, principally in the evening and in the heat of a room.

Face. Face pale, and sometimes with an expression of suffering.

Teeth. Sharp, shooting pains in the teeth, or drawing, jerking pains, as if the nerve were tightened, then suddenly relaxed, or pulsative, digging, and gnawing pains, often with pricking in the gums, and shivering worse in the evening, or afternoon, in the heat of the bed, or of a room, mitigated by cold water or fresh air.

Mouth. Tongue loaded with a thick coating of a whitish or yellowish color.

Throat. Pain, as if from excoriation in the throat, as if it were all raw, with sensation as if these parts were swollen, principally when swallowing, or accumulation of tenacious mucus, which covers the parts affected.

Appetite. Bitter or sour taste in the mouth, immediately after having eaten; sensation of derangement in the stomach, similar to that caused by fat pork or rich pastry; after eating, nausea, and pressure in the pit of the stomach, and many other sufferings.

Stomach. Nausea and vomitings take place in the evening or at night, and after eating or drinking, with shivering, paleness of face, colic; pressive, spasmodic, contractive, and compressive pains in the stomach and precordial region, after a meal or in the evening; pulsations in the pit of the stomach.

Fæces. Loose evacuations, with colic and cuttings, of greenish, bilious, or watery matter; blind and bleeding hemorrhoides, with itching, smarting, and pain, as if from excoriation.

Genital Organs. Inflammatory swelling of the testes, and of the spermatic cord (sometimes only on one side), with pressive and drawing pains extending into the abdomen; metrorrhagia; black menstrual blood, with clots of mucus, or discharge of pale and serous blood; menses irregular, too tardy, or entirely suppressed, with colic, hysterical spasms in the abdomen; nausea, and vomitings, shiverings, and paleness of face; leucorrhea thick, like cream.

Larynx. Shaking cough in the evening, at night, aggravated when lying down, accompanied with a desire to vomit, or by a choking, as if caused by the vapor of sulphur; moist cough, with expectoration of white, tenacious mucus, or of thick yellowish matter.

Chest. Spasmodic constriction of the chest, or larynx, in the evening, or at night when lying horizontally; frequent and violent palpitation of the heart.

Trunk. Rheumatic, tensive, and drawing pain in the nape of the neck.

Arms. Sharp, jerking, and drawing pains in the shoulder-joint, as well as in the arms, hands, and fingers.

Legs. Pain, as from subcutaneous ulceration in the legs and soles of the feet; swelling of the knees, with sharp, drawing, and shooting pains; great fatigue in the legs and in the knees, with trembling.

30. Rhus Toxicodendron.

Rheumatic affections, with swelling; vesicular erysipelas; bad effects from a strain, dislocation, concussion, and other mechanical injuries, especially when attended with sufferings in the joints and synovial membranes; gastric affections; diarrhea and dysentery; coxalgia and spontaneous dislocation.

General Symptoms.—Rheumatic and arthritic drawings, tension and tearing in the limbs, increased to the highest degree during repose, in bad weather at night, and in the heat of the bed; red and shining swellings.

Sleep. Disturbed sleep, with anxious and frightful dreams.

Fever. Malignant fever, with loquacious delirium, violent pains in all the limbs, excessive weakness, dry or black tongue, dry, brownish or blackish lips, heat and redness of the cheeks.

Head. Heaviness and pressive fullness in the head; beating and pulsations in the head, especially in the occiput; balancing and sensation of fluctuation in the head at every step, as if the brain were loose.

Eyes. Inflammation of the eyes and lids; swelling of the whole eye and surrounding parts.

Ears. Swelling and inflammation of the parotids, with fever.

Face. Erysipelatous inflammation and swelling of the face, with pressive and tensive shootings, and burning crawling; vesicular erysipelas, with yellow serum in the vesicles; humid eruption and thick scabs on the face.

Mouth. A yellow and sometimes also a sanguineous saliva flows from the mouth at night.

Appetite. Thirst from a sensation of dryness in the mouth.

Fæces. Loose, sanguineous, serous, or slimy evacuations; obstinate diarrhea.

Larynx. Cough, excited by a tickling in the ramifications of the bronchi, short and dry.

Chest. Shootings and lancinations in the chest and its sides.

Trunk. Pains in the loins, as if beaten; stiffness of the nape and neck.

Arms. Warts on the hands and fingers.

31. Secale.

Gastric and bilious affection; Asiatic and sporadic cholera; diarrrhea, especially in old men; metrorrhagia of weak women.

Sleep. Great desire to sleep, and deep, lethargic sleep.

Eyes. Eyeballs sunk deep in the sockets.

Face and Teeth. Face pale, discolored, yellow, wan, with the eyes hollow and surrounded by a blue circle.

Fæces. Loose, frequent evacuations, with serous or slimy fæces, and sudden prostration of strength; involuntary evacuations.

32. Sepia.

General Symptoms. — The symptoms disappear during every violent exercise, except on horseback, and are aggravated during repose, as also in the evening; uneasiness and throbbing in all the limbs, violent ebullition of blood during the night, with pulsation in the whole body; great tendency to take cold, and sensitiveness to cold air.

Skin. Itching in different parts, which changes to a burning sensation; brown, reddish, and livid spots on the skin; deformity of the nails.

Fever. Profuse perspiration from the slightest movement; sadness and dejection with tears; susceptibility and peevishness.

Head. Attacks of headache, with nausea and vomiting when shaking or moving the head, and also at every step; semi-lateral headache; violent congestion of blood to the head.

Eyes. Pressure on the eyeballs; inflammation, redness, and swelling of the eyelids, with sties.

Ears. Shooting in the ears.

Nose. Scabby and ulcerated nostrils.

Face. Yellow color of the face; yellow streak on the nose and cheeks in the form of a saddle; yellow color and herpetic eruption around the mouth.

Teeth. Toothache when compressing the teeth, when touching them, and when speaking, as also from the slightest current of cold air.

Throat. Hawking up of mucus, especially in the morning.

Appetite. Putrid, or sour taste; repugnance and dislike to food.

Stomach. Throbbing in the pit of the stomach.

Abdominal Region. Enlargement of the abdomen (in women who have had children).

Fæces. Ineffectual desire to evacuate; greenish diarrhea, often with putrid or sour smell, or especially in children; prolapsus recti; protrusion of hemorrhoides.

Urine. Wetting the bed during the first sleep.

Genital Organs. Bearing down in the uterus; prolapsus uteri; leucorrhea, of a yellowish or greenish red water.

Larynx. Dry cough, which seems to arise from the stomach, especially when in bed in the evening, and often with nausea and bitter vomiting; cough excited by a tickling, and accompanied with constipation, detached with difficulty.

Chest. Dyspnœa, oppression of the chest, and short breath when walking and ascending, as well as when lying in bed, in the evening, and at night; ebullition of blood in the chest, and violent palpitation of the heart.

33. Silicea.

Obstruction, inflammation, induration, and ulceration of the glands; inflammation, softening, ulceration, and other diseases of the bones; ulcers, almost of all kinds; ulceration of the mammæ; chronic coryza and obstinate disposition to take cold in the head; panaritium.

Skin. Mild and malignant suppurations, especially in membranous parts; carbuncles.

Head. Vertigo, with nausea, which mounts from the back to the nape of the neck and head; tearing pains in the head, often semi-lateral; moist scald-head.

Eyes. Redness of the eyes; swelling of the lachrymal gland; black spots before the sight.

Ears. Hardness of hearing; swelling and induration of the parotids.

Nose. Scabs, pimples and ulcers in the nose.

Face. Ulcers on the red part of the lip; herpes on the chin; swelling of the submaxillary glands.

Appetite. After a meal, sour taste in the mouth; pressure in the stomach, water-brash, vomiting.

Stomach. Nausea every morning.

Fæces. Constipation, and slow, hard fæces.

Trunk. Inflammatory abscess in the lumbar region; swelling and deviation of the spine; swelling of the glands of the nape of the neck, on and under the axillæ, sometimes with induration; suppuration of the axillary glands.

Arms. Burning sensation in the ends of the fingers; panaritium.

Legs. Inflammatory swelling of the knee; caries in the tibia; offensive smell from the feet.

34. Sulphur.

General Symptoms. Great sensitiveness to the open air and to the wind; the majority of the sufferings are aggravated, or appear at night, or in the evening, and also during repose, when standing for a long time, and by exposure to cold air; they disappear when walking or moving the parts affected, and also in the warmth of a room; but the heat of the bed renders the nocturnal pains insupportable.

Skin. Itching in the skin, at night in bed; scabious eruptions, with burning itching; desquamation and excoriation of the skin in several places; ulcers, with elevated margins, surrounded by itchy pimples; inflammation, swelling, and induration, or suppuration of the glands.

Fever. Frequent and profuse perspiration day and night; aptness to perspire when working, partial perspiration, principally on the head.

Head. Fullness, pressure, and heaviness in the head, principally in the forehead; congestion of blood to the head, with pulsative, clucking, hammering sensations, and feeling of heat in the brain; quotidian, periodical, and intermittent headaches, appearing principally at night, or in the evening in bed, or in the morning; movement, walking, the open air, and meditation often excite or aggravate the headaches.

Eyes. Itching, tickling, and burning sensation in the eyes and eyelids; inflammation, swelling, and redness of the sclerotica, conjunctiva, and eyelids; pustules and ulcers round the orbits, as far as the cheeks; great sensitiveness of the eyes to the light.

Ears. Obstruction and sensation of stoppage in the ears, on one side only; humming and roaring in the ears.

Nose. Inflammation, ulceration, and scabs in the nostrils.

Face. Heat, and burning sensation in the face, with dark redness of the whole face, circumscribed redness of the cheeks.

Teeth. Appearance or aggravation of toothache, principally in the evening, at night, or in the open air, and also from a current of air, from cold water, eating and masticating.

Mouth. Aphthæ in the mouth and on the tongue.

Throat. Pressure, as if from a plug, or from a tumor in the throat.

Appetite. Dislike to sweet and acid things.

Abdominal Region. Shootings in the abdomen, principally in the left side when walking; pains in the abdomen, principally at night, or after eating and drinking, mitigated by bending forward.

Fœces. Constipation, and hard, knotty, and insufficient evacuations; hemorrhoids.

Genital Organs. Excoriation between the thighs and groins.

Larynx. Moist cough, with profuse expectoration of thick, whitish, or yellowish mucus; when coughing, pain as if from excoriation, or shootings in the chest.

Chest. Obstructed respiration, dyspnæ and attacks of suffocation, principally when lying down at night, and also during sleep; periodical spasms in the chest; shootings in the chest or sternum, or extending as far as the back, or into the left side.

35. Veratrum.

Sporadic or Asiatic cholera; diarrhea, of different kinds, also those produced by cold drinks, when one is over-heated.

General Symptoms.—Pains in the limbs, which are rendered insupportable by the heat of the bed, and disappear completely when walking; sudden, general, and paralytic prostration of strength.

Fever. General coldness of the whole body, and cold, clammy perspiration; fever, with external coldness; pulse slow, and almost extinct.

Head. Attack of headache, with paleness of the face, nausea and vomiting; cold perspiration of the forehead.

Nose. Icy coldness of the nose.

Face. Face pale, cold, hippocratic, wan, with the nose pointed, and a blue circle round the eyes ; cold perspiration on the face ; lips dry, blackish, and cracked.

Teeth. Grinding of the teeth.

Mouth. Sensation of coldness on the tongue ; tongue dry, blackish, cracked.

Appetite. Immediate vomiting and diarrhea, however little is eaten.

Stomach. Violent nausea, with desire to vomit, with excessive thirst ; violent vomiting, with continued nausea, great exhaustion and desire to lie down ; vomiting of black bile and blood ; vomiting, with diarrhea ; the least drop of liquid and the slightest movement excites the vomitings ; burning sensation in the pit of the stomach.

Abdominal Region. Excessively painful sensitiveness of the abdomen when touched ; cramps in the abdomen, and cuttings, as if from knives ; burning sensation through the whole extent of the abdomen, as if from hot coals.

Fæces. Loose, blackish, greenish, brownish evacuations ; unnoticed evacuation of liquid fæces.

Urine. Retention of urine ; urine diminished.

Genital Organs. Menses suppressed, with delirium.

Chest. Chest very much oppressed ; cramp in the chest, with painful constriction ; violent palpitation of the heart, which causes heaving of the chest.

Arms. Icy coldness in the hands ; cramps in the fingers.

Legs. Violent cramps in the calves of the legs and feet icy coldness of the feet.

36. Apis Mellifica.

Dropsical affections ; suppression and translation of acute and chronic eruptions, catarrhs and erysipelas ; nettlerash and its consequences ; swelling and inflammation of the tongue, mouth and throat ; hydrocephalus ; apoplexia ; iritis, corneitis, staphyloma, sty on the eye-lid; chronic diarrheas, inflammation of the abdominal and pectoral organs; œdema of the extremities; scarlatina; measles.

General Symptoms.—General feeling of lassitude with trembling; sudden prostration of the vital force, vomiting, diarrhea, cold extremities, paleness of face and feebleness of pulse.

Skin. Eruption like nettlerash, with burning and itching, blotches on the body and back of the hands; large, hard, elevations like musquito bites upon the back and legs, with stinging, itching and burning; furuncles and large swellings with stinging pains; œdematous swelling of the extremities.

Moral Symptoms. Irritable disposition; unfitness for mental exertion; dread of death, feels as if he should not be able to breathe again.

Head. Oppressive headache when in warm room and reading.

Eyes. Burning, stinging itching in the eye, eyelids, with swelling and pricking sensation as if from a foreign body; smoky opacity of the cornea, with almost entire loss of sight.

Nose. Violent sneezing (coryza?).

Face. Burning, biting, stinging heat with a purplish hue, erysipelas on cheek and nose; swelling under the eye.

Mouth and throat. Scalding of the mouth and throat; feeling of contraction in the throat with difficult deglutition; tongue feels as if burnt (glossitis).

Stomach. Violent eructations; nausea and inclination to vomit, with rumbling in the abdomen and threatening diarrhea.

Abdominal region. Sickly feeling; dull pain, and soreness of the bowels when sneezing or pressing upon them; enlargement of the abdomen, with swelling of the feet, and scanty urine.

Fæces. Frequent yellow watery evacuations; painful diarrhea.

Anus. Hemorrhoids with constipation; biting, boring, stinging pain; urging to stool.

Urine. Scanty, with burning pain, highly colored.

Menstruation. Profuse, with faintness; ovaritis (ovarian dropsy?).

GLOSSARY OF MEDICAL TERMS.

Abortus. Miscarriage; abortion.

Abscess. A collection of pus seated in any particular organ or tissue.

Adhesion. In surgery, the direct union of parts, that have been divided. This union is often attended by inflammation, which is thence called

Adhesive Inflammation, which attends the union of surfaces, separated by a wound; it is synonymous with union by the first intention.

Adypsia. The absence of natural thirst.

Alkali. A substance which unites with acids in definite proportions, so as to neutralize their properties more or less perfectly, and to form salts. It changes vegetable blues to green.

Allopathy. A term used by homœopathic writers to designate the old practice of medicine in contradistinction to their own, now generally employed by both parties; literally implies, curing a disease with a medicine which produces a dissimilar one.

Amenorrhœa. Absence or stoppage of the menstrual flux.

Anasarca. Dropsy of the cellular tissue, or membrane, immediately under the skin.

Angina. Sore throat. The term is also applied to diseases with difficult respiration.

Angina Membranacea. Croup.

Angina Parotidea. Mumps.

Angina Pharyngia. Inflammation of the membrane which lines the pharynx.

Anorexia. Want of appetite.

Anthrax. Carbuncle.

Antiphlogistic. Applied to remedies employed in the old system against inflammation; literally, against heat.

Antrum Highmori. The maxillary sinus. A hollow or cavity above the teeth of the upper jaw, in the middle of the superior maxillary bone.

Anus. The inferior opening of the rectum.

Apoplexia. Apoplexy; a loss of voluntary motion and consciousness. See *Diagnosis* under this head.

Apyrexia. The intervals between febrile paroxysms.

Arthritis. Gout.

Ascaris, plur. Ascarides. Pin-worms.

Asphyxia. Absence of pulsation.

Asthenic. Low; applied to disease; literally, want of strength.

Astringents. Medicaments used in the old practice to contract the animal fibre.

Atony. A want of tone or energy in the muscular power.

Atrophy. A morbid state of the digestive system, in which the food taken into the stomach fails to afford sufficient nourishment. A wasting of the whole, or of individual parts of the body.

Auscultation. The detection of symptoms by the ear in disease.

BILIOUS. Connected with the secretion of bile.

BLEPHARITIS. Inflammation of the eyelids.

BORBORYGMUS. Rumbling in the intestines, caused by flatus or wind.

BRONCHIA; BRONCHI. The tubes into which the trachea or windpipe divides.

BRONCHITIS. Inflammation of the ramifications of the windpipe.

BULIMY; BULIMIA. Canine, or excessive hunger.

CADAVEROUS. Resembling a corpse.

CÆCUM. The blind gut; so called from its being perforated at one end only.

CARCINOMA. Cancer, adj. *Carcinomatous.*

CARDIALGIA. Pain in the stomach.

CARDITIS. Inflammation of the heart.

CARIES. Ulceration of the bones.

CAROTIDS. The name of two large arteries of the neck.

CARPOLOGIA. Picking at the bed clothes.

CARTILAGE. Gristle.

CATAMENIA. The menstrual flux.

CATARRH. Cold; used, also, to express inflammation of the mucous membrane.

CATARRHAL OPHTHALMIA. Simple inflammation of the conjunctiva.

CATHARTIC. Purgative.

CELLULAR TISSUE. The fine, net-like membrane enveloping or connecting most of the structures of the human body.

CEPHALALGIA. Headache.

CEREBRAL. Appertaining to the brain.

CERVICAL. Belonging to the neck.

CESSATIO MENSIUM. Discontinuance of the menstrual flux.

CHLOROSIS. Green sickness.

CHRONIC. Long continued, in contradistinction to acute.

CICATRIX. A scar left after the healing of a wound.

CLAVI PEDIS. Corns.

CLONIC SPASM. A spasm which is not of long duration. It is opposed to *tonic* spasm, which see.

COAGULA. Clots of blood.

COAGULABLE LYMPH. The term given to the fluid which is slowly effused into wounds, and afterward forms the uniting medium or cicatrice.

COLIC. Griping in the intestines.

COLLAPSE. Failing of vitality.

COLLIQUATIVE. Excessive discharge of any secretion.

COMA. Drowsiness.

COMA SOMNOLENTUM. Drowsiness, with relapse thereunto on being roused.

COMATOSE. Drowsy.

COMPRESS. Soft lint, linen, etc., folded together so as to form a pad, for the purpose of being placed, and secured by means of a bandage, on parts which require pressure.

CONGESTIO AD CAPUT. Determination of blood to the head.

CONGESTIO AD PECTUS. Determination of blood to the chest.

CONGESTION. Overfullness of the blood-vessels of some particular organ.

CONJUNCTIVA. The membrane lining the eyelids, and extending over the forepart of the eyeballs.

CONTAGION. Propagation of a disease by contact.

CORNEA. The anterior transparent portion of the eye. It is of a horny consistence.

CORYZA. Cold in the head.

COXAGRA. Inflammation of the hip-joint. Literally, seizure or pain in the hip.

COXALGIA. Literally, pain in the hip; inflammation of the hip-joint.

CRANIUM. The skull.

CREPITATION. Grating sensation, or noise, such as is caused by pressing the finger upon a part affected with emphysema; by the ends of a fractured bone when moved; or by certain salts during calcination.

CREPITANT RHONCHUS, or RALE.—The fine crackling noise heard in consequence of the passage of air through a viscid fluid. It is heard in the first stage of inflammation of the lungs.

CREPITUS. Crackling or grating.

CUTANEOUS. Appertaining to the skin.

CUTICLE. The outer or scarf-skin.

CYSTITIS. Inflammation of the bladder.

DEGLUTITION. The act of swallowing.

DELIRIUM. Derangement of the brain, raving.

DEPLETION. Abstraction of the fluids; generally applied to venesection.

DESICCATION. A drying up.

DESQUAMATION. Falling off of the epidermis in form of scales.

DIAPHRAGMITIS. Inflammation of the diaphragm (muscular partition between the thorax and abdomen.)

DIAGNOSIS. Distinction of maladies.

DIARRHEA. Looseness of the bowels.

DIATHESIS. Constitutional tendency.

DIETETIC. Relating to diet.

DIPLOPIA. Affection of the eyes, in which objects appear double or increased in number.

DIURETIC. Medicines which increase the secretion of urine.

DORSAL. Appertaining to the back.

DRASTIC. Powerful purgatives.

DUODENUM. The first intestine after the stomach, so called from its length; the twelve-inch gut.

DYSCRASIA. A morbid condition of the system; adj. *Dyscrastic.*

DYSECOIA. Deafness.

DYSMENORRHŒA. Painful menstruation.

DYSPEPSIA. Indigestion; literally, difficulty of appetite.

DYSPNŒA. Difficulty of respiration. Shortness of breath.

DYSURIA. Difficulty in passing urine.

EFFUSION. A pouring out, or escape of lymph or other secretion.

EMACIATION. A falling off in the flesh.

EMETIC. Provoking vomiting.

ENCEPHALITIS. Inflammation of the brain and membranes.

ENDEMIC. Peculiar to a particular locality.

ENDOCARDITIS. Inflammation of the internal parts of the heart.

ENTERALGIA. Colic.

ENTERITIS. Inflammation of the intestines.

EPHEMERAL. Of a day's duration

EPHIALTES. Nightmare.

EPIDEMIC. Diseases arising from general causes.

EPIGASTRIUM. The region of the stomach.

EPILEPSY, EPILEPSIA. Falling sickness.

EPISTAXIS. Bleeding from the nose.

EPITHELIUM. The cuticle.

ERYSIPELAS. St. Anthony's fire. Rose. A disease of the skin.

ERYSIPELAS PHLEGMONODES. Phlegmonous erysipelas.

ERYSIPELAS ŒDEMATODES. Œdematous erysipelas.

ERYSIPELAS ERRATICUM. Wandering erysipelas.

ERYSIPELAS GANGRENOSUM. Gangrenous erysipelas.

ERYSIPELAS NEONATORUM. Induration of the cellular tissue in infants.

EXACERBATION. Aggravation of fever, etc.

EXANTHEMA. Eruption terminating in exfoliation.

EXPECTORATION. Discharge of any matter: phlegm; pus from the chest.

EXUDATION. Discharge of fluid from the skin, etc

FÆCES. Alvine excrement.

FASCIÆ. In anatomy, dense fibrous expansions, which either attach or invest muscles.

FAUCES. The throat.

FEBRIS. Fever

FEBRIS NERVOSA. Nervous fever, or typhus.
FEMUR. The bone of the thigh.
FIRST INTENTION. See *Union by the.*
FISTULA. An obstinate, tube-like sore, with a narrow orifice; adj. *Fistulous.*
FISTULA LACHRYMALIS. An ulcerated opening in the lachrymal sac.
FLATUS. Wind in the intestines. Flatulency.
FŒTUS. The infant in the womb.
FOMENTATION. The application of flannel wet with warm water.
FUNCTIONAL DISEASES. Those in which there is supposed to be only derangement of action.
FURUNCULUS. A boil.
FURUNCULUS MALIGNANS. Carbuncle.
GANGRENE. Incipient mortification. Adj. *Gangrenous.*
GASTRALGIA. Pain in the stomach.
GASTRIC. Belonging to the stomach.
GASTRITIS. Inflammation of the stomach.
GASTRODYNIA. Vide *Cardialgia.*
GLAND. A small body met with in many parts of the body, and consisting of various tissues, blood-vessels, nerves, etc.
GLOSSITIS. Inflammation of the tongue.
GLOTTIS. Opening of the windpipe. The superior opening of the larynx.
GRANULATION. See *Incarnation.*
HEMATEMESIS. Vomiting of blood.
HEMOPTYSIS. Discharge of blood from the lungs. Spitting of blood.
HEMORRHAGE Discharge of blood.
HEMORRHOIDES. Piles.
HECTIC FEVER. Habitual or protracted fever.
HELMINTHIASIS. Worm disease.
HEMIPLEGIA. Paralysis of one side of the body, longitudinally.
HEPATITIS. Inflammation of the liver.
HEPATIZATION. Structural derangement of the lungs, the result of inflammation, changing them into a substance resembling the liver; hence its name.
HERNIA. Rupture.
HERNIA CONGENITAL. Congenital hernia. Literally, hernia from birth.
HERPES CIRCINNATUS. Ringworm
HORDEOLUM. Stye.
HYDROCEPHALUS. Water in the head.
HYDROPHOBIA SYMPTOMATICA. Symptoms resembling those arising from hydrophobic virus, appearing during the course of other diseases.
HYPERTROPHY. A morbid increase of any organ, arising from excessive nutrition.
HIPPOCRATIC. Sunken and corpse-like.
HYPOCHONDRIUM. Region of the abdomen, contained under the cartilage of the false ribs.
HYPOCHONDRIASIS. Spleen disease; great depression of spirits, with general derangement; adj. *Hypochondriacal.*
HYPOGASTRIUM. The lower anterior portion of the abdomen.
HYSTERIA. Nervous affection; almost peculiar to females.
ICHOR. A thin, watery discharge secreted from wounds, ulcers, etc.; adj. *Ichorous.*
ICTERUS. Jaundice.
ICTERUS NEONATORUM. Jaundice of infants.
IDIOPATHIC. Original or primary disease.
IDIOSYNCRASY. Individual peculiarity.
ILIUM. The haunch-bone; it, together with the pubis, sacrum, and ischium, contributes to form the pelvis.
ILEUS MISERERE. A form of colic, a twisting pain in the region of the navel.
INCARCERATED. Strangulated or constricted; a term applied to rupture.
INCARNATION. The process by which abscesses or ulcers are healed;

this takes place by means of little grainlike, fleshy bodies, denominated granulations, which form on the surface of ulcers or suppurating wounds, etc., and serve the double purpose of filling up the cavities and bringing closely together, and uniting, their sides.

INCUBUS. The nightmare.

INFECTION. Propagation of disease by effluvia.

INFILTRATION. Diffusion of fluids into the cellular tissue.

INTEGUMENTS. The coverings of any part of the body. The skin, with the adherent fat and cellular membrane, form the common integuments.

INTENTION. See *Union by the first.*

ISCHIAS. Pain in the hip.

ISCHURIA. Suppression of urine.

LACHRYMATION. Tear-shedding.

LACTATION. Suckling; also the process of the secretion of milk.

LACTEAL. Appertaining to the process of the secretion of milk.

LACTIFEROUS. Conducting or conveying the milk.

LARYNGEAL. Belonging to the larynx.

LARYNGITIS. Inflammation of the larynx.

LARYNX. Upper part of the windpipe.

LESIONS. Injuries inflicted by violence, etc.

LESION, ORGANIC. Structural derangement or injury.

LEUCO-PHLEGMATIC. Torpid or sluggish; mostly applied to a temperament characterized by want of tension of fibre; with light hair, and general inertness of the physical and mental powers.

LEUCORRHŒA. Female sexual weakness; vulg. *whites.*

LOCHIA. Discharge from the womb after delivery.

LUMBAGO. Rheumatism in the loins.

LUMBAR. Appertaining to the loins.

LUMBRICUS. The round or long worm.

LUXATION. Dislocation.

LYMPH. A colorless liquid, circulating in the lymphatics.

LYMPHATIC. As applied to temperament; same as leuco-phlegmatic.

LYMPHATICS. Absorbent vessels with glands and valves distributed over the body.

LYMPHATIC GLANDS. CONGLOBATE GLANDS. These are composed of a texture of absorbents, or lymphatic vessels, connected together by a cellular membrane.

MAMMA. The breast in the female; adj. *Mammillary.*

MANIA. Insanity; madness.

MARASMUS. A wasting away of the body.

MATERIA MEDICA PURA. The title of that splendid work of the immortal HAHNEMANN, in which the true properties of medicaments are given, as determined by experiment upon the healthy body.

MAXILLARY. Appertaining to the jaws. The superior and inferior *maxillary bones* from the upper and lower jaws.

MEGRIM. A pain affecting only one side of the head.

MEIBOMEAN GLANDS. Small glands within the inner membrane of the eyelids.

MENORRHAGIA. Excessive discharge of blood from the uterus.

MENSES AND MENSTRUAL FLUX. The monthly period.

MENINGITIS SPINALIS. Inflammation of the spinal membranes.

METASTASIS. The passing of a disease from one part to another.

METEORISMUS. Extreme inflation of the intestines.

METRORRHAGIA. Discharge of blood from the womb.

MIASM, or *Miasma* (*Marsh*). Peculiar effluvia or emanations from swampy grounds.

MICTURATION. Urination.

MILIARIA. Eruption of minute transparent vesicles of the size of millet seeds; miliary eruption.

MILIARIA PURPURA. Scarlet-rash.

MORBUS COXARIUS. Disease of the hip; hip-disease.

MUCOUS MEMBRANE. The membrane which lines the sides of cavities which communicate with the external air, such as that which lines the mouth, stomach, etc.

MUCUS. One of the primary animal fluids; secretion from the nostrils.

MYELITIS. Inflammation of the spinal marrow.

MYOPIA. Short-sight; near-sightedness.

NARCOTIC. Having the property of inducing sleep.

NASAL. Belonging to the nose.

NASAL CARTILAGES. The cartilages of the nose.

NEPHRITIS. Inflammation of the kidneys.

NEURALGIA FACIALIS. Face-ache.

NODOSITIES. Swellings; nodes, a swelling of the bone or thickening of the periosteum.

NOTALGIA. Pains in the loins.

OCCIPUT. The posterior part of the head.

ODONTALGIA. Toothache.

ŒDEMA. Swelling; dropsical swelling; adj. *Œdematous.*

OLFACTION. The act of smelling.

OMENTUM. The caul. The viscus consists of folds of the peritoneum connected together by cellular tissue; it is attached to the stomach, lying on the anterior surface of the bowels.

OPHTHALMIA. By this term is now usually understood simple inflammation of the *Conjunctiva.* Catarrhal Ophthalmia.

OPHTHALMIC NERVE. The first branch given off from the Gasserian ganglion of the fifth pair of nerves; it divides into the lachrymal, frontal, and nasal nerves.

OPHTHALMITIS. Inflammation of the entire ball of the eye.

ORGANIC DISEASE. In pathology, diseases in which there is derangement or alteration of structure, are termed organic.

OS UTERI. The mouth or opening of the womb.

OSSICULA AUDITORIA. The small bones of the ear. They are situated in the cavity of the tympanum, and are four in number: termed the malleus, incus, stapes and os orbiculare.

OTALGIA. Earache.

OTITIS. Inflammation of the ear.

OTORRHEA. A discharge, or running from the ear.

OZÆNA. An ulcer situated in the nose. See *Ozæna.*

PALATE BONES. These are placed at the back part of the roof of the mouth, between the superior maxillary and sphenoid bones, and extend from thence to the floor of the orbit.

PALPITATIO CORDIS. Palpitation of the heart.

PANARIS. Whitlow; panaritium; parenychia.

PANCREAS. A gland situated transversely behind the stomach.

PARALYSIS. Palsy.

PARALYSIS PARAPLEGICA. Paralysis affecting one-half of the body transversely.

PARENCHYMA. The connecting medium of the substance of the lungs.

PAROTITIS. Inflammation of the parotid gland; the *mumps.*

PAROXYSM. A periodical fit of a disease.

PARTURITION. The act of bringing forth.

PATHOGENETIC. The producing or creating of abnormal phenomena.

PATHOGNOMIC. Characteristic of, and peculiar to, any disease.

PATHOLOGY. The investigation of the nature of disease.

PECTORAL. Appertaining to the chest.

PECTUS. The chest.

PELVIS. The basin-shaped cavity below the abdomen, containing the bladder and rectum, and womb in woman.

PERCUSSION. The act of striking upon the chest, etc., in order to elicit sounds to ascertain the state of the subjacent parts.

PERICARDITIS. Inflammation of the Pericardium (sac containing the heart).

PERINÆUM. The space between the anus and the external sexual organs.

PERIOSTEUM. The membrane which envelops the bones.

PERITONÆUM. The serous membrane which lines the cavity of the abdomen, and envelops the viscera contained therein.

PERITONITIS. Inflammation of the peritoneum.

PETECHIÆ. Spots of a red or purple hue, resembling a flea-bite.

PHAGEDENIC. A term applied to any sores which eat away the parts, as it were.

PHARYNX. The throat, or upper part of the gullet.

PHASE. Appearance, or change exhibited by any body, or by *disease.*

PHLEBITIS. Inflammation of the veins.

PHLEGMATIC. Vide, *Leuco-Phlegmatic.*

PHLEGMON. An inflammation of that nature which is otherwise termed *healthy inflammation.*

PHRENITIS. Inflammation of the brain.

PHTHISIS (Pulmonalis). Consumption, abscess of the lungs.

PHYSIOLOGY. The branch of medicine which treats of the functions of the human body.

PLETHORA. An excessive fullness of the blood-vessels.

PLEURA. The serous membrane which lines the cavity of the thorax or chest.

PLEURITIS or PLEURISY. Inflammation of the pleura.

PLEURODYNIA. Pain or stitch in the side.

PNEUMONIA, PNEUMONITIS, PERI PNEUMONIA. Inflammation of the parenchyma of the lung.

POLYPUS. A tumor most frequently met with in the nose, uterus, or vagina.

PORRIGO SCUTULATA. Ring-worm of the scalp.

PRÆCORDIAL REGION. The fore-part of the chest.

PROGNOSIS. The act of predicting of what will take place in diseases.

PROLAPSUS ANI. Protrusion of the intestines.

PROSOPALGIA. Face-ache.

PRURIGO. Itching of the skin.

PSOAS MUSCLES. The name of two muscles situated in the loins.

PSOITIS. Inflammation of the psoas muscles.

PUBIS. The pubic or share-bone.

PUERPERAL FEVER. Appertaining to childbed.

PURIFORM. Pus-like, resembling pus.

PURULENT. Of the character of pus.

PUS. Matter. A whitish, bland, cream-like fluid, found in abscesses, or on the surface of sores.

PUSTULE. An elevation of the scarf-skin, containing pus or lymph, and having an inflamed base.

PYROSIS. Heart-burn; water-brash.

QUINSY. Inflammatory sore throat.

QUOTIDIAN. Intermittent, about twenty-four hours intervening between the attacks.

RABIES. Madness arising from the bite of a rabid animal, generally applied to the disease showing itself in the brute creation.

RACHITIS. The rickets.

RAUCITAS. Hoarseness.

RECTUM. The last of the large intestines, terminating in the anus.

REMITTENT. A term applied to fevers with marked remissions and generally subsequent exacerbation.

REPERCUSSED. Driven in.

RESOLUTION. A termination of in

flammatory affections without abscess, mortification, etc. The term is also applied to the dispersion of swellings, indurations, etc.

Rheumatic Ophthalmia. Inflammation of the tunica albuginea, and of the sclerotica.

Rose. A term applied to erysipelas, from its color.

Rubeola. Measles.

Sacrum. The bone which forms the base of the vertebral column.

Saliva. The fluid secreted by the salivary glands into the cavity of the mouth.

Sanguineous. Consisting of blood.

Sanies. A thin, greenish discharge of fetid matter, from sores, fistulæ, etc., adj. sanious.

Scabies. Psora. Itch.

Scapula. The shoulder blade.

Sciatica. A rheumatic affection of the hip-joint.

Sciatic Nerve. A branch of a nerve of the lower extremity.

Scirrhus. Indolent, glandular tumor, generally preceding cancer in an ulcerated form.

Sclerotica. The hard membrane of the eye; it is situated immediately under the conjunctiva.

Scorbiculus. Pit of the stomach.

Scorbutus. Scurvy.

Scrofulous Ophthalmia. Inflammation of the conjunctiva, with slight redness, but great intolerance of light, and the formation of pimples, or small pustules.

Secretory Vessels, or Organs. Parts of the animal economy, which separate or secrete the various fluids of the body.

Semi-lateral. Limited to one side.

Sinus. A cavity or depression.

Solidification. Vide *Hepatization*.

Somnolence. Disposition to sleep.

Specific. A remedy possessing a peculiar curative action in certain diseases.

Spleen. A spongy, viscous organ, of a livid color, placed on the posterior part of the left hypo chondrium.

Splenitis. Inflammation of spleen.

Splints. Long, thin pieces of wood, tin, or strong pasteboard, used for preventing the extremities of fractured bones from moving so as to interrupt the process by which they are united.

Sputa. Expectoration of differen kinds.

St. Anthony's Fire. Erysipelas.

Stertorous. Snoring.

Stomacace. Canker or scurvy of the mouth.

Strabismus. Squinting.

Strangury. Painful discharge of urine.

Sternum. The breast-bone.

Stethoscope. An instrument to assist the ear, in examining the morbid sounds of the chest.

Stricture. A constriction of a tube or duct of some part of the body.

Struma. Scrofula. The king's evil; adj. *Strumous*.

Sty. An inflammatory small tumor on the eyelid.

Sub-maxillary. Under the jaw.

Sub-maxillary Glands. Glands on the inner side of the lower jaw.

Sub-mucous Tissue. Placed under the mucous membrane.

Sudorifics. Medicines which produce sweating.

Sugillation. A bruise, or extravasated blood.

Suppuration. The morbid action by which pus is deposited, in inflammatory tumor, etc.

Syncope. Fainting or swooning.

Synocha. Continued inflammatory fever.

Synovia. A peculiar, unctuous fluid secreted within the joints, which it lubricates, and thereby serves to facilitate their motions.

Synovial Membrane. The membrane which lines the cavities of the joints, and secretes the synovia.

TÆNIA. Tape-worm.
TARTAR. A concretion incrusting the teeth.
TEMPORAL. Appertaining to temples.
TENDON. The white and shining extremity of a muscle.
TENESMUS. Painful and constant urging to alvine evacuations, without a discharge.
TETANUS, adj. *Tetanic.* A spasmodic rigidity of the parts affected.
THERAPEUTICS. That branch of medicine describing the action of the different means employed for the curing of diseases and of the application of those means.
THORAX. The chest, or that part of the body situated between the neck and the abdomen.
THRUSH. Numerous small, white vesicles in the mouth. See Thrush.
TIC DOULOUREUX. Face-ache.
TINEA ANNULARIS. TINEA CAPITIS. Ringworm of the scalp.
TINEA FACIEI. Milk-crust; milk-scab.
TITILLATION. Tickling.
TONIC. Medicines which are said to increase the tone of the muscular fibre when debilitated and relaxed.
TONSILS. The oblong, sub-oval glands placed between the arches of the palate.
TONSILITIS. Inflammation of the tonsils.
TRACHEA. The windpipe.
TRACHEOTOMY. An operation by opening the windpipe.
TRAUMATIC. Appertaining to wounds; arising from wounds.
TREMOR. Trembling.
TRISMUS. Lock-jaw.
TRITURATION. The reduction of a substance to minute division, by means of long-continued rubbing.
TUBERCLE. A small, round, eruptive swelling, anatomically speaking. In pathology, the name is applied to a peculiar morbid product occurring in various organs or textures, in the form of small, round, isolated masses of a dull whitish yellow, or yellowish gray color, opaque unorganized, and varying in shape and consistence according to their stage of development and the texture of the part in which they are engendered.
TYPHOID. Applied to diseases of a low character.
UMBILICAL CORD. The navèl-string.
UMBILICUS. The navel.
UNION BY THE FIRST INTENTION. The healing of wounds by adhesion; the growing together of the opposite surfaces of a wound, when brought into close approximation, without suppuration or granulation. The latter process of healing is sometimes designated the *second intention.*
URETHRA. The urinary canal.
URTICARIA. Nettle-rash.
UTERUS. The womb.
VARICELLA. Pimples, quickly forming pustules, seldom passing into suppuration, but bursting at the point and drying into scabs. Chicken-pock.
VARIOLA. Small-pox.
VARIOLA. SPURIA. (*Varicella.*) Chicken-pock.
VARIX, plur. *Varices.* Swelling or enlargement of the veins.
VENESECTION. The abstraction of blood by opening a vein.
VERTIGO. Giddiness, with a sensation as if falling.
VESICLE. A small, bladder-like eruption; an elevation of the cuticle containing a transparent, watery fluid.
VICARIOUS. Acting as a substitute.
VIRUS. Contagion or poison.
VISCID. Glutinous and gelatinous.
VISCUS, plur. *Viscera.* Any organ of the system. A bowl.
VOMICA. An abscess of the lungs.
ZYGOMATIC PROCESS. A thin, narrow projection of bone, defining the squamous portion of the temporal bone at its base.

INDEX.